Other Books By Tom Bisio

A Tooth From The Tiger's Mouth: *How to Tr*
with *Powerful Healing Secrets of the Ancient Chinese Warriors*

The Essentials of Ba Gua Zhang
By Gao Ji Wu and Tom Bisio

The Attacking Hands of Ba Gua Zhang
By Gao Ji Wu with Tom Bisio

Zheng Gu Tui Na: *A Chinese Medical Massage Textbook*
By Tom Bisio and Frank Butler

Strategy and Change: *An Examination of Military Strategy, The I Ching and Ba Gua Zhang*

Nei Gong: The Authentic Classic. *A Translation of the Nei Gong Zhen Chuan* Translated by Tom Bisio, Huang Guo-Qi and Joshua Paynter

Ba Gua Circle Walking Nei Gong: *The Meridian Opening Palms of Ba Gua Zhang*

Coming Soon!
The Ba Gua Nei Gong Series: Vol. 1-6

Disclaimer
The author and publisher of this book **are not responsible in any manner** for any injury or illness which may result from following the instructions or performing the exercises contained within the book.

The activities described in this book, physical or otherwise, may be too strenuous or dangerous for a given individual.

Before embarking on **any** of the physical activities described in this book, the reader should consult his or her physician for advice regarding their individual suitability for performing such activity.

Decoding the Dao:
Nine Lessons in Daoist Meditation

A Complete & Comprehensive

Guide to

Daoist Meditation

Outskirts Press, Inc.
Denver, Colorado

The opinions expressed in this manuscript are solely the opinions of the author and do not represent the opinions or thoughts of the publisher. The author has represented and warranted full ownership and/or legal right to publish all the materials in this book.

Decoding the Dao: Nine Lessons in Daoist Meditation
A Complete and Comprehensive Guide to Daoist Meditation
All Rights Reserved.
Copyright © 2013 by Tom Bisio v2.0

This book may not be reproduced, transmitted, or stored in whole or in part by any means, including graphic, electronic, or mechanical without the express written consent of the publisher except in the case of brief quotations embodied in critical articles and reviews.

Outskirts Press, Inc.
http://www.outskirtspress.com

ISBN: 978-1-4787-0394-5

Outskirts Press and the "OP" logo are trademarks belonging to Outskirts Press, Inc.

PRINTED IN THE UNITED STATES OF AMERICA

Acknowledgements

Endless thanks to my wife Valerie Ghent for helping me teach the original nine lesson course that provided the inspiration for this book and for her ongoing collaboration on books, photos, videos and articles on Ba Gua Zhang, Xing Yi Quan and Daoist practices. She also assisted me in proofreading and did not laugh too much when I said the thirtieth time "I just need to add one more thing to the book." Valerie, thank you for your love and support.

Thanks to the students who took the first nine lesson course for their patience and understanding as we ironed out the teaching method. And a great thank you to all of the Ba Gua and Xing Yi students whose questions stimulated me to delve deeper into the material.

To Huang Guo Qi, for being a wonderful friend and for translating and guiding me through so many trips to China over the last 20 years. Huang's translations of documents and his ability to research and find the answers to arcane questions on Daoism, Nei Gong and internal martial arts helped make this book possible. Thank you Huang for always being there and for your indefatigable spirit.

My thanks to Finbar McGrath and Wes Tasker. Aside from being friends and colleagues, Finbar and Wes have a great interest in Daoist practices. We exchanged books and ideas on Daoist meditation over several years leading up to the publication of this book. Both Wes and Finbar proofread the book and caught numerous errors and inconsistencies. Any that remain are my fault, not theirs.

Thanks to Frank Butler for sharing the knowledge of Daoism he gleaned from his teacher Kenneth Gong.

Contents

Introduction to Daoist Meditation — 1
Preface — 2
Daoism and Daoist Meditation — 5
Methods of Daoist Meditation — 9
How to Use this Book — 9
Your Meditation Toolbox — 11
Romanization of Chinese Characters — 11
Why Meditate? — 13

PART I: The Nine Lessons — 21
Lesson 1: The Breath — 23
The Importance of the Breath — 24
The Physiology of Breathing — 26

Lesson 1: Practice - Attending to the Breath — 29
Postures for Meditation — 29
Why Nasal Breathing? — 34

Lesson 2: Kidney Breathing, Qi & Dantian — 37
What is Kidney Breathing? — 38
Back Pain, Neck Pain and Shallow Breathing — 39
The *Qi*-Breath Connection — 40
Qi/Breath and *Dantian* — 44
The *Mingmen* — 46

Lesson 2: Practice - Kidney Breathing — 49
Preliminary Exercises — 49
Kidney Breathing — 51

Correcting Difficulties in Kidney Breathing ... 56
The Three Harms ... 57

Lesson 3: Quieting the Mind & Gathering the Qi ... 59
Qi/Breath, Thought and Emotion ... 60
Ordering the Mind & Gathering the Qi ... 63
Stillness, Harmony & Engagement ... 65
Holding Fast to the "One" ... 66
The Inadequacy of Words ... 67

Lesson 3: Practice - Counting The Breaths ... 70
Counting the Breaths ... 70
Observing Your Thoughts ... 71
Adjusting the Mind ... 71

Lesson 4: Returning to Emptiness - Wu Ji ... 75
Chinese Cosmogony and Wu Ji ... 76
Wu Ji and Daoist Meditation ... 82
The Wu Ji Posture & the Martial Arts ... 84
The Wu Ji Posture ... 84

Lesson 4: Practice - The Wu Ji Posture ... 85
Assuming the Wu Ji Posture ... 85
The Alignments Work Synergistically as Parts of a Whole ... 86
Images, Exercises & Points for Attention ... 87
Exercise 1: Rocking and Rooting ... 88
Exercise 2: Progressive Sinking ... 90
Practice the Wu Ji Posture Daily ... 91

Lesson 5: Wu Ji and Song (Relaxation) ... 93
The Concept of Song ... 95

Lesson 5: Practice - Song   96

Lesson 6: Dissolving & Clearing Blockages   101
What is a Blockage?   102
What Causes the *Qi/Breath* to Block?   103
The Importance of Clearing Blockages in Daoist Meditation   105
The Dao De Jing on Desire and the Dao   106
Dissolving and Clearing Blockages   107

Lesson 6 Practice - Dissolving Blockages   108
Auxilary Exercise: Pour the Cream on Top   109
Dissolving Blockages Method 1: Heavenly Qi/Breath Meditation   112
Dissolving Blockages Method 2: Body Breathing   113

Lesson 7: The Three Treasures and Circulation of Water & Fire   115
The Three Treasures: *Jing, Qi & Shen*   116
Inter-Penetration and Inter-Transformation of *Jing, Qi* and *Shen*   118
The Inseparability of the Three Treasures   120
Kan-Water & Li-Fire   121
The Circulation and Inter-Transformation of Kan and Li   123
The Story of the Weaving Maiden and the Cowherd   126
Chen Tuan's Diagram Revisited   127
Reverse Breathing: Connecting the Kidney and the Heart   128

Lesson 7: Practice - Connecting Heaven & Earth,
Circulating Fire & Water   130
Exercise 1: Connecting Heaven and Earth   130
Exercise 2: Circulating Fire & Water   133
Supplementary Exercises to Assist the Circulation of Water & Fire   139
Exercise 1: The Triple Heater Exercise   139

Exercise 2: Connecting the Kidneys and the Heart — 141

Lesson 8: Golden Fluid & The Micro-Cosmic Orbit — 147
Saliva: Elixir of Immortality — 148
Science & Saliva — 149
Ren and *Du* & the Micro-Cosmic Orbit — 150
Circulation of the Micro-Cosmic Orbit — 154
Waxing and Waning of Yin & Yang and the Micro-Cosmic Orbit — 155
Hormones, *Jing* and the Endocrine System — 159

Lesson 8: Practice - The Micro-Cosmic Orbit — 161
Assist the Micro-Cosmic Orbit: Deer, Crane & Tortoise Breathing — 164
Deer Exercise: Activating *Du Mo* — 167
Crane Exercise: Enabling the *Qi/Breath* — 168
Tortoise Exercise: Activating *Ren Mo* — 168
The Story of the Tortoise Exercise — 168
Special Section: Women's Practice and the Crane Exercise — 170

Lesson 9: Golden Fluid Returning to Dantian Meditation — 173
Su Dong Po and the Golden Fluid Meditation — 174
Li Ching Yun: "Immortal" of the Modern Era — 176
The Three Passes — 177
The Image of the Waterwheel — 179

Lesson 9: Practice - Golden Fluid Returning to Dantian — 181
1. Sit Upright and Concentrate the Mind — 182
2. Knead the Ears — 183
3. Press the Eyes with Warm Hands — 183
4. Rub the Nose — 184
5. Wash the Face; Cultivate the Heavenly Palace; Comb the Hair — 185
6. Knock Teeth; Clench Fists; Concentrate Mind; Swallow Saliva — 186

7. Regulate Respiration for Nine Breaths; Embracing Kun Lun	186
8. Strike the Heavenly Drum and Listen to the Sound 24 Times	187
9. Shake the Heavenly Pillar Slightly; Stir the Golden Fluid	188
10. Hold the Breath, Chafe the Hands, Exhale and Rub the Back	189
11. Regulate Respiration for Nine Breaths Focusing on *Dantian*	190
12. Shake/Rotate the Two Shoulders to Regulate the Ren and Du	191
13. Extend the Two Legs, Bend the Head and Pull the Feet	192
14. Count Nine Breaths; Rinse the Mouth and Swallow Saliva	192
Cool-Down: Rubbing the Meridians	193
Golden Fluid Returning to *Dantian* – Summary	195

Beyond the Nine Lessons – The Macro-Cosmic Orbit — 197

Exercise 1: Combining Wu Ji and Tai Ji: Nezha Stirs the Sea	199
Exercise 2: Uniting the Original *Qi*	201
Exercise 3: Heel Breathing	204
The Macro-Cosmic Orbit and the Eight Extraordinary Vessels	205
The Circulation of *Qi*/Breath in the Eight Extraordinary Vessels	209
Great Heavenly Circulation: Macro-Cosmic Orbit Meditation	210

Taoist Nourishing Life & Longevity Methods — 213

Living in Harmony with the Seasons and Climate	215
Spring	218
Summer	219
Fall	220
Winter	221
Regulating the Emotions	223
Diet & Eating Habits	225
Basic Eating Habits	225
More Dietary Advice	225
Eating with the Seasons	226

Work and Rest: Balancing Activity and Inactivity	229
Li Dong Yuan on Economy of Speech	229
Sexual Activity	230
Supplementary Life Nourishing Exercises	232

PART II: Cracking the Code - Understanding Daoist Meditation   237

Dao De Jing on Daoist Meditation: Hidden Messages Within the Text   241

Chapter 1: How to Embody the Dao	243
Chapter 2: How to Cultivate the Personality	244
Chapter 5: How to Use Emptiness	245
Chapter 6: How to Complete the Idea	246
Chapter 10: How to be Able to Act	248
Chapter 11: How to Make Use of Non-Existence	251
Chapter 12: How to Keep Off Desires	252
Chapter 78: How to Trust in Sincerity	254
Chapter 59: How to Guard the Dao	255
Chapter 42: On the Changes of the Dao	255

Diagram of the Inner Circulation of Qi/Breath: *Nei Jing Tu*   257

The Weaving Maiden and the Cowherd	263
The Ocean in the Lower Abdomen	263
The Boy and Girl and the Treadmill	265
The Cauldron and the Four Tai Ji Diagrams	265
The Plow and the Ox	266
The Spinal Cord (the Mountain Path) and the Three Gates	266
The Grove of Trees	266
The Pagoda	268
The Eyes (Sun and Moon)	269
The Mountains and the Head as the Vault of Heaven	270

The Brain and the Marrow	271
The Two Monks	272
The Rainbow	272
The Bridge, the Spring and the Pool	273

Keys to the Code: Understanding Daoist Symbolism — 275

Keys to the Code	276
The Five Powers	283
Dragon and Tiger	286
The Shen: The Five Psycho-Spiritual Faculties	288
Alchemy: Lead and Mercury	293
Reversing the Movement of the Five Powers	298
Daoist Numerology	309
Images of Sages and Immortals	320
The *Ren* and *Du* Vessels	321

Daoist Meditation and the Image of the Gen Diagram — 325

Image and Name	326
The Gen Ideogram	329
Gen Judgment and Line Commentary	329
The Gen Diagram and Daoist Meditation	332
Gen: The Inner Hexagram	334

Conclusion: The Message in the Code — 337

Appendix I: Reactions to Meditation and Qi Gong — 341

Reactions to Meditation and Qi Gong	342
Sensations You Might Experience When Practicing Qi Gong & Daoist Meditation	343
Other Considerations	345

Appendix II: Body Configurations for Daoist Meditation & Nei Gong — 347

Yi Jing Body Images: The Dui Trigram and the Jie Hexagrams — 349

Supplemental Method for Strengthening the Kidneys and Restraining Leakage to Nourish the *Qi-Breath* — 350

Yi Jing Body Images: The Zhen and Gen Trigrams — 350

Traditional Mnemonic for the Body Alignments in Nei Gong & Daoist Meditation — 354

Appendix III: Extract on Daoist Meditation from Sun Xi Kun's Ba Ga Quan Zhen Chuan — 357

About Sun Xi Kun — 358

Part 1: Authentic Cultivation of the Dao — 358

Part 2: The True Formula of the Dao Elixir Secret Treasure — 363

Part 3: The Method of Quiet Sitting - Oral Instruction — 370

Part 4: Discussion of the Medicine Collecting Method — 374

Part 5: Women's Seated Meditation for Cultivating the Dao — 376

Part 6: Women's Aperture Closing Gong — 380

Chapter Notes: — 387

Bibliography — 411

Introduction To Daoist Meditation

Preface

I first encountered Daoist (Taoist) meditation as part of martial arts training, specifically in the internal art Xing Yi Quan. When learning Xing Yi Quan, the student employs breathing, intention and posture to engage with the movement of the vital force and breath through the central meridians of the body. In this way one learns to relax while developing a subtle, flexible power for combat. At the same time, the mind must be empty without thought and intention in order to let the vital force move unobstructed through the body. During the early years of my study of Xing Yi Quan, much of what various teachers told me seemed abstract and contradictory. The body should move, but spontaneously, without thought and intention. Concurrently our training involved specific exercises that utilized breath and movement to facilitate this spontaneous movement. It seemed impossible to perform exercises that employed very specific intention in order to have "no intention," and to perform very specific, controlled movements in order to generate spontaneous movement. When I mentioned this dilemma, the answer was an exasperated, "Keep practicing." I did keep practicing and in time watched spontaneous movement occur in my own body as though I were an outside observer. Similarly, the imagery used in Daoist texts is confusing and often seems to be contradictory. Yet within the contradiction, within the imagery and symbolism, lies a means of by-passing the ordinary mind, a means of going beyond the ordinary movements of body and mind to engage with a deeper internal movement, a deeper part of oneself.

Daoist meditation maintains an appearance of complexity, while underneath it is fairly simple. What confuses the beginning practitioner is the vast network of images, symbols and metaphors that overlay what are actually a few basic and yet profound concepts. These symbols, images and metaphors have a twofold purpose:

1. The symbols deliberately obfuscate the correct methods of practicing Daoist meditation by acting as a kind of code within which these methods are hidden. In this way only the initiated will understand the practice methods.
2. The symbols aid the meditator, giving him or her an alternative and imagery-rich language, a departure from ordinary language. Through this departure the everyday mind is by-passed, allowing one to engage with another, more subtle mode of perception. In this way one is able to perceive the subtle movements and changes taking place within the body.

In this book, I hope to aid the reader in decoding Daoism's unique language so that the practice method can be clearly understood, while simultaneously demonstrating how to employ this language as a practical guide. Properly understood, Daoist imagery aids the meditator in perceiving, understanding and modulating the internal landscape of the body during meditation. Each of the nine lessons that follow present one or more aspects of Daoist symbolism and imagery that are then integrated into the actual practice of meditation. This creates an interweaving of Daoist theory, Daoist symbolism and imagery with the actual practice of meditation. Each aspect informs and is informed by the others.

In *Daoism Explained,* Hans-Georg Moeller uses the image of a wheel as an analogy of the *Dao*. Mueller points out that the hub is an empty space in the center of the wheel. At its very center, the hub is empty and still, yet around it there are spokes radiating outward in all directions. There is only one hub, but there are many spokes. The spokes have material form, while the very center of the hub does not. The very emptiness at the center of the hub is what gives the wheel the ability to turn and move. As it moves, the spokes continuously change position relative to the center, which is constant and unchanging. Change, movement and transformation are inextricably linked to the unchanging center.[1]

This book follows a linear progression through nine lessons. This progression is largely because a step-by-step format is the easiest way to learn, in effect, to construct a wheel. Once constructed, once moving, the wheel can be accessed at any point. One can engage with any part of it, at any time, as the individual parts are all equal, all extensions of the unchanging center

Daoism And Daoist Meditation

This is not a book on Daoism in general, nor is it a book on the history of Daoism. Daoism is a broad and multilayered tapestry that has many branches and manifestations which have developed over centuries. Some historical background and discussion of Daoist ideas is useful in helping the reader to understand the practice method and purpose of Daoist meditation. These discussions are sprinkled throughout the book, occurring within the context of practical application of Daoist theories with regards to the practice of meditation. Theory informs practice and practice elucidates theory.

Daoism started in China's pre-history and over the centuries has had a profound influence on all aspects of Chinese culture. Literally meaning the "Path" or the "Way", Daoism (particularly in the West), is usually associated with the writings of Lao Zi (Lao Tzu), the author of the *Dao De Jing* (Tao Te Ching), and Zhuang Zi (Chuang Tzu). Their works, and the teachings that flow from them, are often erroneously referred to as "Philosophical Daoism." However Daoism, like many things Chinese, is rooted in practicality. *Dao* or "Way" as a philosophical idea was not just concerned with abstract questions about truth and reality, but with patterns of human behavior and practical knowledge.[2]

Daoist meditation has much common ground with Buddhist methods of meditation such as Zen and Vipassana, as well as Yogic methods of meditation and breath control. It is not surprising then, that Daoist Meditation has sometimes been called "Daoist Yoga." Through the centuries, there has been an interpenetration of Daoist, Buddhist and Confucian ideas. Daoist ideas influenced the development of Chan Buddhist meditation methods, and these methods in turn contributed to Daoist meditation practices. Despite these crossovers, Daoist meditation retains its own unique methods and goals.

In Daoism there are many kinds of meditation. All involve clearing the mind of distractions and focusing the mind-intention in some way. Many people today are familiar with Qi Gong exercises which involve coordinating mind-intention with breath and movement. These exercises are used to promote health and rejuvenate the body. Daoist meditation, sometimes called *Nei Gong* or "inner exercise", is often considered to be more efficacious in replenishing the vital essences of the body and was traditionally seen as a kind of internal alchemy that changed the body from the inside-out. These practices were employed by many adepts as a means of attaining so-called physical "immortality." The premise of much of Daoist meditation is that as people interact with the world, they do so on the basis of their desires and emotions, intellectual distinctions and appetites. As a result they activate and expend their vital essence and begin to lose their primordial *Qi* or vital force.[3] As they expend essence and *Qi*, they decline, become sick and eventually die, often not even living out their allotted lifespan. Healing then means that there is a recovery of essence and a replenishing of *Qi*. Promoting longevity is the next step. Once a state of good health is achieved, Daoist longevity practices known collectively as *Yang Sheng* or "life nourishing" methods can be employed to replenish one's primordial *Qi* up to, and even beyond, the level one had at birth. This allows people to attain their natural lifespan and live to old age in good health. The Daoist idea of immortality is a step beyond, an attempt to transform all of one's *Qi* into primordial *Qi* and ultimately refine it to become spirit, eventually becoming transcendent and by-passing death.[4]

In fact, some early Daoists like Ge Hong (283-343 CE) urged the necessity of prolonging life and becoming immortal by laborious action and the employment of a wide variety of techniques and methods throughout one's lifetime.[5] Whether such immortality is possible is a matter of some debate, but regular practice of Daoist meditation has been shown to improve the body's health and functioning on both the physical and mental levels, improving mental acuity, health longevity, vigor, sexual potency and emotional balance.

How does meditation accomplish this? By attaining a state of quiescence, of stillness where one regains connection with the primordial energies. Wang Chuan Shen, a philosopher in the Ming Dynasty, explained this succinctly when he said: *the quiescent state is actually quiescent movement. It is not motionless. Therefore quiescent exercise is essentially quiescent movement. So entering the quiescent state is essentially quiescent movement.*[6] It is movement within stillness. This movement within stillness is different from ordinary movement and can bring about psychological and physiological changes: one of which is that energy consuming processes change to energy storage, thereby retarding the aging process.[7]

Daoist meditation also focuses on the breath as one of the key elements in engaging with this movement within stillness. Breathing exercises (*Tu Na*) are some of the oldest recorded medical exercises in China. Regulating the breath is an indispensable part of meditation, Daoist alchemical longevity practices and health promoting exercises such as Qi Gong.

Meditation, which focuses on quiescence or "movement within stillness", is often viewed as being a compliment to movement-based exercises such as Tai Ji Quan (T'ai Chi Ch'uan), Ba Gua Zhang, Qi Gong exercises and other internal exercise systems. By practicing both movement within stillness and stillness within movement, a balance is created. Da Liu, a well-known Tai Ji exponent, expresses this dynamic in the following way:

T'ai Chi Chu'uan and meditation should compliment one another. The relationship between them manifests a subtle interweaving of opposite (yin and yang) tendencies. This relationship can be seen in the famous diagram known as the T'ai Chi Tu (Diagram of the Supreme Ultimate). This diagram consists of two fishlike figures within a circle: one black, and the other white. T'ai Chi Ch'uan, essentially a form of movement is yang, the white fish. Meditation, which involves standing or sitting quietly, is yin, the black fish. But this distinction takes into account only the external aspects of the two activities. To perform T'ai Chi Ch'uan exercise correctly, one must be very peaceful and quiet inside while executing correctly the externally visible movements. Conversely, the meditator must use the breath and the mental concentration to move the vital energy through the psychic channels while remaining externally at rest. Thus the inner aspect of each of these practices is opposite its outer aspect, just as the white fish contains a black circle or "eye", and the black fish, a white circle.[8]

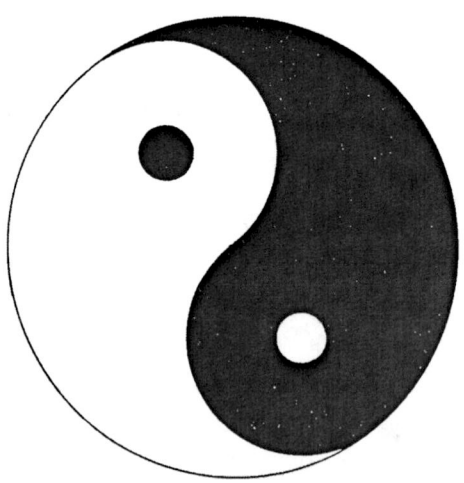

Diagram of the Supreme Ultimate

Bodhidharma (Da Mo), a Buddhist monk from southern India who traveled to China in the early 5th century, had a similar viewpoint. Bodhidharma is credited with transmitting Zen (Chan) Buddhism to China. Legend has it that after noticing that many of his students were so weak and sickly that they fell asleep during meditation, he created exercises to strengthen their bodies and their concentration. These exercises are believed by some to be the forerunners of the Shaolin martial arts.

Methods of Daoist Meditation

There are many methods of Daoist meditation. They can be done standing, sitting, or lying down. So-called "sleep exercises," associated with the 10th century sage and "immortal" Chen Tuan, involve lying on one's side in a near catatonic state.[9] Daoist meditation can involve focusing the mind inwardly or outwardly:

- Focusing the mind on body parts or on the internal organs
- Following the breath with the mind
- Counting breaths
- Visualizations of light, colors or beautiful objects
- Focusing on objects in nature such as trees or water
- Absorbing the energy of the sun or the moon by meditating at certain periods of the lunar or solar cycle
- Feeling or visualizing the breath and qi moving through the meridians
- Focusing on or "holding fast to **The One** - experiencing the "mind within the mind" while revolving the breath through the body[10]

How to Use this Book

In these nine lessons we will explore meditation methods that focus on the breath, the movements of the internal body, and on inner stillness. We will also explore some methods of standing meditation as a means to get in touch with this intention-less state through the alignment of the body, through relaxing the body's tensions, and by dissolving blockages that hinder and interrupt the flow of *Qi* or vital force. Finally, we will explore meditation as a kind of internal alchemy that rejuvenates and replenishes the body's innate energies. These methods have been used for over two millennia by Daoist adepts to promote and prolong life. The trajectory of the book will follow the methods listed above, culminating in the Golden Fluid Returning to Dantian Nei Gong - a unique internal exercise that combines ancient *Dao Yin* (guiding and leading the *Qi*) health exercises with Daoist alchemical meditation. Each lesson builds upon the previous lesson, but can also stand alone as its own practice method. Thus the nine lessons do double duty, giving a step-by-step progression while at the same time providing you with a toolbox of different practices that can be used in different situations.

Each lesson contains both practice exercises and discussions of relevant topics to flesh out the reasoning behind the various methods of meditation and help the reader/practitioner more deeply understand the principles and theories that underlie the practice. Rather than hitting the reader with the theory behind the practice all at once, relevant theory is discussed with each lesson, building on the previous lessons. In this way key concepts are repeated and approached from a variety of angles, making them easier to assimilate.

The lessons can be done for ten days each, so that the course is completed in ninety days, or one can slow down the progression and spend a month or more on each lesson. The general rule for internal exercises is that one should practice for one hundred days without missing a day in order to make a significant change in the body, mind and spirit. So after the 90 days or nine months just keep practicing. At the end of Part I are two chapters that take you beyond the nine lessons, offering other thoughts about Daoist meditation, as well as presenting other Chinese methods of promoting health and longevity. Part II of this book delves into the symbolism and theory behind Daoist meditation. Part II "cracks the code," giving you access to the metaphors and images that may have previously been obscured, but now can enhance your meditation practice.

Your Meditation Toolbox

There is no one method of Daoist meditation, yet all methods have a common thread. In the lessons ahead you will learn a number of variations of the practice of Daoist meditation. Although there is a clear progression, each lesson preparing you for the ones that follow and each building upon what came previously, one method is not better than another. Each method is like a tool in a toolbox. The tool may be more or less useful at certain times or in certain circumstances. Some methods can easily be done sitting on a crowded bus, others require a quiet space in which to practice. Each method approaches the same goal in a different way. You may want to spend more time with some of the lessons than others or continue with the practice method in one lesson even as you begin to work on the next lesson. You may want to use one method in the morning and another at night. Remember there is no one correct way or progression. Follow the progression and the guidelines but do so in a flexible and practical manner.

Romanization of Chinese Characters

When using Chinese terms in an English text, it is easy to forget that they are a Romanization of pictographs or Chinese characters. The Chinese read the pictographs, they do not use Romanization methods such as *pinyin* to write. Romanization helps westerners to learn Chinese and can impart a basic understanding of speech and pronunciation. Therefore, there is ultimately no one way to Romanize a character. Different methods have been used in the past, and convention often dictates which Romanization method is used in a specific case. For example the martial art *Tai Ji Quan* is most often known to Westerners as "T'ai Chi Ch'uan," or just Tai Chi Chuan; *Qi* - often mistranslated as "energy" - is often written as "Chi," and *Daoism* as "Taoism." There are many debates about this in scholarly circles, but for purposes of this book we will use *Pinyin*, the method officially adopted in mainland China for the Romanization of Mandarin. The following is a short list of terms and names that will appear in the book. In most cases the first appearance of a Chinese word or name will feature both spellings.

Pinyin		**Other Romanization Methods**
Qi	=	Chi or Ch'i
Qi Gong	=	Chi Kung
Dao; Daoism	=	Tao; Taoism
Tai Ji Quan	=	Tai Chi Chuan
Ba Gua Zhang	=	Pa Kua Chang
Xing Yi Quan	=	Hsing-I Chuan
Dantian	=	Tantien
Dao Yin	=	Tao Yin
Jing	=	Ching
Lao Zi	=	Lao Tzu
Zhuang Zi	=	Chuang Tzu
Dao De Jing	=	Tao Te Ching
Wu Ji	=	Wu Chi

It is also important to keep in mind that because Chinese is a tonal language, Romanized words that are spelled the same are often actually two different words represented by two different Chinese characters. Therefore context is important when trying to understand Chinese concepts through *Pinyin* and translation.

For example:

Jing (Essence): is a Romanization of the character: 精, while *Jing* (Still; Quiescent; Calm) is a Romanization of the character: 静.

Why Meditate?

Why meditate at all? Does this "navel gazing" have a functional purpose? What does meditation actually do, and why has this withdrawal into the interior for centuries been a cornerstone of Eastern mysticism? To understand meditation and particularly Daoist meditation we must look at the meaning of the Dao (Tao) itself.

Lao Zi's classic text, the *Dao De Jing* (Tao Te Ching), literally means "the classic of the virtue of the Dao."

道德经 Dao De Jing

道 Dao

Dao means path or way. It is derived from

> 首 Head (*shou*)
>
> 辶 Go (*chuo*)

德 De

The character *De* (德) was originally a combination of:

> 彳 Footstep (*chi*) and Straight 直 (*zhi*).
>
> Later 心 Heart (*xin*) was added.

De is usually translated as virtue; morality; ethics.

经 Jing

Jing here means a cannon or scripture, but *Jing* originally meant a warp in a loom.

Although *De* is often literally translated as virtue or ethics, its meaning in Daoism is more complex. Originally in both meaning and usage, the word *De*, conveyed an idea of potential or power. Arthur Waley says that for the early Chinese, *De was bound up with the idea of potentiality. Fields planted with corn represent potential riches; the appearance of a rainbow, potential disaster; the falling of "sweet dew," potential peace and prosperity. Hence De means a latent power, a virtue inherent in something.*[11] However *De* is not just potential or latent power, but the ability to freely exercise our natural ability. That natural, inherent ability is our *De* and in effect makes us who or what we are. Being connected with who we are is what fulfills us as human beings.[12]

In Chinese Cosmogony, Heaven comes before (*xian*) and Earth, after (*hou*). Heaven and Earth develop from the *Wu Ji* (Wu Chi), an undivided potential without limit. *Wu Ji* (literally "no polarity") is sometimes referred to as emptiness, or the void - essentially it is matter that is undifferentiated, undivided, non-polarized. Movement occurs within this non-polarized, undifferentiated matter. The movement is like wind, like a breath. It is an inhalation and an exhalation, or an opening and a closing. This movement is the *Breath-Energy* or the *Qi/Breath* (see Lessons 3 and 4 for more detailed discussions of the *Wu Ji* and *Qi*). This movement, this polarity created by the *Qi/Breath* is the *Tai Ji* (Tai Chi), the "great pole", or "extreme polarity." With the *Tai Ji*, the lighter transparent *Qi/Breath* rises and the heavier opaque *Qi/Breath* sinks down. The light and yang aspect produces Heaven and the yin and heavy aspect produces Earth. The yang diffuses and the yin receives. The potential that opens into life is rooted in Heaven, but the breath through which Heaven's forms are accomplished is rooted in Earth. Using imagery dervied from the *Yi Jing* this can be expressed as follows: the strong unbroken lines of the Heaven Trigram flow downward to be received by Earth's softer "receptive (broken) lines." Earth in turn responds, actualizing Heaven's potential into form and sending the *Qi/Breath* back upward.

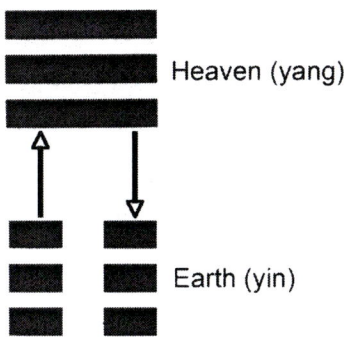

> *Heaven abides so that we have virtue [potential].*
> *Earth abides so that we have Qi/Breath.*
> *When virtue [potential] flows and Qi/Breath is blended, there is life.*[13]

The crossing of Heaven and Earth is life (*Sheng*). The ideogram for *Sheng* (life; growth; to engender; birth) is a picture of a growing plant pushing up through layers of earth:

生 Sheng

Like the plant in the ideograph above, human beings are rooted in the Earth, but stretch upward toward Heaven. We are between Heaven and Earth, and everything within us is in some way a reflection of their interaction:

> *Everything we live with under Heaven is the outpouring of heavenly virtue; streaming down upon us is the gift that never runs dry. Our heart beats in response to the life offered to it. We call it virtue and attribute it definitely to Heaven. The existence of "I" is virtue expressed. Normally virtue is placed in dependence on the heart within a Being. The heart shelters Heaven. Illuminated by Heaven's radiance, the heart is able to recognize the correctness and authenticity of conduct. Why? Because the Heaven within us is our virtue [our De], just as the Heaven outside of us is the virtue [De] of all virtue [De].*[14]

It should be mentioned that Heaven here refers to a natural operating system, organic and all-encompassing that governs and abides in all things. It is important to remember that in this context, virtue (*De*) includes, but is not equivalent to, morality and ethics. The term also implies an effective force or power, an efficacy or potency.

Earth carries and receives Heaven's virtue and embodies it in form. Heaven can only be spoken of as a compliment to Earth, and only observed through its interpenetration with Earth's *Qi/Breaths* and its ever-evolving forms. Through Earth's *Qi/Breaths*, Heaven's creative spark, its virtue, is observable.

> *Earth in me, is the presence of diversity, of varied and multiple aspects, under the authority of the celestial unity that forges a being. It is also the ceaseless transformations. The breaths extend everywhere; they occupy available space without encumbering it; they are light and fluid, which permits their junction and co-penetrations and also their rising to meet Heaven. The breaths of Earth are not imprisoned; all they ask is to intersect each other under the impulse of Heaven. Thus all that is breaths in me is Earth, breaths projected toward the one Heaven, for Heaven makes these breaths those of one particular being, with its own destiny and nature.*[15]

Human life is a manifestation of the all-encompassing respiration of Heaven and Earth, and the yin and yang flux that flows between them. Therefore, life for human beings in the natural world is expressed through movment and change. This *Qi/Breath*, born of the interaction between Heaven and Earth, flows and circulates everywhere; it flows through the body as it would through a landscape or a painting.[16] The body is a living landscape in which the forces of Heaven and Earth are always present, always operating. Life is a result of concentration of the *Qi/Breath*, and death is its dissolution. *Thus it is said that what courses through the entire world and causes it to communicate is the unitary breath, yi qi* (literally: the "One Qi").[17]

> *Through this breath-energy, I am connected to the primordial current, the generous progenitor from which life stems directly and permanently. That is why "wisdom" consists "solely" in returning to the primordial flow.... This re-incites my life. More succinctly put, wisdom is a matter of freeing myself from all internal obstructions and focalizations in order to recover the communicative aptitude of the qi that produces me. This qi can neither mature nor stagnate but must be kept alert.*[18]

Meditation in Daosim is considered to be a method of nourishing life (*Yang Sheng*, 养生). *Yang Sheng* practices aim at both preserving health and leading a fuller life. In Daoist meditation, focusing on our breath allows us to connect with the "One Breath." Meditation in this context becomes a way of going inside, a disengagement from the world in order to re-connect with the unitary *Qi/Breath* that is at the core of our life force. By connecting with the endless, limitless flux between Heaven and Earth, by re-connecting with Heaven's virtue and Earth's breaths, we reconnect and replenish from the well of life itself and recover the authenticity and wisdom which was implanted within us at our inception. Worldly affairs - our wants, desires, likes, dislikes, obsessions, and fixations - pull us away from the unity into countless divisions and differentiations that disperse our own *Qi/Breath*. The ultimate dispersal of *Qi/Breath* on a physical plane is death, but in another sense these fixations create impediments that impair our connection to the limitless changes of Heaven and Earth, thereby creating another kind of "death."

Although Daoism and life nourishing practices frequently reference long life and immortality as goals, it is implied that the real goal is to live life as a fully integrated human being. In his wonderful book, *Vital*

Nourishment: Departing From Happiness, Francois Jullien distinguishes between "living to live"[19] and living.

> *He who worries about prolonging and preserving life and who is therefore preoccupied with his own life, who values and clings to it, does not live. He who thinks only of his own life does not live, not so much because this tiresome concern with his own life interferes with his joy of living but, more radically, because it obstructs and corrupts the very source of his vitality. By contrast, he who achieves the "transparency of morning" after treating life as external no longer fears life and death but finds peace and tranquility in whatever happens to him. His vitality unfolds on its own and avoids becoming bogged down in any form of attachment, including the attachment to life. He is free to respond only to the stimuli that come his way and thus he lives in the "cool transparency of morning."*[20]

When confronted with Daoist tales of immortality and special powers, one is reminded of the famous Sufi parable:

> *One day Hassan, a Sufi mystic, went to Rabiya, the great Sufi woman. He had just learned how to walk on water, so he told Rabiya, "Let us go and walk on water and have a little spiritual discourse, discussion." That spiritual discussion was just an excuse; he wanted to show Rabiya that he could walk on the water.*
>
> *Rabiya said, "On the water? That does not appeal to me. Let us go to the clouds! We will sit on the clouds and have spiritual discourse."*
>
> *Hassan said, "But I don't know how to go to the clouds and sit on the clouds."*
>
> *Rabiya said, "Neither do I! But what is the point? Why can't we have a religious discourse here? Why go to the water or to the clouds?" All great mystics have been against miracles, and all fools are interested in miracles.*[21]

Daoism maintains that being (*You* 有) and non-being (*Wu* 無) are concrete, and therefore experienceable states of the "real." Reality then, is an ongoing process of change, transformation and movement which is neither *You* or *Wu*, but can more accurately be described as an interpenetration of *You* and *Wu*.[22] Therefore one's perception and participation in the world is intimately connected with one's reality, and therefore with "reality" as a unitary concept. The knower and the known are one whole.[23] *Reality in the Chinese experience is an experience and vision of the creative unity exemplified in the unity and totality of life as an everlasting process of productive transformation.*[24] In Daoism and Daoist meditation, life and death are merely points of change within an ongoing cycle of change. Neither is privileged. Both are equally valid or real, just as all phases of cyclical change are equally valid and real.[25] There is no heroic defiance of death or ecstatic celebration of life, but instead an ongoing experience of change and transformation of which life and death are but a part. In this context, meditation becomes a tool to connect with that change and transformation.

Meditation as a life nourishing practice is something that must be done slowly and constantly. Like nurturing a delicate growing plant, it is a series of small steps performed carefully and at the right time. We want to move quickly; we want to see progress, but like the farmer in the Chinese fable who pulled on rice shoots to help them grow more quickly only to succeed in killing the plants, excessive enthusiasm can cause great harm. Instead adopt a natural attitude, like a small boat without paddles or sail that leisurely follows the course of a meandering stream.[26] Things evolve slowly. Change occurs constantly but manifests slowly. It is our ongoing engagement with the process without seeking immediate results that actually produces the results.

It is appropriate to end this chapter with the inspirational words of a Daoist adept:

Therefore, take a bold resolution and start to train seriously. As from today you should dwell in singleness of thought; your eyes and ears should disengage from objects; regulate your diet; reduce your sleep; refrain from futile talk and jokes; stop thinking and worrying; cast away soft comfort and cease to discriminate between the handsome and the ugly so that you can be like the cicada feeding on dew to preserve its unsullied body and like the tortoise absorbing the vitality from sunlight to enjoy long life.[27]

PART I

The Nine Lessons

LESSON 1:

THE BREATH

吐纳
Tu Na

Lesson One: The Breath

The Importance of the Breath

Breathing "is" life. While we can survive for days without eating, drinking or sleeping, we cannot live for more than a few minutes without breathing. Most of us pay attention to what we eat and drink. We are aware of how food affects our physical and mental well-being, yet we tend to take breathing for granted. Respiration is one of the body's most basic rhythms. This is why breathing exercises can have profound effects, both physical and psychological, on the entire human organism. Paying attention to our breath is as important as brushing our teeth, getting enough sleep and eating right.

The movements of the diaphragm and ribs in inhalation and exhalation help the vena cava to return blood to the heart. Additionally, as the organs of digestion have direct and indirect attachments to the diaphragm, its piston-like action in breathing aids digestion and peristalsis. Even the kidneys move slightly with every breath. It is no surprise that impaired breathing can have profound affects on the functioning of the internal organs.

The effect of regular practice of breathing exercises had been shown to have a broad range of physiological effects:

- Hypertensive patients practicing Qi Gong breathing exercises along with drug therapy were shown to have a lower incidence of stroke and were able to reduce drug intake.[1]
- Asthma patients who practiced breathing exercises or Qi Gong regularly, reduced their medication, and took less sick leave due to lung problems.[2]
- Improvements in micro-circulation were noted in patients who practiced Qi Gong and breathing exercises regularly.
- Several research studies have indicated that breathing exercises can produce beneficial effects on cardiovascular function such as

increased cardiac output, oxygen uptake and adaptation to higher altitudes.
- Deep diaphragmatic breathing has been shown to widen the scope of action of the muscles of the diaphragm, freeing the rib cage and enhance pulmonary ventilation.
- Diaphragmatic breathing rhythmically massages the internal organs and stimulates the brain.
- Slow, deep breathing in a situation previously demonstrated to provoke gastric problems such as tachygastria, prevented the development of stomach symptoms and decreased the symptoms of motion sickness.
- Deep breathing allows the body to take in more oxygen and release more carbon dioxide. This leads to many health benefits: a lowering of blood pressure, slowing of heart rate, and relaxation of the muscles.
- Slow, deep breathing has been shown to calm the mind, reducing anxiety and stress and reducing insomnia.
- Slow and regular breathing, below 10 breaths per minute, is known to affect reflex control of the cardiovascular system and to modulate blood pressure. More specifically, lung inflation increases with decreasing breathing rate, stimulating pulmonary stretch receptors.
- Blood lactate levels fall sharply during the first 10 minutes of meditation. Increased lactate is instrumental in producing attacks of anxiety.[3]

It has been clinically shown that slow, regular breathing at a rate of less than ten breaths per minute not only modulates blood pressure, but **reverses the vascular pathology associated with hypertension**. Regular practice of slowed breathing actually produced a drop in BP of 20-30 points. The Food and Drug Administration approved RESPeRATE, a biofeedback-like device that helps slow breathing in order to treat hypertension. Physiologically this "slow" breathing appears to result in significant and sustained reductions in blood pressure by reducing the body's sympathetic neural activity and relaxing the muscles surrounding small blood vessels. This allows for a slight dilation of the blood vessels so that blood flows more freely, thereby lowering the blood pressure. The effects have been shown to be cumulative. [4]

The Physiology of Breathing

During inhalation the diaphragm muscle contracts, causing it to move downwards. Its curved shape flattens, thereby increasing the air space inside the thoracic cavity and decreasing the pressure in the thorax region. This creates a negative pressure in the lungs, allowing the air in the atmosphere around us to come into the lungs. When the diaphragm relaxes on exhalation, pressure in the thoracic region increases and air space is reduced, pushing air out of the lungs.

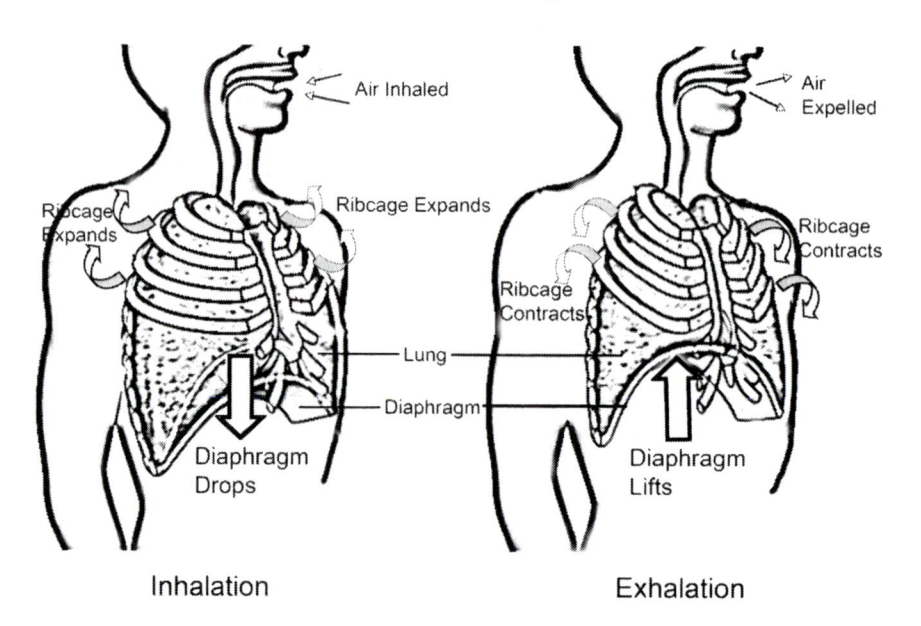

Inhalation | Exhalation

From a structural standpoint alone, the movement of the diaphragm has ramifications throughout the body. Although there is little effect on the aorta, these movements act as a pump for the vena cava, assisting return circulation to the heart. Anything affecting the tonus of the muscular fibers of the diaphragm can affect gastro-intestinal physiology due to the connective tissue relationship between the esophagus and the diaphragm. The pleural dome, the connective tissue layer that caps the pleura of the lungs, essentially forming the "top" of the lungs, is suspended by fibers of the scalene muscles of the neck and fibrous muscular fasiculi which attach to the thorax. Other surfaces of the pleura attach to the diaphragm, sternum, ribs and vertebral column. Many of the viscera also attach to the diaphragm. The liver, the stomach, the flexures of the colon coincide directly with the diaphragm, while other viscera have ligamentous connective tissue attachments to the diaphragm. Even the psoas muscle, a deep abdominal muscle that supports the spine and flexes the hip, blends with the crura and other posterior attachments of the diaphragm, all of which in turn blend with the anterior longitudinal ligament that runs up the front of the spine, connecting the vertebral bodies and the discs.[5] **All of these structures are influenced by the movements of the diaphragm and respiration**.

Osteopath Jean-Pierre Barral has shown that the piston-like action of the diaphragm influences the mobility and "motility" of the viscera. In studies involving patients with infectious lung diseases and those treated with therapeutic pneumothorax (collapsing of the lung), he observed that if the lungs and pulmonary system are attacked, the natural axes of rotation of the viscera and the intra-thoracic pressure are changed. Musculoskeletal structures of the thorax may then move along different axes. Such changes can have widespread effects. *For example, the Kidney moves 3 cm with each breath, which cumulatively amounts to 600 meters per day. With extremely forced respiration it will move as far as 10cm. A minor disturbance in response of the kidney to breathing can therefore cause a major problem over time.*[6]

Respiration oxygenates the blood and expels waste products like carbon dioxide. At a cellular level, oxygen is the indispensable key that unlocks the stored energy of ATP. The breaking of ATP's chemical bonds provides the energy for mechanical work, electrical impulses, cell division secretion, etc. *Like a fountain, the living organism retains its improbable configuration by borrowing sources of energy from the world around it and by configuring and reconfiguring organization upon the matter which is ceaselessly flowing through it, and in order to do this, to exploit the energy resources of the substances it borrows from the outside world a cell must have oxygen.*[7]

This description sound remarkably like traditional Chinese cosmological and medical concepts. As we shall see in future lessons, the connection of oxygen and ATP has many overlaps with the Chinese concept of *Qi* (vital force), which is itself intimately connected with the breath. Sheldon Paul Hendler MD, stresses the importance of ATP:

Without ATP there is no energy, no life. It is ATP that we utilize to act, feel, think. It provides the energy we use every time we "fire" a brain cell, contract a muscle, repair a cell, reproduce our kind. Not surprisingly it takes a lot of ATP to make all of this happen If you are active physically, you are making/using an amount of ATP close to your ideal body weight each day. The body and brain are sensitive to even very small reductions in ATP production. This sensitivity is expressed in terms of aches and pains, confusion, intermittent fatigue and greater susceptibility to infection, and finally, chronic fatigue and persistent illness.[8]

Dr. Hendler suggests that improper breathing can actually result in progressive damage to the heart through the cumulative effect of repeated arterial spasms.[9] Hendler advocates maximizing oxygen flow and ATP production through the very same basic breathing exercises that form the foundation of Daoist meditation - what the Chinese call "Kidney Breathing" (see Lesson Two).

Lesson 1: Practice – Attending to the Breath

Postures for Meditation:
- Sitting cross legged on a pillow
- Sitting on a chair

If you have not meditated before it might be easier to start sitting on a chair as it is easier to set the alignments. Correct alignment is important for the air pathways to open correctly and for the diaphragm to move freely.

When sitting keep the spine vertical, with the head floating. The acu-point *Bai Hui* ("hundred meeting point") is at the top of the head in line with the ears. *Bai Hui* should feel as though it is pulled upward, while the body weight is released downward into the tailbone. This creates a gentle traction of the vertebrae, aligning them one on top of the other. As you sit, feel as though each vertebrae is stacked and aligned with the other vertebrae that are above and below it.

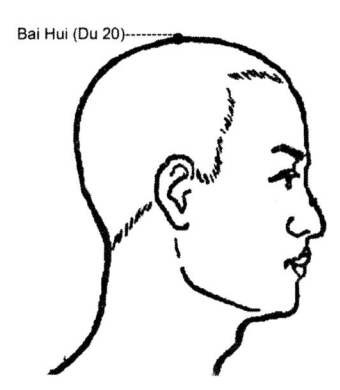

Bai Hui (Du 20)

As you sit, check your alignment. Proper alignment allows the meridians to open and the breath to move without obstruction. Proper alignment relaxes the body, allowing the mind to attend to what is happening inside you and around you.

1) Set Your Alignment

Sitting in a Chair

- The feet are flat are on the floor with the knees over the ankles.
- Ideally choose a chair height that allows the knees to be bent 90 degrees and the thighs to line up with the hips.
- The hips, knees and feet are lined up.
- The hips must be open and relaxed.
- Ideally sit towards the front of the chair so that your buttocks are on the seat of the chair, but your thighs are, for the most part, not touching the chair.
- If you feel your back needs support, then sit farther back in the chair with a small pillow supporting your low back area.

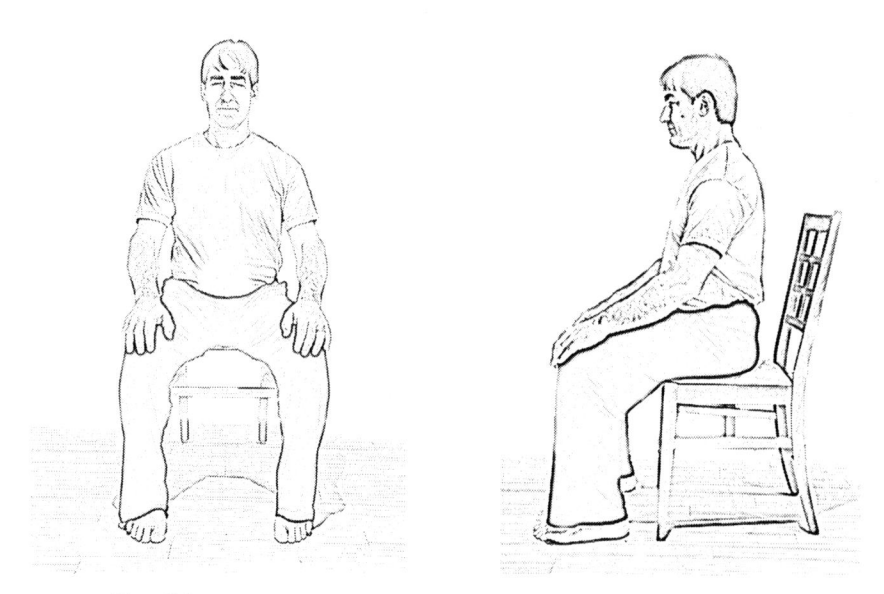

Sitting on a Cushion

- Make sure the cushion is sufficiently high that the *kua* (inguinal area) is open and the back is straight rather than slumped.
- The hips must be relaxed and open.

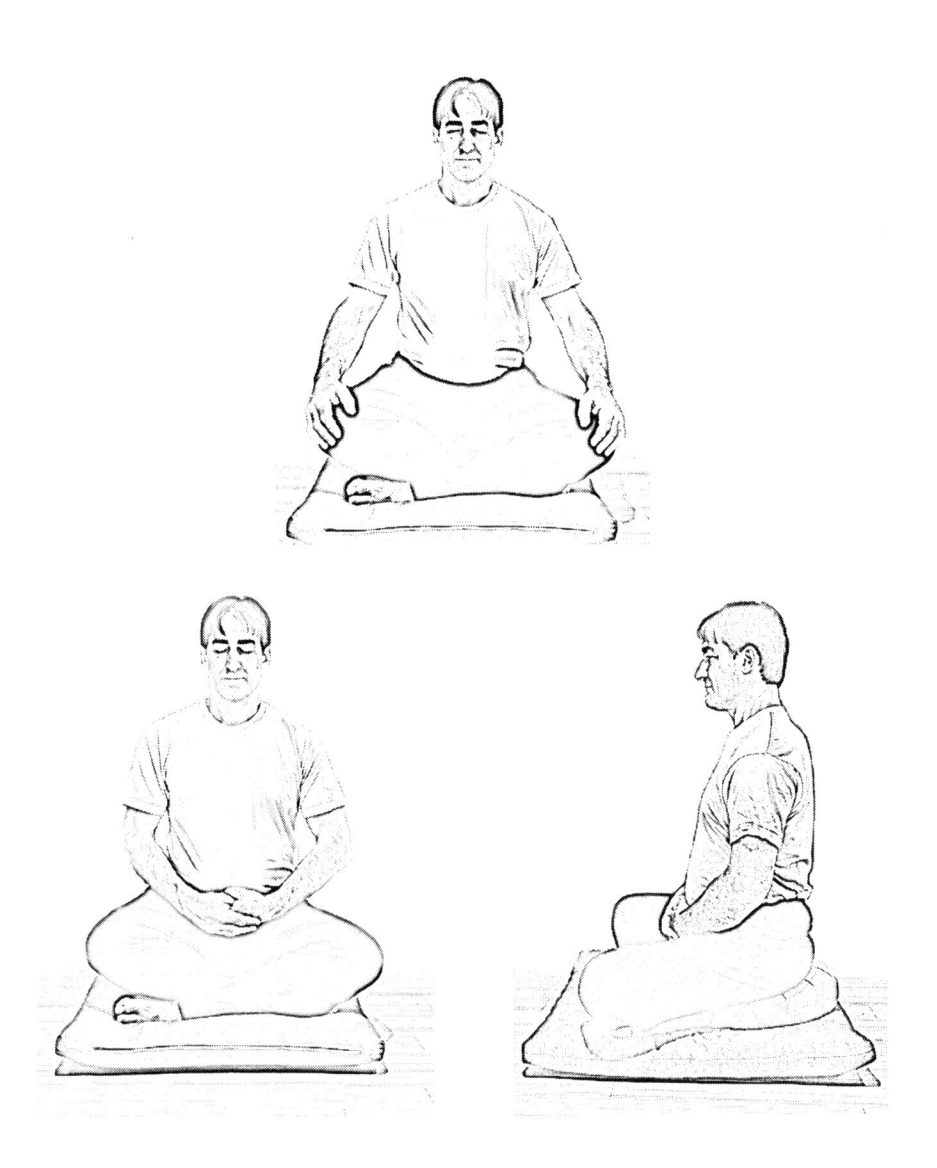

General Alignments (Chair or Cushion)
- The back is relatively straight from the tail to the vertex. The lumbar area is relatively flat, not arched.
- The head and upper thoracic spine are lifted while the shoulders drop.
- The head is suspended from the vertex, but draw the chin in slightly in order to lengthen the neck.
- The hands are palm-down on the knees with the elbows bent.

- Alternatively, the hands can be palm-up on the knees or enclosed within each other in either the yin-yang "hand knot" configuration (shown below) or placed palm up on top of each other, with the little finger side of the hands touching *Dantian*.

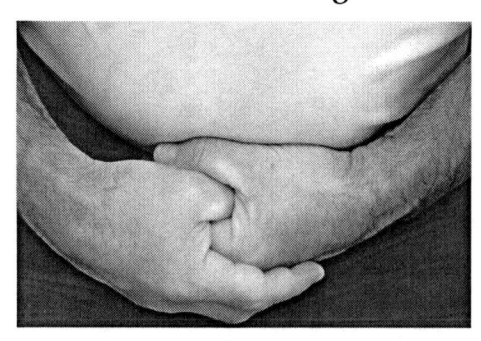

Yin Yang "Hand-Knot"

- Keep space under the armpits as though there is a ball under each armpit.
- Lift the ribs of the upper back without lifting the shoulders.
- Drop and soften the chest muscles.
- Relax and loosen the shoulders.
- Let the tailbone sink down and slightly under.
- Lift the *kua*. The kua is the area in the front portion of the hip known as the inguinal area. It must be lifted and open, rather than collapsed or contracted.
- The vertebrae are stacked one upon the other.
- Touch the tip of the tongue lightly to the upper palate just behind the upper teeth. This connects two important energetic vessels (meridians). We will discuss this in detail in subsequent lessons.
- Relax your face and jaw.

2) Observe the Breath

In the beginning, take the time (even one or two minutes if necessary) to check your alignment at each practice session. With practice this will become automatic and the process will be quick.

Read the following as you begin to focus on the breath:

Now that you are sitting in correct alignment, **pay attention to the breath**.
- Breathe slowly in and out of the nose, softly, slowly and without sound.
- Become aware of both the inhalation and exhalation, looking at each individual breath one at a time.
- Pay attention to the flow of air in and out of the nostrils, feeling the movement of air in and out of the nose. Let the breath fill your awareness by noticing the flow of air in and out of your nostrils.
- Thoughts may come and go, you may become distracted, but your attention inevitably returns to the breath, observing it one breath at a time.
- The breath has a rhythm. Observe the rhythm, the inflow and outflow.
- Remember when we inhale, the diaphragm drops, creating a negative pressure inside the lungs relative to the air pressure in the atmosphere around us. We do not suck air into our lungs, it enters the nose, and comes into our lungs, seamlessly and effortlessly.
- It takes no effort to breathe, we do it all the time, every day. Just observe your breath, neither emphasizing the inhale nor the exhale, simply watching, feeling, connecting with the rhythm.
- Notice the space between the inhale and the exhale. When does one end and the other begin?
- Notice the breath without influencing it, without judging it. You are just sitting and breathing.

Do this for as long as you like. Try to start with at least five minutes. Although it is perhaps ideal to set aside a practice time that is the same each day, this exercise can be practiced anytime and anywhere. If you find the exercise difficult, do it several times a day, even for just a minute or two. You can practice focusing on the breath almost anywhere - riding a bus or train, walking down the street or just sitting quietly for a few minutes in your office. Each time you practice, take a minute or more to set your alignment and then focus on the breath. In this way proper alignment will become second nature. Practice whenever you like and notice how the body and mind respond to the practice.

Observing the Breath is the first step, but it is the key step.

Why Nasal Breathing?
- The nostrils cleanse the air and trap dust particles and bacteria.
- The blood vessels in the nose warm the air.
- The nerve endings of the tunica-mucosa-nasi are stimulated as air flows over them. This in turn stimulates the organs and regulatory mechanisms of the body, especially heartbeat, blood pressure and the movement of the respiratory muscles.
- There are small bones in the nose called the turbinates. They are curved boney plates that function like turbines to churn the air as it passes through the nasal cavity. As the air circulates, it is warmed, moistened and cleaned by the respiratory mucosa that cover the surface of the turbinates.
- The turbinate bones increase the surface area of the inside of the nose. By directing and deflecting airflow across the maximum mucosal surface of the inner nose, they are able to propel the inspired air. This action, coupled with the humidity and filtration provided by the turbinate bones, helps to carry more scent molecules towards the higher, and very narrow regions of the nasal airways, where olfactory nerve receptors are located. This has an immediate and direct effect on the brain.

- The turbinate bones create a spiral movement in the airflow. The *Qi/Breath* also moves in spirals, churning and tumbling through the meridians, vessels and cavities of the body. Breathing through the nose facilitates this internal movement.

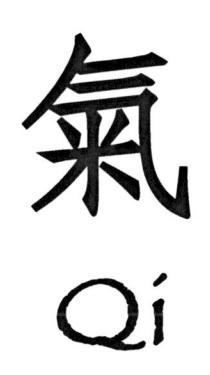

LESSON 2:

KIDNEY BREATHING, QI & DANTIAN

氣
Qi

Lesson Two: Kidney Breathing, Qi & Dantian

What is Kidney Breathing?

"Kidney Breathing" is essentially diaphragmatic breathing. Obviously we use the diaphragm every time we breathe, so why make a big deal about diaphragmatic breathing? In these lessons and in general, the term "diaphragmatic breathing" - what the Chinese call *Dantian* Breathing or simply "Kidney Breathing" - refers to letting the lower abdomen expand on inhalation and contract slightly on exhalation. This facilitates breathing that is slow and deep. Why is slow, deep breathing important? Many of us primarily use only the top part of the diaphragm and lungs to breathe. This results in shallow chest breathing that does not fully utilize the diaphragm or the muscles of the ribcage, the upper back and the deep back muscles that all have attachments to the diaphragm. The richest blood flow and perfusion of oxygen occurs in the lower lungs. If airflow to the loweer lungs is not optimal, then perfusion of oxygen into the blood is reduced.[1] Only by ventilating the lower lungs can we optimize the flow of oxygen to the cells.

The diaphragm is a strong dome-shaped muscle that divides the chest cavity from the abdominal cavity. As we saw in Lesson One, many of our internal organs have direct or indirect attachments to the diaphragm, so that its movement in breathing directly effects the functioning of the organs, aiding venous return, peristalsis and digestion, and the diffusion of fluids through the body cavities. The diaphragm also has attachments to the spine, the lower ribs, and the psoas muscle, which in turn connects to the upper leg. The more fully the diaphragm moves, the more these structures also move and are massaged and exercised.

The deeper and longer our breaths, the more oxygen is conveyed to our blood and our cells. The chemical bonds of ATP – the body's basic energy unit – are unlocked on a cellular level by oxygen. We can optimize our energy and health by making sure we fully oxygenate our cells.[2] This is achieved through Kidney Breathing. Numerous studies have shown that Kidney Breathing:

- Widens the scope of action of the muscles of the diaphragm, freeing the rib cage and enhancing pulmonary ventilation.
- Allows the body to take in more oxygen and release more carbon dioxide which leads to many health benefits, including a lowering of blood pressure, slowing of heart rate, and relaxation of the muscles.
- Calms the mind, helping to reduce insomnia.
- Increases energy and reduces fatigue.
- Reduces anxiety and stress.

Back Pain, Neck Pain and Shallow Breathing

Chronic back pain is often associated with shallow breathing. If you don't breathe into your lower abdomen and lower back, your back can lose its pliability and resiliency and become stiff. In the acupuncture clinic we often see patients with low back pain who breathe shallowly. When your back hurts, it hurts to breathe in the lower abdomen as the back expands with each breath. Yet the connective tissue attachments of the diaphragm with the ribs and lower back can be employed to help the back relax and regain normal functioning. The first breaths are usually painful, but after a little while, Kidney Breathing helps the pain subside and the tight muscles begin to relax.

Because some of the neck muscles also attach to the top of the lungs via the pleural dome, lower back pain and shallow breathing can lead to tight neck muscles and neck pain. Once you no longer breathe into the low back, the body seeks to balance the situation by using the muscles of the neck and upper ribs to lift the upper part of the lung in an attempt to ventilate the lungs more fully. This often causes them to become chronically tight.

The Qi-Breath Connection

What is *Qi (Chi)*? There is no single word in the English language that adequately expresses the concept of *Qi*. It can be translated to mean a gas or a vapor, or understood as electromagnetic waves or fields of force. The famous Chinese scholar Joseph Needham felt that the term: "Matter-Energy"[3] may most appropriately express the idea of *Qi*. For simplicity, *Qi* is often erroneously referred to as "Energy" or "Vital-Energy" in medical discussions. Webster's Dictionary defines "Energy" as follows:

- Vitality or affective force
- The capacity of acting, operating or producing an effect
- Inherent power
- Vigorousness
- Activity and the product or effect of activity
- The capacity for doing work or the equivalent, as in a coiled spring (potential energy) or a speeding train
- Having existence independent of matter (as light or X rays traversing a vacuum)[4]

Qi is simultaneously all and none of these things. To understand the concept of *Qi* more clearly it is helpful to study the ideogram itself and to look at how the Chinese have conceptualized *Qi* throughout the centuries. The Chinese character for *Qi* depicts vapors, curling and rising from the ground to form clouds above. The ancient oracle bone, bronze or seal form of the character depicts this very clearly:

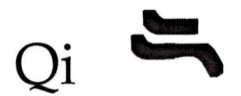

Qi

Later the ideogram was expressed showing vapors rising to form a layer of clouds. This is also part of the character for steam:

Qi 气

The ancient form of the ideogram for Qi adds the character *mi* (rice) which is depicted as: 米. This creates an image of steam or vapor rising from cooking rice.

气 + 米 = 氣 Qi

This rendering gives us the image of steam or vapor rising from cooking rice. Various interpretations may be made. It may depict the nurturing energies of rice reduced to their smallest component, a vapor, or, as Needham indicates, the changing states of energy and matter.

In early Chinese Texts, *Qi* is used to refer to various phenomena:
- Air
- Mists and Fog
- Moving Clouds
- Aromas
- Vapors
- Smoke
- Breathing - Inhalation and Exhalation

By the time of Confucius, (551-479 BCE) *Qi* also referred to physical powers or physical vitality, as well as vapors which could congeal and gather to coalesce, forming liquids or solids. Zhang Zai (Chang Tsai), who lived from 1020-1077, was an important thinker who synthesized Buddhist and Daoist ideas with Confucian thought. He regarded *Qi* as a constantly changing vital force, from which new forms emerged. *When the Qi condenses, its visibility becomes apparent so that there are then the shapes (of individual things). When it disperses, its visibility is no longer apparent and there are no new shapes. At this time of condensation can one say otherwise than that this is but temporary? But at the time of its dispersing, can one hastily say that it is non-existent?*[5]

In the 12th century, Zhu Xi (Chu Hsi) took these ideas a step further by positing that the hard and tangible and the imperceptible and intangible were but two sides of the same coin. On the surface, this seems much like theories about the interchangeability of matter and energy in modern physics. *Qi is therefore the vital principle of all things. At the same time, all things are only a state of qi. Qi is also present in all things, but it is present under diverse forms and in diverse states.*[6] Qi therefore cannot be identified as a specific thing - it is the movement, but not the form. The form is only realized through the *Qi*. It is a manifestation of *Qi*. Qi only reveals itself in the change, movement and transformation of things. For centuries *Qi* has been understood as:

> *A force that expands and animates the world in a turning motion by which it spreads and distributes itself into every corner of space and time. It has no detectable existence outside of the forms it takes and their transformations; the instruments or beings that reveal it are its particularized forms, and when they disappear they become Qi again. Qi does not "persist" alongside these manifestations. They **are** the forms it takes, and what it is. When they disappear, the Qi passes into another form. It is both a principle of coherence and unity that connects all things and a potential, a immanent life force in the world that is knowable only in the various chaging aspects it assumes.*[7]

In common usage, *Qi* can refer to air, gases and vapors, smells, spirit, vigor, morale, attitude, the emotions (particularly anger), as well as tone, atmospheric changes, the weather, breath and respiration. In the body *Qi* is often discerned by its actions, *the balanced and orderly vitalities, partly derived from the air we breathe, that cause physical changes and maintain life.*[8] When we say that someone is healthy, it is because the functioning of the their body (the manifestation of the their *Qi*) is orderly and without dysfunction.

Benjamin Swartz adds an important element to the definition of *Qi* when he says:

> *It is also clear, however that Qi comes to embrace properties which we would call psychic, emotional, spiritual, numinous and even "mystical". It is precisely at this point that Western definitions of "matter" and the physical which systemically exclude these properties from their definition do not at all correspond to Qi.*[9]

This aspect of *Qi* is particularly important in understanding Daoist meditation, because on a fundamental level, meditation is simply one of a number of Daoist methods in which the *Qi* is cultivated for the purpose of psycho-spiritual transformation.

In Chinese medicine, the term *Zheng Qi* ("correct" or "upright" *Qi)* refers to the harmonious, smooth and active flow of the *Qi* in the body. This creates a state of balance and adaptability. *"Zheng" is not limited to the medical context, but also indicates the correct rhythm of nature, the proper way of living in society, the orthodox attitude of conforming with the government and the upright position of a proper citizen and family member.*[10] *Qi* that is dysfunctional and inharmonious is called *Xie Qi*. It is sometimes rendered as "evil *Qi*" because it violates the normative order of things. In the human body the presence of *Xie Qi* leads to pain, dysfunction, mental and spiritual confusion, and premature death. The *Qi* can become disordered due to disease, injury, imbalanced emotions, over-thinking, working too hard, improper diet, and an unharmonious lifestyle that is not in tune with the natural order of things. Daoist practices such as meditation attempt to prevent the influence of *Xie Qi* by connecting to and balancing the universal energies of Heaven and Earth and returning our interaction with them to the primordial state. The first step in this process is the practice of diaphragmatic or "Kidney" Breathing.

It should be obvious by now that there is no single English word that can substitute for the character *Qi*. In context of Daoist meditation, translating *Qi* as "energy" is both unhelpful and misleading. Because of the indivisible connection of *Qi* and breath, some scholars substitute "vapor" or "vital breath" for *Qi*. In this book from now on we will refer to *Qi* by using the term *Qi/Breath*, the exception being when quoting other authors.

Qi/Breath and Dantian

The *Dantian* is generally considered to be the area 2-3 inches below the navel. Rather than being an area on the surface of the abdomen the *Dantian* is actually just in front of the spine. Medical texts locate *Dantian* 1.3 inches below the navel, while Daoist alchemical texts locate it 1.3 inches behind the navel at the intersection of *Chong Mo* and *Dai Mo* two of the Eight Extra Meridians (more information on the Extra Meridians is discussed in "Beyond the Nine Lessons: the Macro-Cosmic Orbit"). If the body is lying flat and this intersection is projected on the belly it resembles the character for field (田).[11] Effectively *Dantian* is said to be "between the kidneys," denoting a place where rarified energy moves, gathers and coalesces.

Dantian 丹田

The term *Dantian* literally means "Cinnabar Field", but in Daoism it also has the following names:
- **Elixir Field**
- **Gate of Destiny**
- **Original Pass** (referencing the *Guan Yu* acu-point which lies body inches below the navel) this point is also sometimes called *Dantian*.
- **Terminal Exit**

- **Sea of Qi** (referencing the *Qi Hai* acu-point (REN 6) which is 1.5 body inches below the navel).

Some commentaries describe the Terminal Exit as a rock in the ocean that radiates heat. Water that comes into contact with the rock turns to vapor immediately.[12] This image will be useful later when we talk about the role of saliva in *Qi/Breath* and transformation.

More generally, any place where the *Qi/Breath* gathers can be described as *Dantian*. Therefore, other areas of the body such as the navel, the center of the chest ("middle *Dantian*") and the area between the eyebrows ("upper *Dantian*"), can also be referred to as *Dantian*. However, unless specified otherwise in this book, *Dantian* generally refers to the area below the navel and just in front of the spine.

"Cinnabar Field" alludes to Chinese alchemical practices in which metals and other substances were smelted and refined in order to transform them into gold, or practices in which substances like Mercury and Cinnabar were transformed into an "elixir of immortality." In Daoist meditation, this is a metaphor for transforming the *Qi*-Dynamic of the body through relaxation and focusing on the *Qi/Breath*, so that the Primordial *Qi* (*Jing* or "essence") which resides in the lower abdomen, is transformed.

The *Dantian* is the fountainhead of the *Jing* (essence), an aspect of the *Qi/Breath* (stored in the kidneys), that is related to the reproductive generative energies in human beings. Therefore *Dantian* is sometimes referred to as "the palace that keeps the essence." In traditional Chinese medicine, *Jing* is the material basis for the physical body, its physical infrastructure. Therefore it nourishes, moistens and fuels the body. *Jing* produces the bone marrow and is the foundation of the blood and fluids of the body. It is energetically related to semen in men and the uterus and ovum in women. On a simple level, *Jing* can be thought of as a form of potential energy, like the fluid in a battery, from which the body can draw on as required. *Jing* can be depleted by imbalances in the smooth functioning of the body. Therefore, the energies of the other organs have their root in the kidneys and the *Dantian*.

The Mingmen

The *Mingmen*, is considered to be the area between the two kidneys. It is also known as the "Cinnabar Field," so there is considerable overlap between the concepts of the *Dantian* and *Mingmen*. *Mingmen* means literally the "Life Gate" or "Gate of Destiny." The word *Ming* can also refer to the idea of issuing an order or a command. The acupoint DU 4, Governing Vessel 4 (GV 4), is also known as *"Mingmen."* DU 4 lies between the 2nd and 3rd lumbar vertebrae. Although the Life gate (*Mingmen*) is actually inside the body, the *Mingmen* acu-point is the major acu-point for directly accessing the Life Gate.

Mingmen　命門

The trigram Kan, which is associated with the water element in Chinese cosmology and the kidneys in Chinese medicine, is often used to represent *Mingmen*. Kan consists of two broken (yin) lines enclosing a single (yang) solid line. This yang line is the "moving *Qi*" between the two kidneys, or the "hidden fire within water."

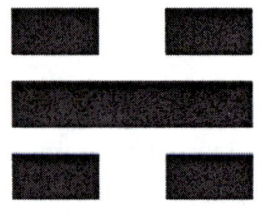

Kan-Water

This hidden fire or hidden yang is the original yang, the first true *Qi* of heaven, the eternal yang that creates and produces things. Without creation there is cessation of movement and life. *Mingmen* has a doorway which is the gate of consolidation for the whole body.[13] Therefore *Dantian* and *Mingmen* access the deepest regions of the body. Zhuang Zi refers to these two areas metaphorically as an ocean *which is the greatest of the world's waters, the ten thousand rivers spill into it endlessly and yet it is never too full. Its waters escape through the Terminal Exit and yet it never empties.*[14] Zhao Xianke, medical expert of the Ming dynasty, described the *Mingmen* as follows:

> *Mingmen dominates all twelve channels. Without it the kidneys would be weak, the spleen and stomach cannot digest food; the liver and gall*[bladder] *would not give even the greatest general the energy to think and plan; the urine and feces would not be moved, and the heart would malfunction causing dizziness and endangering life. During the lantern festival, for example, many families hang at the gate a lantern with a candle surrounded by paper figures. When the candle is lit, the figures start revolving, as the flame grows stronger, they move faster; as it weakens or goes out, they slow or come to a stop. The figures may remain on the lantern, but they are actually dead. This is Mingmen's role in Qi transformation.*[15]

From a medical standpoint, the *Mingmen* dynamic must be balanced by cultivating yin. Zhu Dan Xi (1281-1358), a famous doctor of the Jin-Yuan Dynasties, felt that *Mingmen* Fire (Ministerial Fire) is generated out of emptiness caused by our daily actions to maintain life. This is observable in any movement. Movement is yang. This includes work, leisure activities, our thoughts and desires. Any movement beyond a certain limit which is repeatedly overstepped, whether internal or external, has the potential to stir up fire and thereby imbalance yin and yang. Zhu often advocated yin supplementation to counteract this tendency. Quiescent meditation is one way to cultivate yin and counteract this tendency.[16]

The kidneys, *Mingmen* and *Dantian* are effectively the hub for the many channels and vessels through which the *Qi/Breath* and blood flow. They set in motion and distribute the *Qi/Breath*, continuously producing and promoting growth, movement and transformation. *Jing* is to some degree interchangeable with the blood, and can transform into *Qi/Breath*. It is therefore not surprising to know that focusing the mind and the *Qi/Breath* on the *Dantian* and the kidneys has been shown to stimulate the endocrine and nervous systems, and to regulate the functions of some of the internal organs. It should be noted that the Chinese idea of the kidneys is not equivalent to just the two organs we call the kidneys. It incorporates to some extent functions that modern science attributes to the bladder, the sexual organs, the adrenal glands and other parts of the endocrine system.

Although we know that it is the lungs that inhale the air, in Chinese medicine breathing is also considered a be a function of the kidneys. The kidneys are said to "grasp" the *Qi/Breath* that is inhaled by the lung. Without this enclosing and absorption of the air-vapor, the *Qi/Breath* is not fully taken in by the body. This is why diaphragmatic breathing is often referred to as "Kidney Breathing." One manifestation of asthma is a result of the kidneys not "grasping the *Qi/Breath*", and it is treated with herbs that nourish and strengthen the kidney, rather than herbs that aid dilation of the bronchioles. In this lesson we will allow the *Qi/Breath* to "sink down to the *Dantian*," a common aspect of many Qi Gong and martial arts exercises. This does not mean forcing the air down into the lower abdomen or the low back. It means that by deep diaphragmatic breathing, a sense of fullness is created in the lower abdomen and low back, letting you know that your *Qi/Breath* really is sinking down to *Dantian*.

Lesson 2: Practice - Kidney Breathing

Preliminary Exercises

Many people find Kidney Breathing difficult in the beginning. This may be particularly true if you have had abdominal surgery or have a history of asthma or bronchitis. If you have never tried to breathe into the lower abdomen or find it difficult to do so, it may be useful to practice a few preliminary exercises first.

Preliminary Exercise #1
- Lie on your back with your knees bent and your palms on your lower abdomen.
- Tuck the chin very slightly to lengthen the neck and gently tuck your tailbone so that the lower back is pressed into the floor.
- Focus your awareness on the *Dantian* (the general area between the navel and the pubic bone).
- Inhale through the nose, letting the lower abdomen expand against your hands. At the same time feel your lower back expand outward against the floor.
- Exhale and feel what happens in these areas as the air goes upward from the lower abdomen to be expelled from the nose.
- Breathe like this for several minutes using the bent knee position, the hands and floor as aids to help you.

If you still have difficulty breathing easily into the lower abdomen and kidney area, you may find it helpful to gently press down just below the solar plexus with the hands one on top of the other as you inhale. This mechanical method of sinking the *Qi/Breath* can help you tune in to Kidney Breathing.

Preliminary Exercise #2

- Exhale and bend forward at the waist, sitting back on your right leg with your left leg straight and just the heel of the left foot resting on the floor. Place your hands on your lower back.

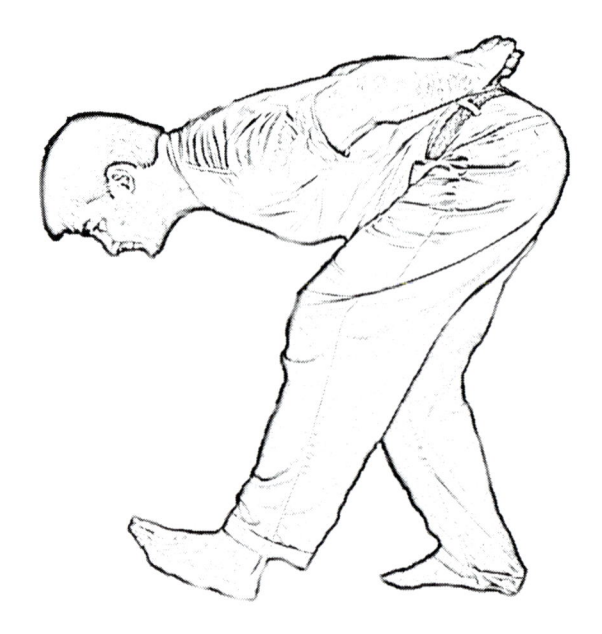

- Inhale and feel your lower abdomen expand against the lower leg. In this position, with the lower back open and stretched, it is also possible to feel your back and sacrum and even your hamstring muscles expand with the *Qi/Breath*. Use your hands to sense this expansion.
- Exhale and feel what happens in the abdomen and low back as the *Qi/Breath* move upward and outward.
- Hold this position for 3-4 cycles of inhalation and exhalation.
- Switch legs and repeat on the other side.
- The exercise can be repeated 2-3 times, switching legs each time.

If you find it difficult to balance when performing this exercise, you can rest your hands on a chair or stool as shown below:

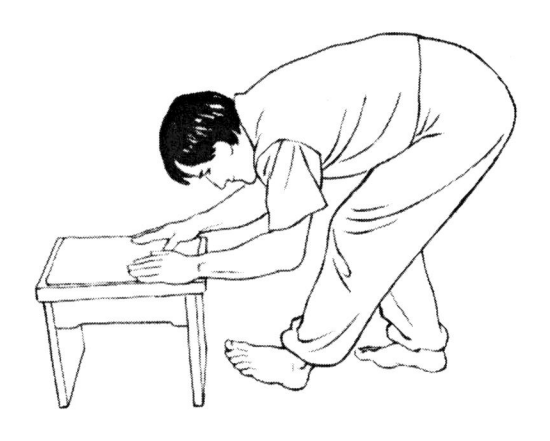

Kidney Breathing

1) Posture

Review the sitting posture from Lesson One. You will be using the same posture for this lesson. The body alignments are important because the *Qi/Breath* moves easily through areas that are open and relaxed, rather than sharply bent or tense. That is why the shoulders and arms must be relaxed and curved, and hips and legs open. It is much like a hose. The flow of water will be blocked anywhere it is kinked or sharply bent.

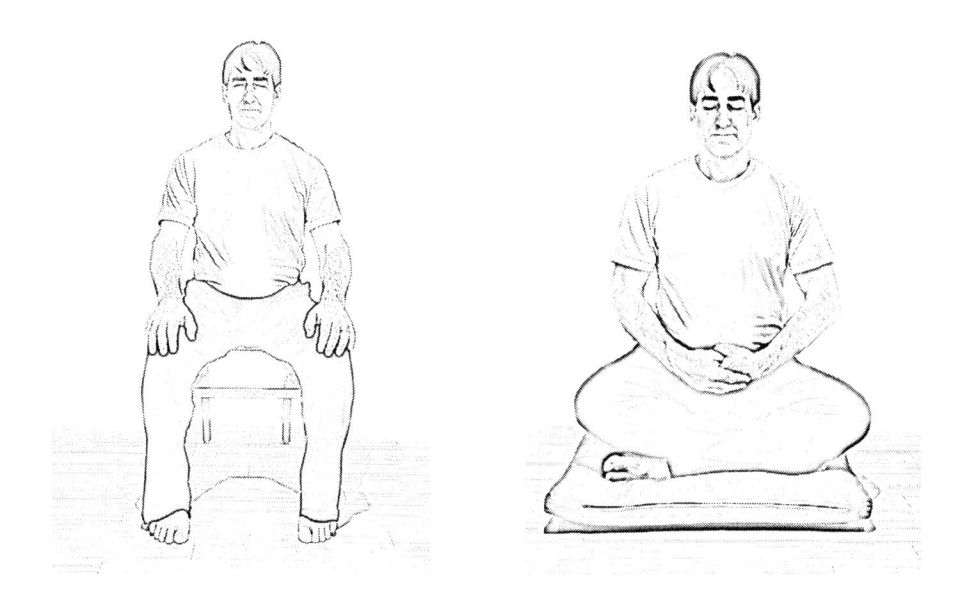

2) Adjusting The Body

This is a good time to make adjustments in the body position and posture. Adjusting the body step-by-step can help empty and calm the mind. Setting everything up properly from the beginning each time you meditate and practice Kidney Breathing ensures that the practice will be correct. Make sure that the place and position that you will sit in is comfortable and that you will be undisturbed.

1. Arrange your feet and legs so that you are comfortable and aligned.
2. Make sure that your clothing is loose and comfortable, that it protects you from drafts and that it will not be too hot or insufficiently warm.
3. Arrange the hands either on your knees or in the yin-yang hand knot.
4. Make sure the limbs and body are symmetrical and the alignments of hip and shoulder are correct. Ensure that the body is not crooked or tilted.
5. Line up the nose and the navel and straighten the neck and uplift the top of the head.
6. Gently close or half-close the eyes and look inward.

3) The Tongue and Perineum

The tongue and the perineum (the area between the anus and the genitals) are two points at which the *Ren* (Conception Vessel) and *Du* (Governing Vessel) meridians connect. More will be said later about these very important internal pathways. For now we will employ these structures to aid proper circulation of the *Qi/Breath*.

- Touch the tip of the tongue to the roof of the mouth behind the upper teeth. This connects the *Ren* and *Du* meridians above.
- Gently have a sensation of lifting the perineum upward. Do not tense your anus to do this but rather use the alignments of

suspending the head, sinking the tail and keeping the back straight with the vertebrae stacked one upon the other. At first you may need to consciously tighten the anus and urethra, later they will lift gently without thought.

- Lifting the perineum and closing the anus has another function. It creates an internal upward movement which simultaneously causes the *Qi/Breath* to sink to *Dantian*.
- The perineal area and the anus are like a valve. As the *Qi/Breath* sinks to *Dantian*, it can leak out through this valve. Gently lifting the perineum prevents this from happening.

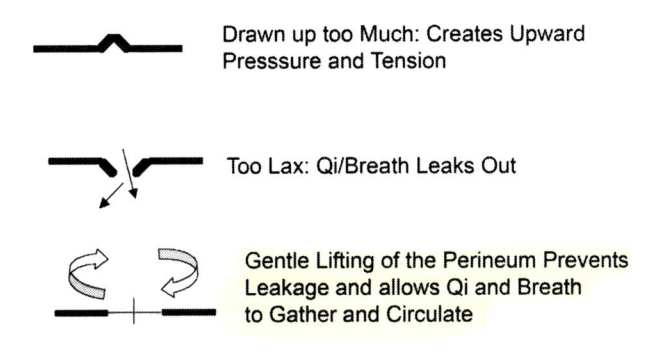

Drawn up too Much: Creates Upward Presssure and Tension

Too Lax: Qi/Breath Leaks Out

Gentle Lifting of the Perineum Prevents Leakage and allows Qi and Breath to Gather and Circulate

The Perineum is Like a Valve

4) Adjusting the Breath

Before each session of Kidney Breathing it is useful to adjust the breath. First, adjust the body as explained above in step two. This paves the way for correctly adjusting the breath, which in turn paves the way for Kidney Breathing. Start with three slow breaths, focusing the attention on *Dantian* and *Mingmen*. Inhale into *Dantian*. As you exhale, release the breath smoothly, imagining that any blockages within the body's energetic pathways move outward wiht the exhalation. Imagine the breath passing outward through all the pores of the body.

5) Kidney Breathing

With the body alignments set and the mind now focused on the breath, bring your attention to the *Dantian*. For our purposes, in this exercise, **the *Dantian* is the general area between the navel and the pubic bone. It is not on the surface of the body, but located just in front of the spine.**

- Breathe naturally and deeply, feeling the lower abdomen expand with each inhalation.
- Feel the area in your back that is directly behind the *Dantian* also expanding.
- The **whole** *Dantian* area - front, back and sides - expands and contracts with each breath.
- Let the breath sink down and back into the sacrum and the kidneys.
- Do not force the air in. Let it naturally and smoothly flow inward.
- Remember that inhaling is effortless: the diaphragm drops, creating a negative air pressure inside the lungs. This **allows** the air outside to enter and sink inward and downward Let the air (the breath) sink in and down to the *Dantian* effortlessly.
- When you exhale, mentally observe or feel the breath rise and move up and out through the nose.
- The breath is like a winding thread or a gentle stream that moves evenly and smoothly down to fill the *Dantian,* and up to be exhaled.
- Again pay attention to the smooth flow of air and its passage in and out of the body. See if you can observe the entire movement of the breath, from the moment it enters the body to the finish of the exhale.

Kidney Breathing

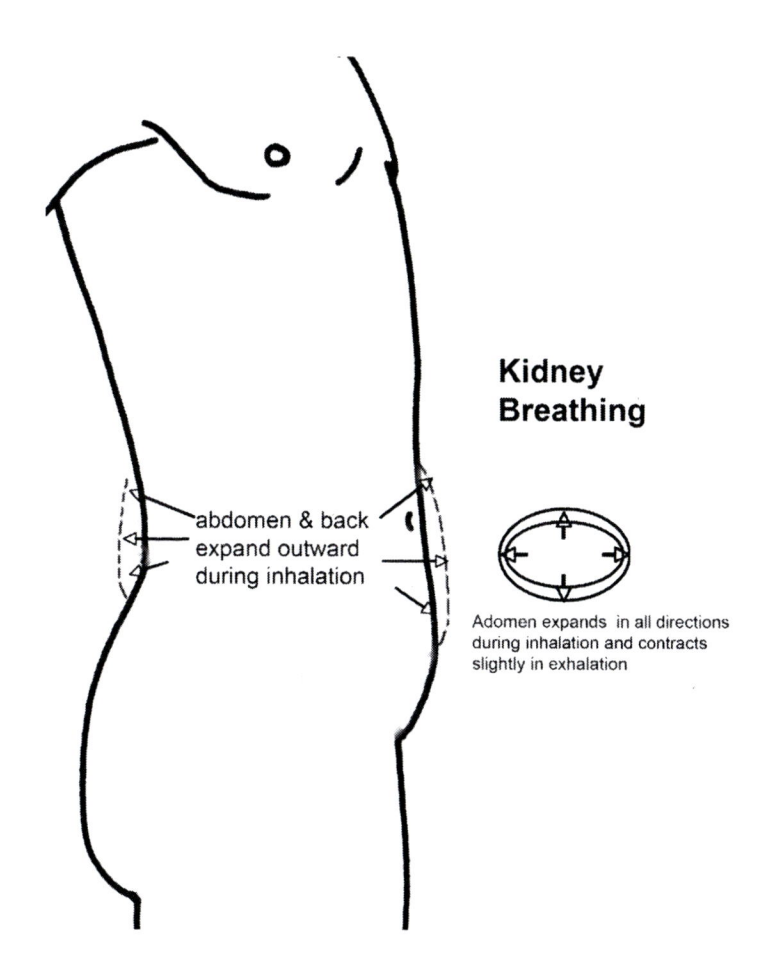

abdomen & back expand outward during inhalation

Adomen expands in all directions during inhalation and contracts slightly in exhalation

Kidney Breathing cannot be forced by pushing the air in and forcing the lower abdomen to expand. **Simply focus your attention on the *Dantian* and the *Qi/Breath* will follow**. Over time, simply by focusing your attention in this way, the breathing will naturally slow, become deeper, longer, smoother and even.

Like sediment sinking to the bottom of a pool of water, *Qi/Breath* will sink to the lower abdomen. Just as the sediment sinks naturally and without effort to the bottom of the pool, the *Qi/Breath* will also sink without physical effort. With practice your breathing will automatically become:

Natural - Easy and unforced

Slow - Unhurried

Deep - Like a bellows, filling completely and fully

Long - Like drawing a thread through cloth

Smooth - Uninterrupted and continuous

Even - Inhalation and exhalation are even and equal in force

Continue Kidney Breathing for 20 minutes, observing the breath throughout each cycle of inhalation and exhalation.

Correcting Difficulties in Kidney Breathing

When practicing Kidney Breathing, you may feel that the breath is not smooth, that it is uneven, catching and halting as you inhale and exhale. This can cause stagnation and blockage (see the Three Harms below). Or you may hear or sense a sound as air passes in and out of your nostrils. This scatters the breath, mind and *Qi*. To correct these difficulties:

1. Stabilize the mind-intention by anchoring it below the navel in the *Dantian/Mingmen*.
2. Relax and release tension by rechecking the alignments of the body.
3. Visualize the breath passing through all the pores of the body, visualize it penetrating through, coming and going, without obstruction, without interruption.

These three corrections help make the breath very fine and subtle allowing the mind to relax and engage with the practice.

The Three Harms

Through centuries of practicing breathing exercises, meditation and other *Nei Gong* exercises, the Chinese have identified three common mistakes that interfere with correct practice and can cause harm to the body. Once one is aware of The Three Harms, it is relatively easy to avoid making these errors.

1. Forced Breathing

Forced breathing can cause the lungs and the muscles of respiration to be tense, creating shortness of breath. Simply focusing your attention on the *Dantian* and the *Qi/Breath* rather than forcing air downward is the key.

2. Labored Use of Strength

Tension in the body, especially if focused on one part of the body, creates blockages in the smooth passage of the *Qi/Breath*. *Qi/Breath* does not travel easily through tense areas. The analogy of a garden hose is useful. The hose fills and expands as water moves through it. A hose is not tense, it does not push the water, it simply acts as an open conduit. If kinked or bent too sharply, the water will not flow smoothly through the hose.

3. Throwing out the Chest and Sucking in the Abdomen

Throwing out the chest and sucking in the abdomen prevents the *Qi/Breath* from sinking to the lower abdomen and the *Dantian*. Soften the chest and let the shoulders drop, while keeping the neck relaxed.

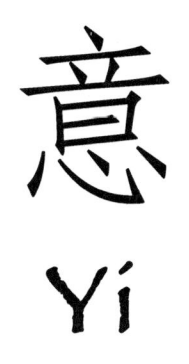

LESSON 3:

QUIETING THE MIND & GATHERING THE QI

意

Yi

Lesson Three: Quieting the Mind & Gathering the Qi

When observing the breath in the first two lessons, you may have noticed that the mind has a tendency to wander. Perhaps a number of breaths passed without you noticing. In this lesson we will work with the mind and the breath together. Our practice will be aided by understanding the relationship of the mind and the *Qi/Breath*.

Qi/Breath, Thought and Emotion

Every movement of the mind is a movement of the *Qi/Breath*. In Chinese medicine, the *Qi/Breath* is the source of all movement, transformation and change, both inside the human body and in the world around us. This means that the *Qi/Breath* is not only intimately connected to the movement inherent in physical processes, but it is also directly connected to our every thought and emotion. In Lesson Two, we saw how atmospheric changes are described as movements and transformations in the *Qi/Breaths* of Heaven and Earth. Similarly, the emotions are understood to be observable expressions of the movements of the *Qi/Breath* within us.

In Chinese thought, anger **is** the *Qi/Breath* rushing upward suddenly. If there is no outlet for this movement, if it is blocked or repressed, anger can be expressed/experienced as frustration (i.e. anger directed inward or downward). Similarly, fear **is** a downward movement of the *Qi/Breath*. This downward movement empties the heart, creating timidity or even terror. Terror is many times accompanied by an involuntary discharge of urine or feces (a sign of the rapid downward movement of the *Qi/Breath*). In Chinese medicine, the emotions are considered to be the internal causes of disease. By fixating on certain thoughts and emotions rather than experiencing them and letting them move through us in an appropriate and seamless way, the *Qi/Breath* can become imbalanced, creating physical illness.

It may seem strange to define emotions in terms of movements of the *Qi/Breath,* yet these movements, although sometimes subtle, are easily perceived. Imagine something that makes you angry and let yourself fully engage with that anger. What do you feel inside the body? There is usually some feeling of fullness or tension in the upper body. It may manifest as a sensation of heat or tension in the head and chest, or an upward surge of energy or blood to the head. There may be tension in the neck, and your face may even get red. Now imagine something sad, or something that makes you sad. You may notice a tightness in the chest accompanied by an emptiness - a kind of hollow feeling inside the chest. Your breath may become shallower and more restrained. Sadness and melancholy prevent the normal movement of *Qi/Breath* so that it stagnates and feels hollow rather than vibrant and full.

Qi/Breath is our connection with the outside world. We experience other human beings and the outside world through the *Qi/Breath*. There is a potential problem in this interaction of the *Qi/Breath* and the senses with the outside world. By obsessing or fixating on things in the world, by interacting with the world on the basis of appetites, desires, emotions and intellectual distinctions, we can upset the internal balance and dissipate essence and *Qi/Breath*. In Daoism, human beings are visualized as being between heaven and earth. Human beings are at the center of the pole which carries vibrations between Heaven and Earth - the *Qi/Breath* of Heaven and *Qi/Breath* of Earth. Our *Qi/Breath* interacts with, and is to some degree a manifestation of, the *Qi/Breaths* of Heaven and Earth.

It is important to understand that in Daoist meditation, "Heaven" does not refer to the Judeo-Christian notion of heaven. Rather, Heaven is a natural operating system, an all-encompassing organic system, that governs everything. Earth in turn responds, realizing Heaven's initiating and creative power.

Heaven

Human Beings

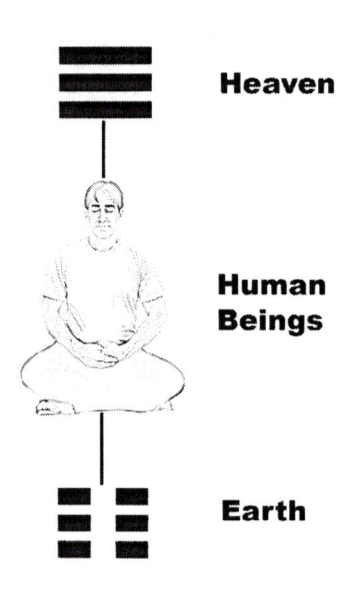

Earth

In their excellent exploration into health and psychology in Chinese medicine, *The Seven Emotions,* Claude Larre and Elisabeth Rochat de La Vallée liken man to a tree growing out of the earth and reaching up to heaven:

> *On the trunk of the tree and the great branches there are a lot of little holes or cavities, and when the wind blows it enters all these cavities and during a tempest you can hear the sound of the resonances inside the wood of the tree and the noise made by the branches, after a while, the wind calms itself and the tree returns to a kind of emptiness without any noise. This is what is called earthly music, which is just music coming through openings and cavities. This is an important point because emotions are always reactions to the world outside by one's inner vitality. It is natural and normal that there are tempests and hurricanes and little showers and great winds, and after that no wind at all, or just a very light rain. The only thing for this tree is to be able to bend with the wind, to follow the violence of the wind in its manifestations and after to come back to a calm, motionless state. This is just an example of the very general use of the human emotions. It is normal for a man between heaven and earth to have stimulations and emotions and sometimes to be very deeply moved by*

them. But the important thing is to be able to restore the balance, and the calm emptiness through all the passages of vitality.[1]

Ordering the Mind & Gathering the Qi

Ordering the *Qi/Breath* with the mind/intention (*Yi*) is the way that one begins to learn to harmonize the emotions and preserve the vital *Qi*. The famous Daoist writer Zhuang Zi advises us to let the mind "fast" in order to experience this calm emptiness. *The Dao gathers in emptiness alone. Emptiness is the fasting of the mind.*[2] *Qi/Breath* is empty, without material form, so it gathers in emptiness and stillness. The generative force (*Jing*) transforms into *Qi/Breath* when the body is motionless, and vitality changes into spirit when the heart is unstirred.[3] In stillness one can harmonize one's *Qi/Breath* with the cosmic *Qi/Breath*. "Fasting the mind" is a way to gather the *Qi/Breath* as opposed to dissipating it; a way of "dwelling in stillness", rather than fixating on things in the outside world.

Zhuang Zi tells us the story of Duke Huan who saw a ghost when hunting in a marsh. When he returned home he became ill and refused to go out. A gentleman of the court said, *"Your Grace, you are doing this injury to yourself! How could a ghost have the power to injure you. If the vital breath that is stored up in a man becomes dispersed and does not return, then he suffers a deficiency. If it ascends and fails to descend, it causes him to be chronically forgetful. And if it neither ascends nor descends, but gathers in the middle of the body in the region of the heart, then he becomes ill."*[4] Duke Huan's illness was a result of his mind fixating on what he had seen. For Zhuang Zi, it is not feelings, thoughts or emotions themselves that separate humans from the Dao, but the human tendency to fixate on specific aspects of the world and to make them part of our goals and desires thus making them absolutes.[5]

Francois Jullien describes this state of inner detachment as one of "blandness," a concept associated with the Dao. Jullien posits that to *honor the bland - to value the flavorless rather than the flavorful - runs counter to our most spontaneous judgment.*[6] Jullien goes on to say that *all flavors disappoint even as they attract, like sound sifted through an instrument that disappears as soon as it is consumed.*[7] In contrast the bland is like:

> *An attenuated sound that retreats from the ear and is allowed to simply die out over the longest possible time. We hear it still, but just barely; as it diminishes, it makes all the more audible the soundless beyond into which it is about to extinguish itself. We are listening then, to its extinction, to its return to the great undifferentiated Matrix. This is the sound that, in its very fading, gradually opens the way to the inaudible and causes us to experience the continuous movement from one to the other. And as it gradually sheds its aural materiality, it leads us to the threshold of silence, a silence we experience as plentitude, at the very root of all harmony.*[8]

In the West, we feel we must express our emotions and a common view is that one who does not express his viewpoints and feelings is uninteresting, inauthentic, a bore or a "cold fish." Jullien cautions us against this assumption:

> *The calm inner world and the intuition of emptiness do not cut us off from emotion. To the contrary, because emotion no longer disturbs us, we apprehend it all the more clearly and are thus able to enjoy it. Fits of passion and its exuberance are charged with making our subjectivity superficial and reducing our sensitivity. When we attain the world of blandness, feelings distract us no longer, and emotive experience is purified, clarified. The mind in keeping with the old metaphor of still water or mirrors, reflects all the better the infinite wealth of life within: not just one particular feeling, lived within the confines of its limitations and contingencies, but all feeling as it becomes whole and inclusive, returned to its virtual state.*[9]

Stillness, Harmony & Engagement

Entering into a state of stillness and emptiness, rather than creating detachment, increases engagement with the world. By using *Qi/Breath*, posture and intention to order and regulate the ongoing changes and transformations of life, by listening with the *Qi/Breath*, one can engage with the undivided primordial state that underlies normal consciousness. This allows one to perform ordinary activities in an outstanding way. Zhuang Zi's story of Prince Wen-Hui's cook illustrates how the brilliance of one's spirit and creativity are released and given free reign upon letting go of desires and wants and engaging with the primordial state.:

> *Prince Wen-Hui's cook was cutting up a bullock. Every touch of his hand, every shift of his shoulder, every tread of his foot, every thrust of his knee, every sound of the rending flesh, and every note of the movement of the chopper was in perfect harmony.* "Ah, admirable," said the prince, "that your skill should be so perfect." [The cook replies that he has applied himself to make "every movement in harmony with the Dao".] *The functions of my senses stop; my spirit dominates. Following the natural markings, my cleaver slides through the great cleavages, taking advantage of the structure that is already there. My skill is now such that my chopper never touches the smallest tendon or ligament, let alone the great bones. A good cook changes his chopper once a year, because he cuts. An ordinary cook changes his chopper once a month, because he hacks. Now my chopper has been used for 19 years; it has cut up several thousand bullocks; yet its edge is as sharp as if it just came from the whetstone.*[10]

The cook goes on to say that he inserts the edge of the chopper into the interstices between the joints where there is space. Then by a gentle movement the part is separated and *yields like earth crumbling to the ground.*[11] He cuts the spaces between things.

This kind of ability is the result of extreme concentration. Yet this concentration is the opposite of obsession, because as Francois Jullien points out, such *exquisite perception* brings with it the ability to guide the *Qi/Breath* in one's physical being and in one's life so that *it is neither thwarted nor dispersed but continues to flow.*[12]

Holding Fast to The "One"

In the *Dao De Jing*, Lao Zi asks:

> *Can you keep the unquiet physical-soul from straying,*
> > *hold fast to the Unity and never quit it?*
> *Can you when concentrating your breath,*
> > *make it soft like that of a little child?*
> *Can you wipe out and cleanse your vision of the Mystery*
> > *till all is without blur?*
> *Can you love the people and rule the land,*
> > *yet remain unknown?*
> *Can you in opening and shutting the heavenly gates,*
> > *play always the female part?*
> *Can you penetrate every corner of the land,*
> > *But you yourself never interfere?*[13]

This passage refers obliquely to Daoist meditation. The physical soul here refers to the semen, or sexual vitality. "Concentrating your breath," refers to the method of breathing in meditation. The breathing must be soft like an infant - a feather in front of the nose would not flutter and more is breathed in than out.[14] The "female part" (i.e.: passive role), and "opening" refer to opening and shutting the mouth and nostrils. "Hold fast to the Unity" means to "hold fast to the One," as opposed to the many, thereby allowing connection and engagement with the undivided primordial state that underlies normal consciousness.[15] "Holding fast to the One" involves stilling mind and body so that thoughts do not arise; allowing the self and the world to seem like "One".

This is a mind in touch with the Dao. As the mind stills, the breath will become soft. This is the "true breath" or cosmic breath.

The *Nei-Yeh* or "Inward Training" is a set of verses from the mid-Fourth Century (the Warring States Period). The *Nei-Yeh* focuses on inner cultivation through breathing and sitting with the body in alignment. It also makes reference to the importance of holding fast to the One:

When you enlarge your mind and let go of it,
When you relax your vital breath and expand it,
When the body is calm and unmoving:
And you can maintain the One and discard the myriad disturbances,
You will see profit and not be enticed by it,
You will see harm and not be frightened of it.
Relaxed and unwound, yet acutely sensitive,
In solitude you delight in your own person.
This is called "revolving the vital breath":
Your thoughts and deeds seem heavenly.[16]

The Inadequacy of Words

The very first chapter of the Dao De Jing tells us that words will not help us to understand the undivided primordial state of the "One."

The Way (Dao) that can be told of is not an unvarying Way (Dao);
The names that can be named are not unvarying names.
It was from the nameless that Heaven and Earth Sprang;
The named is but the mother that rears the ten thousand creatures, each
    after its own kind.
Truly, only he that rids himself forever of desire can see the Secret
    Essences;
He that has never rid himself of desire can see only the outcomes.
These two things issued from the same mold, but nevertheless are different
    in name.

> *This same mould we can but call the Mystery,*
> *Or rather Darker than any Mystery,*
> *The Doorway whence issued all Secret Essences.*[17]

It is clear from this passage that although we need to use words to talk about the Dao (the One), words are inadequate. They are merely stop-gaps. *For what we are trying to express is darker than any mystery.*[18] Images and words are only a means to an end, a way of talking about something. They should not be confused with the end or the thing itself. If one fixes on the words, one cannot grasp the image, fixing on the image the idea cannot be grasped. Once the image and idea are grasped the words and the images can be discarded.[19] In this lesson and the ones that follow, we must use words to understand the images and ideas that enable us to put Daoist methods of meditation into practice. But once set in motion, the ideas can be discarded. Zhuang Zi puts this succinctly and humorously:

> *The fish trap exists because of the fish;*
> *Once you've gotten the fish, you can forget the trap.*
> *The rabbit snare exists because of the rabbit;*
> *Once you've gotten the rabbit, you can forget the snare.*
> *Words exist because of meaning;*
> *Once you've gotten the meaning, you can forget the words.*
> *Where can I find a man who has forgotten the words so I can have a word*
> *with him?*[20]

In *Daoism Explained* Hans-Georg Mueller takes our understanding of Zhuang Zi's allegory of the fish trap one step further. He reminds us that the phrase *de yi* means not only "to get the idea" or meaning, but also "to get what one desires." Mueller points out that having the thing one desires is to be satisfied. The desire disappears once it is satisfied. *Once one has* [consumed] *a pizza or a beer, one cannot have it any longer. The desire is fulfilled when it has disappeared* [been "eaten up"].[21] Therefore, this passage from the *Zhuangzi* is not about understanding thoughts and ideas, but about how to rid oneself of thoughts and ideas so that one can attain an inner silence. In this context, the implication of the final line is that two people who have reached this state of inner silence will have nothing to say.[22]

Lesson 3: Practice - Counting the Breaths

Counting the breaths is one method of quieting and focusing the thoughts that come and go through our consciousness. In this lesson we will count each breath. The first cycle of inhalation and exhalation is counted as "one" and so on up until "nine." When we reach nine breaths we begin again, starting at "one." If we lose count of the breaths before reaching nine, we start again at "one."

Counting the breaths can be difficult. Many people who meditate find it hard to count breaths because as they count, thoughts arise one upon the other and the counting becomes lost. This can create frustration and a feeling of failure. It is important to remember that the goal is not to be good at counting breaths, but to observe the ebb and flow of our thoughts, so that they eventually disappear. The very act of trying to abstain from thought is also a thought and a fixation. Counting the breaths is merely a tool that helps us observe our thoughts and, by that very observation, allows them to disappear. There is no success or failure, there is just the counting and observation.

Counting the Breaths

Review the sitting posture from Lesson One. Use the same posture for this lesson. Then adjust posture and breath as discussed in Lesson Two. With posture and breath adjusted, focus on the breath. Close your eyes and bring your attention to the *Dantian*. Just as you did in Lesson Two, begin Kidney Breathing. Breathe naturally and deeply, feeling the lower abdomen expand with each inhalation. Observe each individual breath, paying attention to the smooth flow of air and its passage in and out of the body. See if you can observe the entire movement of the breath, from the moment it enters the body to the finish of the exhale.

Now with the eyes closed, look inward as you begin to count the breaths, following the airflow, noticing it enter the nose and sink through the throat and chest down to *Dantian*. Then notice it return, moving up from *Dantian* through the chest and throat to be exhaled through the nose. Slowly make the inhale and exhale even as you count the breaths:

- Count from 1 to 9. When you count nine breaths, begin again counting from 1-9.
- If you lose count or your mind wanders, simply begin again starting at 1.
- Count the breaths for as long as you like. A good starting point is to sit and count for 36 breaths – 36 cycles of inhalation and exhalation or 4 sets of 9 breaths.

Observing Your Thoughts

As you look inward and count, thoughts will arise. Look at each thought as it arises. By looking at each thought, we prevent it connecting to another thought and another in an endless chain. By looking at each thought as it arises, it will vanish. Another thought may arise but we use the same method of looking at it and it also vanishes. Gradually thoughts will diminish.

Thoughts are like clouds passing in front of the sun. The sun is still there shining, it is just momentarily obscured by the clouds. When the clouds pass the sun shines again. Similarly when thoughts pass, the mind is still again.

Adjusting the Mind

When entering into meditation the mind can be difficult to regulate. In Lesson Two you learned how to adjust the posture and the breath in order to prepare for meditation, and how to correct the difficulties that can arise in performing Kidney Breathing. These preparations also help to regulate the mental state but often, even when counting breaths, the mind deviates. Sramana Zhi Yi (Chih-i) was one of the most respected figures in

Chinese Buddhism of the *Tian Tai* school who wrote on Buddhist meditation in the Sixth Century CE. Sramana Zhi Yi, passes on to us very specific and practical advice for regulating and adjusting the mental state. He first identifies four mental states that can occur when entering into or abiding in meditation: sinking, floating, laxity and urgency. [23]

Sinking is characterized by a dim mental state, a tendency of the head to droop downward or not remembering anything. It can be corrected by anchoring one's mind on the tip of the nose and holding it there so there is no loss of attention. Once the attention is firm, the mind-intention can return to the *Dantian* and *Mingmen*.

Floating can mean that the mind drifts off and moves about, the body is ill at ease, or that the the mind is drawn to outside conditions or objects. To correct floating, anchor the mind on the *Mingmen* and *Dantian*.

Laxity involves a slackening of the body, coupled with a scattered mind-intention. The body may become slumped. Drawing up the body and lifting the mind-intention upward while attending to the body alignments can correct this.

Urgency means the attention and focus have moved upward. There may be pain in the chest or neck. To correct urgency, relax and release the body letting the mind-intention go downward. *The subtle energetic breath will then flow on down. If one were to do this, then the disturbance would be naturally cured.*[24]

When plagued by distracting thoughts during meditation it can be useful to recall the advice of Hung Ying Ming, a mountain recluse who lived in the 16th Century:

In uneventful times,

The mind is easily distracted.

Then you should make yourself still and let your true nature shine.

When things are happening all around you,

The mind is easily scattered,

Then you should make your true nature shine and allow your center to become still.[25]

LESSON 4:

RETURNING TO EMPTINESS - WU JI

無極
Wu Ji

Lesson Four: Returning to Emptiness - Wu Ji

Chinese Cosmogony and Wu Ji

In Chinese cosmology there was originally *Hun Tun*, an undifferentiated luminous cloud, a void with no boundary, emptiness, a potential state. The *Hun Tun* is sometimes considered a state of chaos in that it is undivided, whole - a state where everything is mixed together. This potential undifferentiated primordial state is also called *Wu Ji*. *Wu Ji* means literally "no limit" or "no polarity." It is the "One," the place we are trying to get close to in meditation.

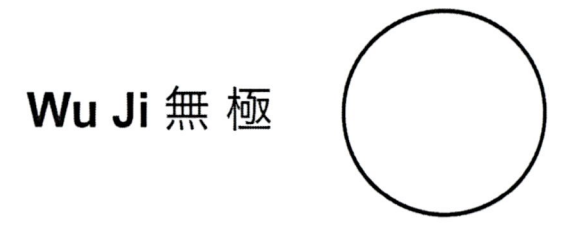

Wu Ji 無極   ◯

Movement occurs within the undifferentiated matter, the non-polarized "stuff" that is the *Wu Ji*. This movement is like the wind, like a breath, like an inhalation and exhalation. It is the primordial *Qi/Breath*, the true *Qi/Breath*. With movement (*Dong*), there is also stillness (*Jing*). With movement, things begin to divide and separate. The lighter transparent *Qi/Breath* rises and the heavier opaque *Qi/Breath* sinks down. The polarity of Heaven and Earth is created. Heaven is yang and Earth is yin. *Qi/Breath* that is influenced by yang floats, rises and moves so it can be characterized as *Yang Qi*. *Qi/Breath* that sinks, falls and is quiescent is influenced by Yin, and can be characterized as *Yin Qi*.

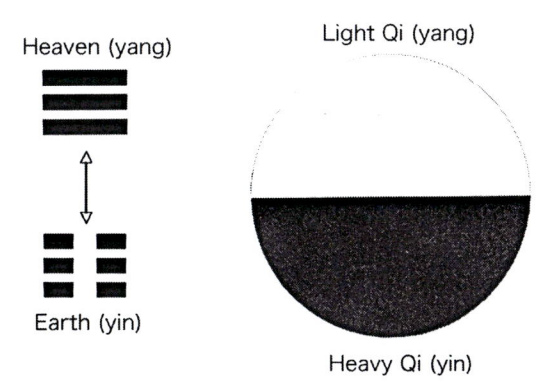

This polarity created by the *Qi/Breath* is called the *Tai Ji*, the "great pole" or "extreme polarity." It can be represented as Heaven and Earth as diagramed above. The *Tai Ji* represents the division of things into *Yin Qi* and *Yang Qi*, movement and stillness, up and down, right and left, etc.

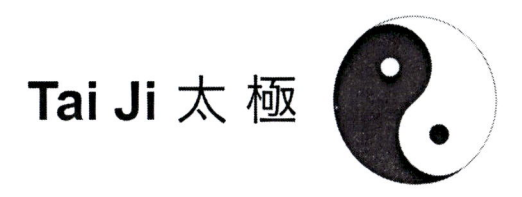

Tai Ji 太極

The polarity represented by the *Tai Ji* is not fixed but relative. Something is only yang relative to yin. Something is said to be "up" only in relation to that which is said to be "down." Additionally, yin contains yang and yang contains yin. This is represented by the white circle within the black fish and the black circle within the white fish. Therefore, nothing can be completely yin or yang; yang contains the seeds of yin and yin contains the seeds of yang. This means that yin and yang can transform into each other, creating an interplay of stillness and movement; of light and dark; of the in-breath and the out-breath.

An alternative Tai Ji Diagram, attributed to Chen Tuan of the Song dynasty, visually conveys the spiraling, circular movement of *Qi/Breath* in the center, initiating the movement which creates polarities of light and heavy; clear and turbid; movement and stillness; yang and yin.

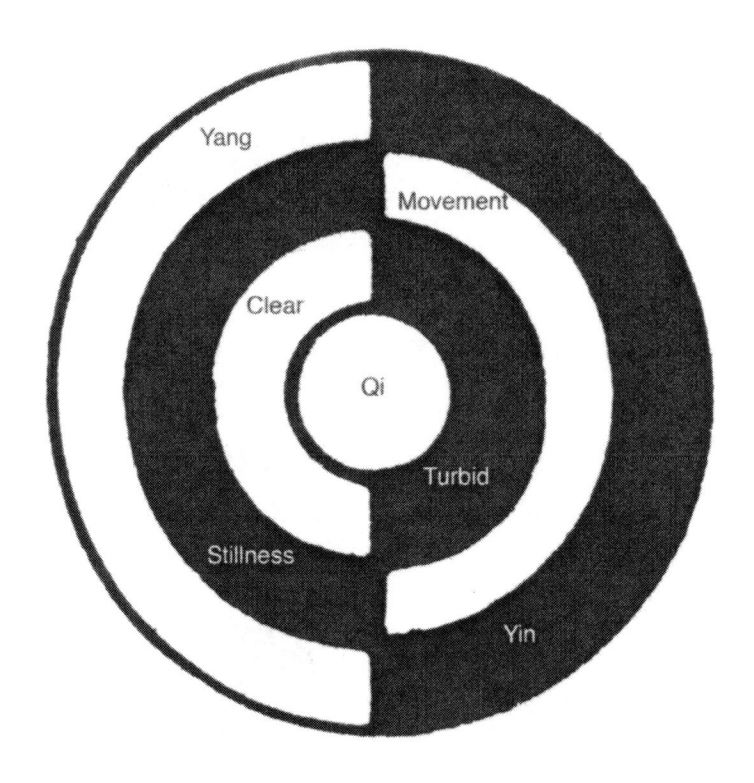

The *Qi/Breath* moving in the center connects yin and yang forming three modalities that complete and compliment each other. From these three, other forces are created. Chen Tuan's larger *Wu Ji* diagram illustrates how *Wu Ji* and *Tai Ji* are the foundation of forms and their interaction.

Wu Ji Diagram of Chen Tuan

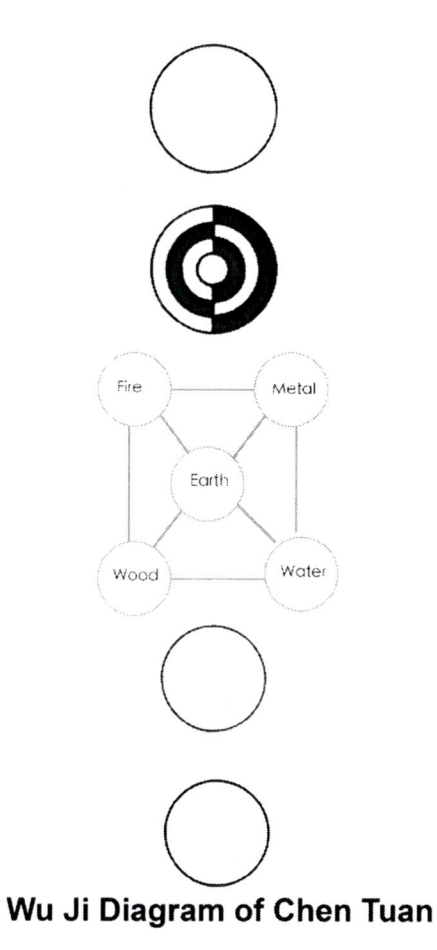

Reading downward, the diagram starts at the top with *Wu Ji* which generates *Tai Ji*. The movement (*Dong*) implicit within the *Tai Ji*, results in the Five Elements (*Wu Xing*). The *Wu Xing* are actually not so much fixed forms as much as dynamic, interacting forces. Thus they are often called the Five Agents, Five Activities or the Five Phases. They are also known as the Five Powers (*Wu Te*).[1] *The nature of Water is to moisten and descend; of Fire to flame and ascend, of Wood to be crooked and straighten; of Metal to yield and to be modified, of Soil to provide for sowing and reaping.*[2]

Wu 五

Xing 形

Wu is the number five. *Xing* is generally used to mean: "to appear"; "to look"; "form"; "shape". However *Xing* can also mean "to act" or "to do."[3] In the 11th Century, Zhu Dan Yi described the interaction of the *Tai Ji* and the *Wu Xing* as follows:

> *Tai Ji moves and produces yang. When the movement reaches its limit it comes to rest. Tai Ji at rest produces yin. When the state of rest comes to a limit, it returns to a state of motion. Motion and rest alternate, each being the source of the other. Yin and yang take up their appointed positions to establish the two forces (Liang Yi). Yang is transformed by combining with yin, producing Water, Fire, Wood, Metal and Earth. Then the five Qi diffuse harmoniously and the Four Seasons take their course.*[4]

The Five Powers are intimately connected with the life of human beings on Earth. The interaction of Heaven and Earth is a fixed, unchanging polarity. It is timeless and immutable. In human beings and the natural world, the breaths of heaven and earth are experienced through the five powers because it is through them, that life takes on material form and shape. Our senses, tastes, sounds, discriminations, even our internal organs, are all considered to be expressions of the Five Powers. The concept of time, cyclical movement and change are also manifestations of the Five Powers, which operate within us in the same way that they operate in the world around us, reflected in the seasons, the weather, and the movements of the planets. The cyclical movement inherent in the Five Powers can be seen in the following diagram.

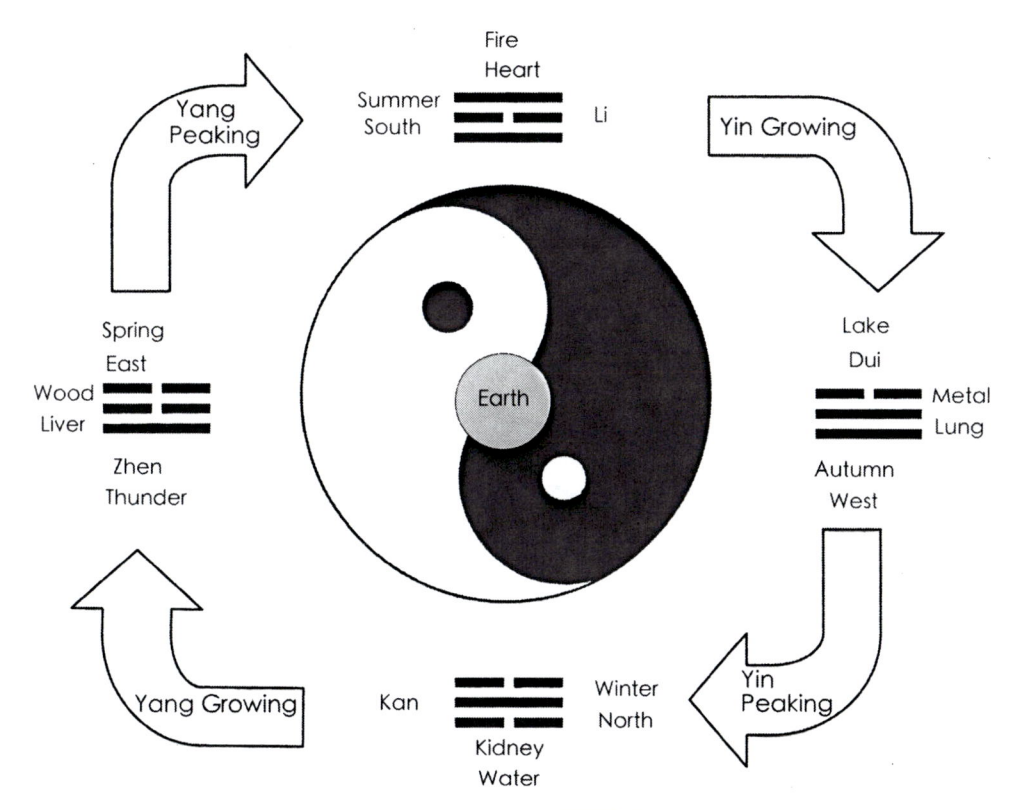

The cyclical interaction of the Five Powers contains the seed of quiescence and stillness. There is dynamic action, but there are also forms and shapes that change and transform. In addition, Earth is the still, receptive center around which the other powers revolve and interact.

As we follow Chen Tuan's diagram to the bottom there is a return or reversion to quiescence and *Wu Ji* (represented by the two empty circles at the bottom). This reversion comes about through the practice of the Wu Ji posture discussed in the practice section of this lesson.

From *Wu Ji*, *Tai Ji* and *Qi/Breath*, everything else (the ten thousand things) comes into being. In the *Dao De Jing* this dynamic is described as follows:

> *The One gave birth successively to two things, three things up to ten thousand. These ten thousand creatures cannot turn their backs to the shade without having the sun on their bellies, and it is on this blending of the breaths, that their harmony depends.*[5]

This idea is often illustrated by using *Yi Jing* (I Ching) diagrams to show how yin and yang change and recombine to create complex forms and interactions.

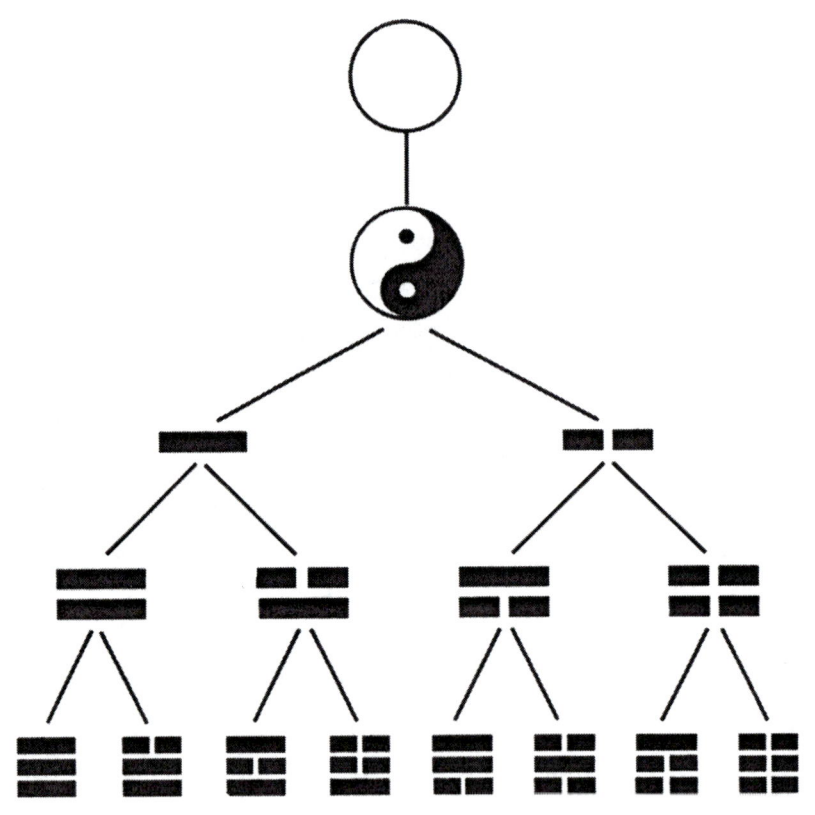

Wu Ji to Tai Ji to Eight Trigrams and Ultimately to the 10,000 Things

Wu Ji and Daoist Meditation

The *Wu Ji*, the place of stillness where the breath begins, is the state we desire to return to in meditation. Standing or sitting with the mind void, without thought and without intention, is the place from which one can experience the spontaneous stirring of a movement; the place where one can experience the interplay of stillness and movement. The *Wu Ji* in meditation is not only a mental state, but a posture, where the body is like a central pole connecting Heaven and Earth. The body posture is unified and undivided. It can be likened to a string on a musical instrument. If it is strung too tight or is too lax it does not resonate and produce the correct pitch. Similarly, if the physical and mental postures are correctly aligned with the poles of Heaven and Earth, they will vibrate in harmony with them. In Lesson Two we saw how human beings are between Heaven and Warth. Yin and yang interact and unite within us. By understanding how they interact, we can experience that unity.

The heavens are like a dome above human beings so the Chinese say that "Heaven is round." The Earth has four cardinal directions in relationship to the roundness of heaven. These directions are delineated by four points - two where the celestial equator meets the elliptic, and two where the equator and the elliptic are are at the maximum distance from each other. These four points mark the spring and fall equinoxes and the summer and winter solstices. *Connecting these points forms a square, and that square is the earth – an idealized earth, bounded by celestial time as defined by the four seasons.*[6] Therefore, "Earth is square." The possessor of the Dao (a human being) sits at the fulcrum of this vibrating dipole, between Heaven and Earth.

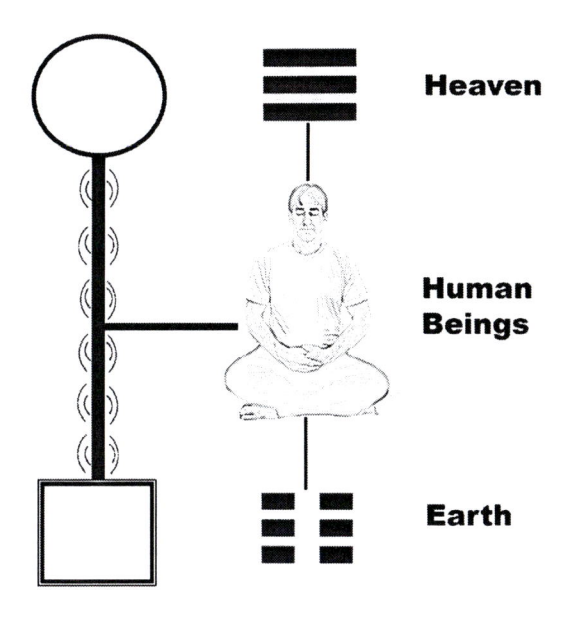

The Wu Ji Posture & the Martial Arts

In the Chinese internal arts, the standing *Wu Ji* (or "void") posture is the place that movement begins. In the martial arts, when one practices the movements of the *Tai Ji Quan* form, *Ba Gua Zhang's* eight palm changes, or *Xing Yi Quan's* five fists – they all begin from the *Wu Ji*; the void; the still place where the breath initiates movement. Each time the movements and forms are practiced, Chinese cosmogony is invoked. The practitioner starts by standing in the void and experiences the first stirring of movement through the breath and the *Tai Ji*. All of the other movements are said to emanate from this posture.

The Wu Ji Posture

Standing in the *Wu Ji* posture with the head toward Heaven and the feet on the Earth, we can feel the head and the upper torso reaching upward to Heaven and the tailbone and the lower body sinking downward toward the Earth. In this way there is a separating force in the body. This separation is clearly felt at the *Mingmen* acu-point which lies opposite the *Dantian* at the 2nd and 3rd lumbar vertebra (see Lesson Two). The bones are heavy and want to sink toward the Earth, so by lifting them up, stacking them one upon the other, a movement toward Heaven is created. The flesh is lighter and wants to rise and float, so by letting the flesh sink, by letting it hang off the bones, a movement toward Earth is created. The tail sinking and head lifting, while the bones lift and the flesh sinks, creates a dynamic tension that fully engages the yin-yang dynamic of Heaven and Earth within us.

Lesson 4: Practice - The Wu Ji Posture

Assuming the Wu Ji Posture

- Start by standing with the feet facing forward and parallel.
- The feet are directly underneath the hips, so that the knees are straight with the kneecaps facing forward.
- Make sure the whole foot is on the floor - that you are not standing more on one part of the sole, such as the heels or the outside of the foot.
- Bend the knees slightly but keep them relaxed.
- The knees are in line with the front of the hip and the space between the first and second toes.
- Bend slightly at hip fold.
- Relax the hip: keep the *kua* open. Although often translated as "hip", *kua* actually refers to the inguinal area in the front of the pelvis going up to the top of the ilium, including both the internal and external structures.
- Round the crotch.
- Relax the waist.
- Sink the tail like a plumb line.
- Gently lift the perineum and anus (this is more an idea and less a physical action).
- Raise the upper back and soften and relax the chest but don't collapse the chest.
- Let the shoulders hang and relax.
- Let the elbows sink and drop.
- Keep space under the armpits. It is as though there is a ball under each armpit.
- Relax the wrists and fingers.

- The head lifts as though suspended by the vertex and the chin is slightly pulled in.
- The eyes look slightly down and forward with a soft gaze.
- The tongue is on the upper palate and the mouth is closed.
- Bring your attention to the *Dantian*. Breathe naturally and deeply, feeling the lower abdomen expand with each inhalation.
- Feel the area in your back that is directly behind the *Dantian* also expanding. Employ "Kidney Breathing."

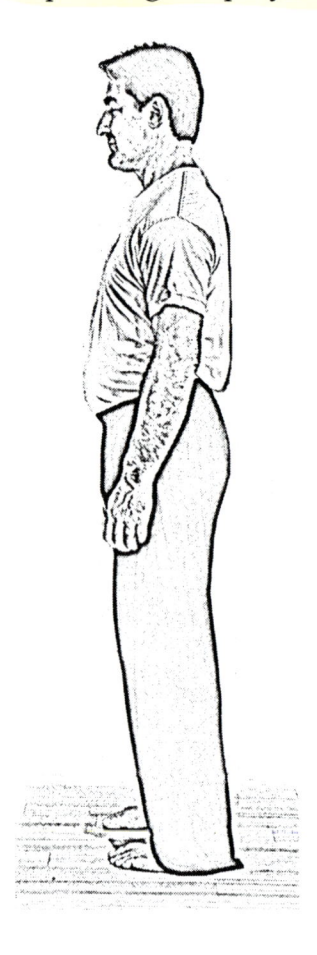

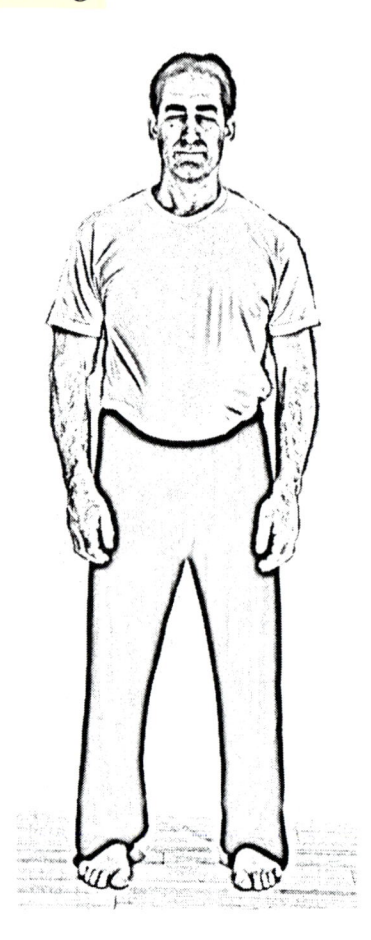

The Alignments Work Synergistically as Parts of a Whole

If you are having difficulty with the posture or some of the alignments, rather than focusing on a single alignment, go through the alignments like a checklist. Each component is part of a whole and works synergistically with the others. For example, a common problem is difficulty in "lifting the perineum" without creating tension. Rather than focusing on the perineum, focus on relaxing and opening the *kua* while rounding the crotch area, sinking the tail and lifting the head and upper back. Attending to these alignments allows the perineum to automatically lift. For quicker reference, Appendix Two gives a synopsis of the key alignments.

Images, Exercises & Points for Attention

As the head and the upper torso gently reach upward, the tailbone and lower body sink downward. This creates a separating force in the body which is most noticeable at the *Mingmen* acu-point, which lies opposite the *Dantian* at the 2nd and 3rd lumbar vertebra.

Let the bones hold the body up, thereby minimizing the work of the muscles in keeping the body erect. By letting the tailbone sink and the head rise a subtle traction is created in the spine - the upper back is gently lifting and the lower back and tail are gently sinking. This allows the spaces between vertebrae to subtly open, and at the same time to stack one upon the other. Inthis way, with minimal effort, the body can maintain this position. The body weight is then transmitted into the ground through the legs. Align the hips, knees and ankles so that they are stacked vertically, one upon the other. At the same time make sure that the bony prominence on the front of the hip, the kneecap, and the space between the big toe and the second toe are in a line. The following exercise can help you feel this alignment.

Exercise 1: Rocking and Rooting

This exercise can help you make sure the skeleton is lined up with the bones stacking up one upon the other.

1) Rock forward toward the toes and back toward the heels - make the motion large. As you rock, notice when the leg muscles begin to tense to keep you from tipping forward or backward. Tune into exactly when the muscles engage and disengage in each direction.
2) Then tune in to where they are not engaged - somewhere in the middle, between the shift, there is a moment where the muscles relax and the bones line up.
3) Now make the motion smaller, still noticing exactly when the muscles engage and disengage. Again also notice the place where nothing is engaged.
4) Gradually reduce the amplitude of the rocking until it is infinitesimal and still see if you can detect the very (almost infinitesimal) start of the tightening of the leg muscles and the very moment they begin to relax. Then see if you can detect the place of relaxation in the middle of the movement.
5) Find the place in the middle where there is no tension. Stop there and stand in the stillness.

Now that the body has found a place of stillness, a place of balance and central equilibrium, notice that the body is like a tree whose roots go down into the earth, while the branches and leaves rise upward reaching toward heaven. Feel the lower body and the feet rooting into the ground while the upper body lifts upward like a tree growing toward the sun.

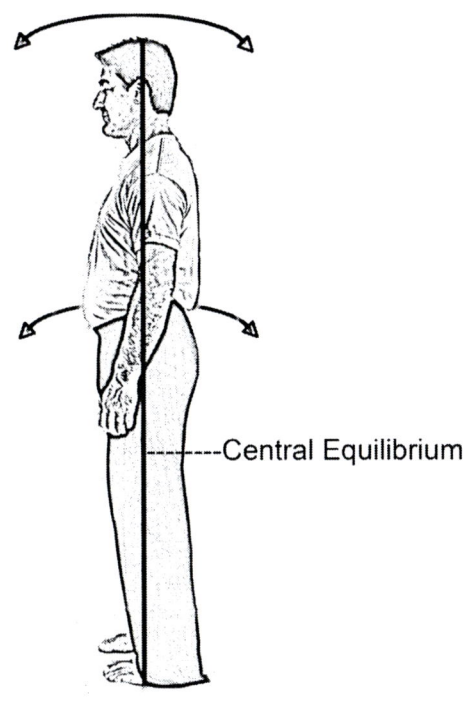

Wu Ji Rocking and Rooting

The body is like a vibrating string on a musical instrument. When it is properly adjusted it vibrates at the "proper pitch," allowing the *Qi/Breath* to flow smoothly throughout the whole body. This can sometimes be perceived as a faint vibration in the body or tingling in the hands.

The bones are heavy and want to sink toward the earth, so by lifting them up, stacking them one upon the other, a movement toward heaven is created. The flesh is lighter and wants to rise to float, so by letting the flesh sink, letting it hang off the bones a movement toward earth is created. The bones can be likened to a clothes hanger hanging on a closet pole, while the flesh is like the clothes on the hanger. Sometimes it is difficult to feel as though the flesh is relaxing and sinking. The following exercise can help with this.

Exercise 2: Progressive Sinking

While standing in the stillness, gradually let the body sink and relax as the bones lift upward. Sinking is effortless, like a stone sinking to the bottom of a pond.

Feel/Imagine:
- The shoulders sinking into the elbows.
- Elbows sinking into wrists.
- Wrists sinking into the hands.
- Hands sinking into the fingers.

Then Feel/Imagine:
- The shoulders sink into the chest and upper back.
- The chest and upper back sinking into the ribs.
- Ribs sinking into waist and lumbar area.
- Waist and lumbar sinking into hips and groin area.
- Hips sinking into thighs and knees.
- Knees sinking into ankles.
- Ankles sinking into the feet and toes.
- Feet sinking into the ground.

You are not sinking in such a way that the body feels as though it is collapsing downward. It is simply a loosening or a "letting go." Simultaneously, while the flesh is sinking, the bones are lifting upward. These two actions are equal, and in a sense cancel each other, so that an equilibrium is created.

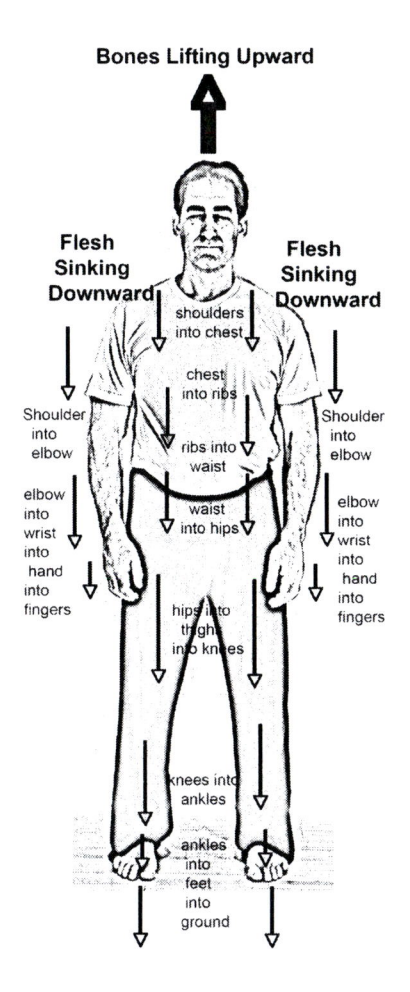

Practice the Wu Ji Posture Daily

The preceding two exercises are aids to achieving the proper posture and alignment. Once you are standing properly in the Wu Ji posture, try and remain there for 20-30 minutes while focusing on the breath. Continue the *Dantian* breathing you learned in Lesson Two. Once you can comfortably hold the posture for 20 minutes or more, Rocking and Rooting and Progressive Sinking do not need to be practiced as individual exercises. Your body will automatically seek to move into the correct alignments guided gently by the mind intention. Standing in the *Wu Ji* Posture can also be combined with counting breaths from one to nine as you did in Lesson Three.

LESSON 5:

WU JI & SONG

(RELAXATION)

松
Song

Lesson Five: Wu Ji and Song (Relaxation)

Qi/Breath flows more easily when the body is relaxed. Tight, tense muscles and joints that are not aligned inhibit the flow of *Qi/Breath* and cause it to block. Since the movements of the *Qi/Breath* are equivalent to the movements of the mind (thoughts, mental images and emotions), if the *Qi/Breath* stops or blocks, the mind also stops and blocks, or fixates. The reverse is also true. If the mind fixes itself on a thought or emotion this upsets the smooth flow of the *Qi/Breath*. When the *Qi/Breath* moves smoothly, thoughts and emotions come and go smoothly, like clouds that momentarily block the sun's light only to pass on. Aligning the body helps the *Qi/Breath* to move freely. When the body is aligned and the flow of the *Qi/Breath* is uninterrupted, then the mind will be stable and clear. The following passage from the *Nei Yeh* (Inward Training) refers to the tranquility and clarity that automatically flow from sitting or standing in an aligned and stable posture while attending to the breath. If you can be aligned and tranquil:

Only then can you be stable.
With a stable mind at your core,
With the ears and eyes acute and clear;
And with the four limbs firm and fixed,
You can thereby make a lodging place for the vital essence.

When your body is not aligned,
The inner power will not come.
When your mind is not tranquil within,
Your mind will not be well ordered.
Align your body, assist the inner power,
Then it will gradually come on its own.[1]

The Concept of Song

In order to learn to relax and let the *Qi/Breath* flow so that the mind can be tranquil and ordered, it can be useful to practice releasing tension and correcting misalignments of the body posture by engaging with the concept of *Song,* or "slackening."

The word *Song* (松) means:

- To loosen: as in loosening one's hair so it falls naturally.
- To slacken: as in releasing a taut rope.
- To release.
- To let go.
- To untie or unbind.

When learning Qi Gong, Chinese teachers often tell their students they need to *fang song* (放松). This phrase is often translated as "relax," however in English "relax" has a connotation of passivity, whereas *Song* connotes an active releasing or unbinding. Therefore it is more useful to mentally use the idea of a slackening, releasing, untying or a loosening. This loosening of tension is not limp. It is an active, potentiated stillness.

In the martial arts the idea of *Song* is sometimes imaged as a pine tree with snow on its branches. The pine boughs bend under the weight of the snow, but if you knock the snow off the boughs they spring back upward. The boughs are loose and supple, but not completely lax and limp.

In engaging with the concept of *Song,* the mind-intention cannot be too forceful. Let the mind gently direct the body so that slackening is slow, natural and unforced. It is a suggestion rather than a command, almost as if you are observing the body form the outside. Let the mind go to each area of the body and suggest that each area loosens, slackens and "lets go." If you cannot feel it *Song/Slacken,* then imagine that it *Song/Slackens* and move on to the next area.

Lesson 5: Practice - Song

1. Assume the Wu Ji Posture and attend to the breath as you begin Kidney Breathing

Take a few moments to set the posture and alignments. Then take several breaths to initiate Kidney Breathing. If you have difficulty with this use the exercises and imagery learned in earlier lessons to correct uneven breathing patterns or unfocused mental patterns.

2. *Song* the Front of the Body

Once you are standing comfortably using Kidney Breathing, bring your attention to the top of the head. Inhale, and then as you exhale, consciously let the top of the head, the scalp and even the hair loosen, slacken and relax. Remember to use Kidney Breathing. There is no need to exert effort. Simply let the top of the head *Song/Slacken* like a rope that is loosened. Say "*Song/Slacken*" or "*Song/Loosen*" to yourself. Then bring your attention to the forehead. Inhale, and then as you exhale let the forehead relax, loosen and slacken. Continue this procedure down the front of body with the:

- Eyebrows
- Eyes
- Nose
- Mouth
- Face
- Jaw
- Front of the neck
- Center of chest
- Sides of the chest
- Solar plexus
- Belly between the sternum and the navel

- Lower abdomen
- Pubic bone and groin
- Front of the hips
- Front of the thighs
- Knees
- Shin
- Ankle
- Top of the foot
- Toes
- Bottom of the foot
- Feel the whole foot settle into the ground

3. *Song* the Sides of the Body

Again, bring your attention to the top of the head. Inhale, and then as you exhale, consciously let the top of the head, the scalp and even the hair loosen, slacken and relax. There is no need to exert effort. Simply let the top of the head *Song/Slacken* like a rope that is loosened. Again, say "*Song/Slacken*" or "*Song/Loosen*" to yourself. Continue this procedure down the sides of the body with the:

- Side of the head
- Side of the neck
- Shoulders
- Elbows
- Hands
- Fingers
- Sides of the torso
- Hips
- Sides of the thighs
- Sides of the knees
- Outsides of the ankles

- Bottom of the foot
- Feel the whole foot settle into the ground

4. *Song* the Back of the Body

Bring your attention back to the top of the head. Inhale, and then as you exhale, consciously let the top of the head say "*Song/Slacken*", or "*Song/Loosen*", to yourself. Continue this procedure down the back of the body with the:

- Back of the head and nape of the neck
- Upper back
- Mid-Back
- Lower Back
- Sacrum and Tailbone
- Buttocks
- Back of the thigh
- Back of the knee
- Calves
- Achilles tendon
- Bottom of the foot
- Feel the whole foot settle into the ground

5. *Song* the Internal Organs

Now bring your attention to the lungs. Inhale, and then as you exhale, consciously let the lungs *Song/Slacken* and soften. Continue this procedure with the:

- Kidneys
- Large Intestine
- Liver
- Gallbladder
- Heart

- Stomach
- Spleen
- *Dantian*

6. *Song* the Entire Body

Finally, expand your awareness to the whole body and let the whole body *Song/Loosen*, soften and relax. Keep standing for several minutes and remain aware of the whole body.

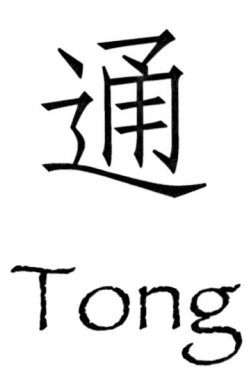

LESSON 6:

DISSOLVING & CLEARING BLOCKAGES

通

Tong

Lesson 6: Dissolving & Clearing Blockages

In the last two lessons we learned that the *Qi/Breath* does not flow easily through tight, tense muscles and joints. Similarly in Lesson Three: Counting the Breaths, we saw how thoughts and emotions can interfere with the harmonious movement of the *Qi/Breath*, causing it to move erratically, to dissipate, or even block. This lesson builds on Lesson Five, by working more directly with dissolving and clearing blockages that can interfere with the movement of the *Qi/Breath*.

What is a Blockage?

A blockage is a place where the *Qi/Breath* does not flow smoothly, where it is interrupted or obstructed. The obstruction is rarely total. The *Qi/Breath* will come up against an obstructed area and attempt to flow around it, just as a river flows around a rock or a log in its path. However, this diversion can mean that the *Qi/Breath* does not circulate smoothly in the area behind the blockage. Similarly, the *Qi/Breath* may trickle rather than flow through a blocked area. In both instances this retards or drags on the smooth uninterrupted flow of *Qi/Breath*. This can create a kind of "dead zone" that always feels "not quite right."

How do we know something is blocked? Pain is one indicator. The following saying from traditional Chinese medicine sums up this idea succinctly:

> 不通這痛 *Bu tong zhe tong* No free-flow, there is pain
>
> 痛則不通 *Tong ze bu tong* Pain, there is no free-flow

If the *Qi/Breath* blocks there is pain. There is no pain when the *Qi/Breath* flows freely. Areas that are tight and painful are blocked. The pain may not be intense. It may be mild or almost unnoticeable. This blockage may be experienced not so much as "pain" but as tension. Tension may be percieved more externally as tight, jumpy muscles, or it may manifest internally as an emotional tension or tightness. Often it is both.

What Causes the Qi/Breath to Block?

1. Physical Injury

Physical injury or trauma can damage tissues and structures leading to reduced penetration of the *Qi/Breath* into the injured area(s).

2. Muscular Tension

Imbalanced neuro-muscular patterns and tight muscles create tension and can lead to the formation of "dead" zones where *Qi/Breath* does not penetrate easily. In these cases, *Qi/Breath* trickles through these areas, or flows around the damaged and tight structures rather than flowing smoothly through them.

3. Sentiments and Emotions

Earlier, in Lesson Four, we became acquainted with the Five Powers and their expression in our earthly existence. This model helps us to understand the effect of our sentiments and emotions on the body. The emotions are considered to be the internal cause of disease in Chinese medicine, yet emotions themselves are not negative. Sentiments and emotions are part of what make us human, able to recognize and celebrate the numinous dimension of our life on earth. The five sentiments are:

> *Vigor (nu) associated with the wood organ, liver; ecstasy (xi), associated with the fire organ, heart; contemplation (si), associated with the earth organ, spleen; nostalgia (bei), associated with the metal organ, lung; and awe (kong), associated with the water organ, kidney. They are part of the physiological movement of the human heart, since 'vigor causes the qi to rise, ecstasy causes the qi to open up, nostalgia causes the qi dissipate, awe causes the qi to descend,...and contemplation causes the qi to congeal.*[1]

In Lesson Three we learned that every movement of the mind is a movement of the *Qi/Breath*. By fixating on certain thoughts and emotions rather than experiencing them and letting them move through us in an appropriate and seamless way, the *Qi/Breath* can become imbalanced. When the five sentiments are indulged to excess, pathologies can develop. *In this case, vigor turns into anger, ecstasy into hysteria, contemplation into worry, nostalgia into grief, and awe into fear.*[2] These pathologies of emotion can create blockages, places where the *Qi/Breath* becomes stuck or compressed, or moves against its natural flow.

Frustration can create a compression or withdrawal of the *Qi/Breath*.

Anxiety, preoccupation and worry affect both the heart and the spleen, leading to a kind of internal emptiness that does not engage fully with the movement of the *Qi/Breath*.

Sadness, grief and melancholy, as in holding onto something negative that occurred in the past, prevents the normal movement, change and transformation of the *Qi/Breath*, causing it to stagnate and become empty or hollow.

Joy and Elation loosen and spread the *Qi/Breath*. However, too much loosening can upset the rhythm of the movement of the *Qi/Breath*, overexciting to a kind of hysterical pitch, and ultimately weakening its movement.[3]

Anger rises upward going against the normal smooth movement of the *Qi/Breath*, creating a kind of counter-current. This counter-current disrupts the flow and transformation of the *Qi/Breath*, creating tension and obstruction.

Fear creates a downward counter-current, an internal sinking of the *Qi/Breath* that can ultimately drain the body's vitality.

Over-thinking or too much reflection can disconnect us from the movement and change inherent in life, creating a compression or stagnanation of the *Qi/Breath*.

4. <u>**Negativity**</u>

Negative thinking is a subcategory of the emotions that can slow down or interrupt the smooth, harmonious movement of the *Qi/Breath*. Statements like: *I can't do it; I won't succeed; I am not making progress; It's a waste of time;* all put a drag on the flow of the *Qi/Breath,* and can lead to a kind of internal stasis.

The Importance of Clearing Blockages in Daoist Meditation

Clearing physical and emotional blockages makes us feel better, promotes health and allows us to access our innate vitality. Additionally, it is a very important step in practicing the more advanced meditation methods in the lessons that follow. Our emotions, desires, frustrations, indulgences, fantasies and longings, our grasping for external objects and stimulation, all interfere with the smooth and unobstructed circulation of the *Qi/Breath*. This includes the *Qi/Breath* of Heaven and Earth that unite and circulate within us. Life's changes and transformation are dependant on the circulation of the *Qi/Breath*. Obstruction and interference with this circulation in turn interferes with the transformation of our consciousness, blocking the ability to connect with the true mind and the authentic self, the dwelling place of a person's inner wisdom. Thoughts and emotions are normal manifestations of the *Qi/Breath,* but if they are inappropriate, or if the mind dwells too much upon them, then they can become obstructions – they can make us physically ill and they can keep us from progressing psychically and spiritually.

When the mind and spirit are calm and tranquil and the body is relaxed, aligned and open, then there is potential for transformation and our natural illumination, originality, creativity and wisdom can come forth. The less energetically rigid and stiff we are, the more soft, flexible and supple we become internally. This internal suppleness, itself a product of smoothly circulating *Qi/Breath,* in turn engenders the ability of the *Qi/Breath* to create internal transformation and change.

Although it is not always possible to clear all our physical blockages, we can work with our emotions and desires as well as the emotional components of physical blockages. The meditation methods and exercises in this lesson all work with clearing and dissolving these blockages. Sometimes people think they cannot go on into advanced meditation practices until they have completely cleared all of their blockages. This is not practical and probably not even possible. Clearing and dissolving to open the way for transformation is an ongoing process, like cleaning your house. Look for signs of progress and change before moving on to Lesson Seven. Clearing and dissolving is something you will return to even as you move on to the other meditation practices.

The Dao De Jing On Desire and the Dao

Nameless it is the origin of all things;
Named it is the mother of the myriad things.
Therefore always be without desire so as to see their subtlety.
And always have desire so as to see their ends.[4]

Our original nature and authentic self are like the Dao - nameless and formless. They cannot be understood with words. We can understand that the Dao bring all things into being, yet we do not know how it happens. Wang Bi's commentary tells us that "subtlety" in this passage means an absolute degree of minuteness. By being without desire and remaining empty we can see the subtlety from which things originate. Yet we should also have desire. Desire that is both rooted and in accord with the Dao. Then we can see the ends to which things arrive.[5]

Dissolving and Clearing Blockages

In Lesson Five we learned how to slacken (*Song*) areas of tension. This is the starting point for clearing obstructions and dissolving blockages of the *Qi/Breath*. Becoming aware that an area is blocked or tight is the first step. By standing in the *Wu Ji* posture, observing and breathing, one becomes aware of these areas bit by bit. By bringing your awareness and attention to an area that is blocked, you bring the *Qi/Breath* to that area. As the mind-intention and the *Qi/Breath* gather, it is possible to slowly disperse, melt, and dissolve the blockage. It does not happen all at once, but little by little over time. Using the mind-intention to force its way through will only make the blockage more resistant. It can be dissolved by cultivating a gentle awareness that slowly diassapates the blockage like water wearing away a rock.

In the martial arts, mind-intention is often likened to a military banner:

Intention like a waving flag,

Also like a lighted lamp.[6]

In ancient times, troops were trained to change battle formations and to advance and to retreat, all guided by waving command flags. At night troop movements were guided by lighted lamps. Similarly the *Qi/Breath* is guided by the intention. In dissolving blockages, the intention and awareness should be applied gently, carefully and precisely. As in guiding troops, attention and awareness should not be applied forcefully and bluntly, or casually and carelessly.

Lesson 6: Practice - Dissolving Blockages

1) Assume the Wuji Posture and perform the step-by-step whole body relaxation (*Song*) practiced in Lesson Five.

2) Remain aware of the whole body as you scan the body section-by-section and note areas of tension.
Notice where things are not *song*, not relaxed; where the breath does not penetrate. These blocked areas may appear to the mind and consciousness as dark spots, or "dead zones."

3) Direct your awareness, your mind-intention, to the blocked areas.
These blocked areas can be cleared by bringing our attention to them one by one. Bring the attention of the mind and consciousness to the area and let it gather there. As it gathers, the blockage begins to melt and then wash away. It may feel like light dispelling darkness or clear air filling a musty room. Dissolving a blockage is like melting ice, or it may simply seem like something muddy and stuck washing away to be replaced by clarity and space. Emotions like anger, sadness, grief and frustration may be associated with blockages. Simply smile inwardly. Smile into these emotions, letting the smile and the mind-intention gather to dissolve these emotions, so that they fade away like smoke dissipating out of the body.

4) Scan down the body. Bring your attention to the blockages one by one and let them dissolve and dissipate.
Don't worry if there are blockages that are difficult to clear. Don't try to force them to dissolve.

Simply let the intention go to the blocked areas and observe without judgment. It does not need to be done all at once. Each day the mind-intention can be gathered and each day these negative energies can be released again, more deeply, more thoroughly.

Auxiliary Exercise: Pour the Cream on Top

Pour the Cream on Top is a very useful auxiliary exercise that can aid you in identifying and dissipating blockages. It can be performed before and after you stand in *Wu Ji* or at any time during the day.

Start: Stand with the feet parallel and shoulder width apart and the arms at the sides.

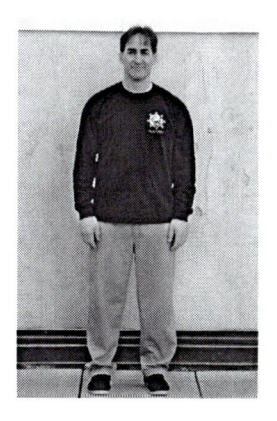

1) Imagine you have dipped your left hand in pure clear, cool water. Feel as though you are scooping water into your palm. Inhale as you slowly raise the left arm to the side, the palm facing upward. You can turn your head to watch the hand as it rises, or look straight ahead. As the arm moves overhead, look straight ahead and let the arm fold inward so that the palm faces the top of your head and imagine pouring the liquid onto your head. When the hand is several inches above the top of the head, begin to exhale and feel the liquid moving down the body as the hand presses downward in front of the body. As the hand moves downward, feel as though the liquid moves downward to the soles of your feet. As you feel the liquid moving downward, tensions and blockages are washed

away with the liquid. When the hand reaches the front of your hip, stand quietly for a moment.

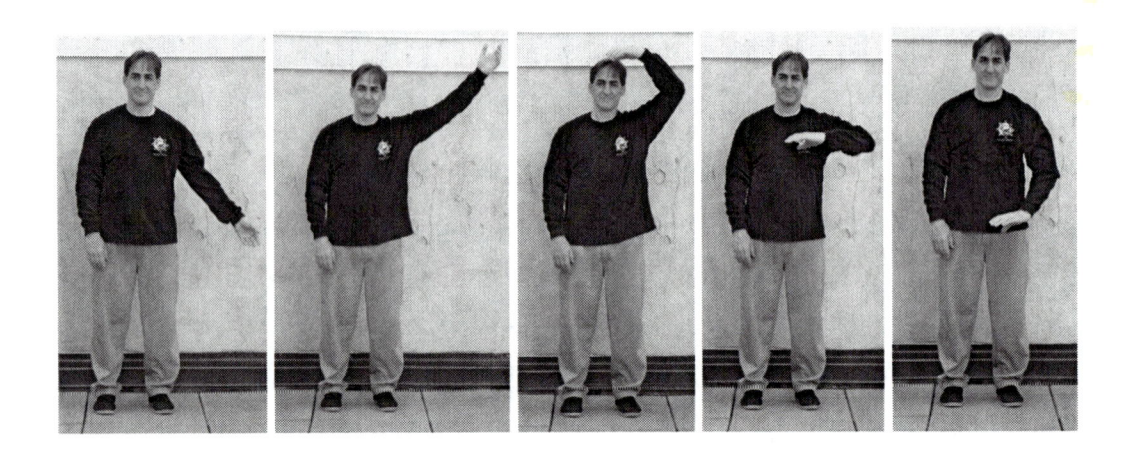

2) Repeat with the right hand.

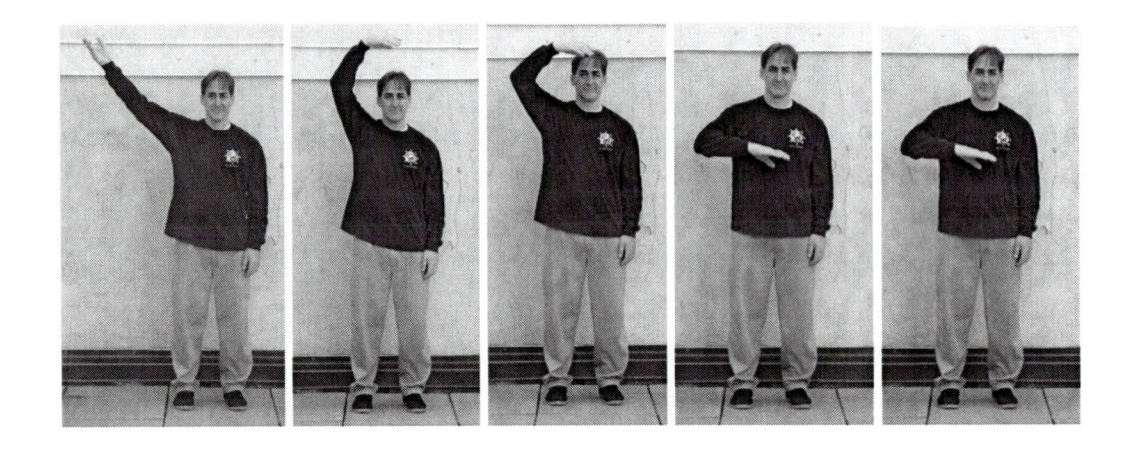

3) Imagine you have dipped both of your hands into pure clear, cool water. Feel as though you are scooping water into your palms. Inhale as you slowly raise the arms, extending them outward to the sides with the palms facing upward. Look straight ahead as the arms rise and move overhead, and then let the arms fold inward as you imagine pouring the liquid onto your head. Let the arms fold inward, with the left palm several inches above the top of the head and the right hand several inches above the left hand. Then begin to exhale and feel the liquid moving down the

body as the hands press downward. As the hands pass the forehead, they become even. As you continue to gently press the hands downward, feel as though the liquid moves downward to the soles of your feet. As you feel the liquid moving downward, let tensions and blockages in the body wash away with it. When the hands reach the front of your hip, stand quietly for a moment.

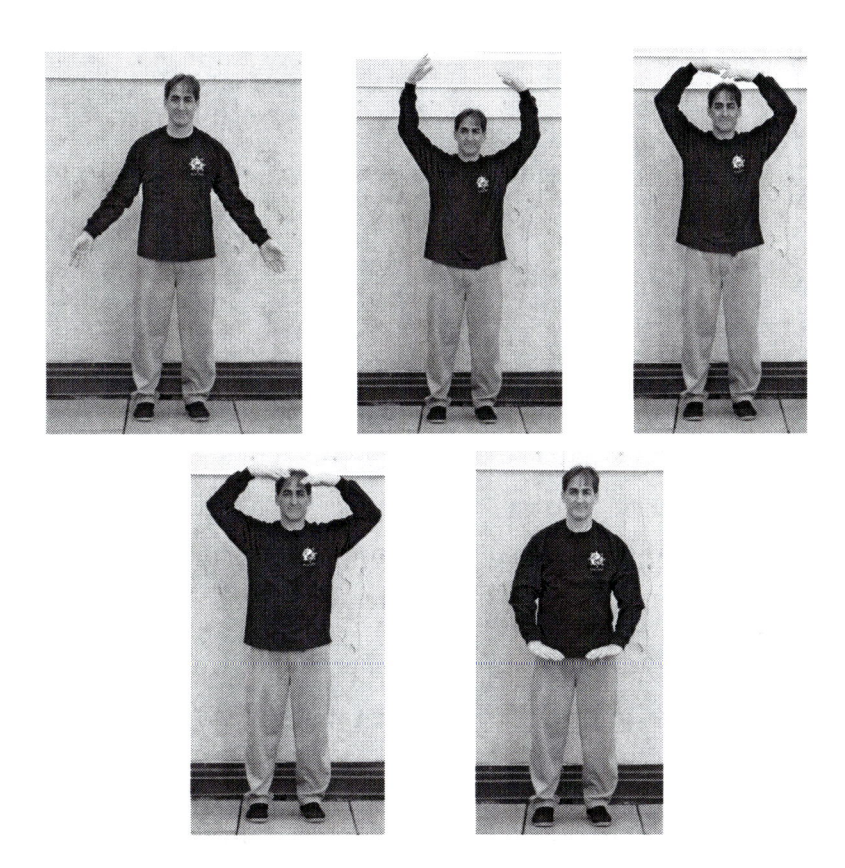

There are two other meditation methods for dissolving blockages. First perform Pour the Cream On Top until you become comfortable with it. Then you can add the following two methods: Heavenly Qi Meditation or Body Breathing Meditation to your practice.

Dissolving Blockages Method 1: Heavenly *Qi/Breath* Meditation

Start: Find a comfortable position. It can be sitting, lying or standing.

1. Sitting: sit either cross-legged on a cushion with the back straight or upright in a chair with the feet flat on the floor.
2. Lying: lie on your back with your arms at your sides, palm down. Lie on something firm but not uncomfortable – for example, a soft rug or mat on the floor. If you like, use a small pillow to make your neck and head comfortable.
3. Standing: stand with the feet shoulder width apart, knees slightly bent and the head erect.

Breathe quietly using Kidney Breathing. Begin by relaxing the body, beginning at the head and going downward to the feet. Mentally tell each body part to relax and then as you exhale feel that part of the body relax. This is essentially an abbreviated version of *Song-Relaxation* that you learned in Lesson Five. Let tension drain out of the body as you relax each part. If you are standing, you can imagine all the tension, pain and negative feelings and emotions drain out through the soles of the feet into the ground.

Now start at the head again and feel the pure clear, light (the *Qi/Breath*) of the heavens wash down through your body, cleansing it of pain and negativity, recharging your tissues and your whole being. The light can be silvery or golden in color. Let the light move downward from the head to the feet, pausing if you wish to spend more time at problem areas. When you have reached the feet, feel the whole body bathed in this pure clear light for several moments, then open your eyes and stretch and move.

Some areas are harder to relax than others. Take your time and don't worry if you cannot completely relax. This will become easier with daily practice.

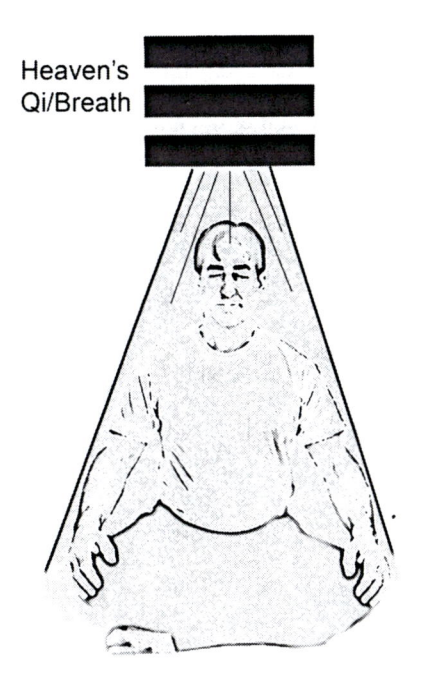

Dissolving Blockages Method 2: Body Breathing Meditation

Body Breathing meditation calms the spirit and regulates the emotions. It is a powerful tool for letting go of negative thoughts and emotions as well as dispelling pain and discomfort.

As in the previous exercise, you can stand, sit or lie on the floor. Close your eyes and look down at the tip of the nose and then into the *Dantian*. Inhale *Qi/Breath* from the natural world around you through the nose and the pores of the skin and let it sink to the *Dantian*. As you exhale, let the *Qi/Breath* flow from the *Dantian* through the whole body and out through the pores and back into nature. As you breathe, whether inhaling or exhaling, feel the *Qi/Breath* moving freely and unobstructed throughout the whole body, and in and out through all of the pores. The breathing is slow, deep, long, continuous and even. Each time you inhale, feel fresh *Qi/Breath* enter the body. Each time you exhale, feel pain and negative thoughts and emotions flow out of the body. Breathe this way for 24 breaths and then return to natural breathing

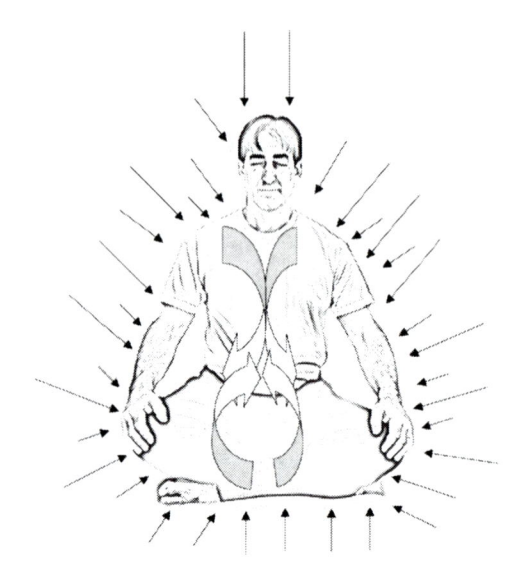

Inhale Qi/Breath Through the Pores Into Dantian

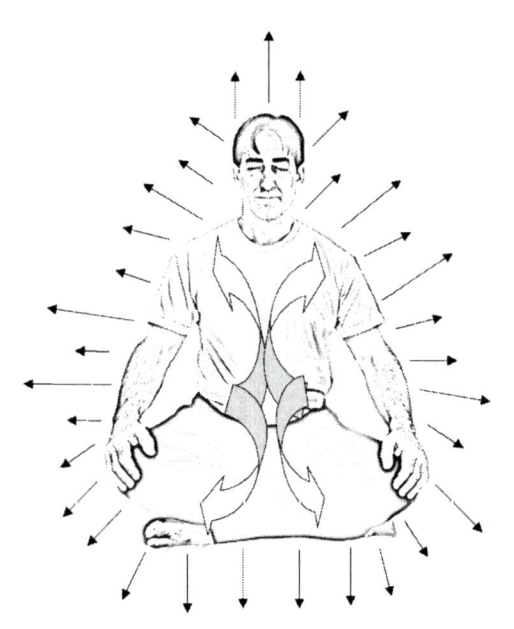

Exhale Qi/Breath Through the Pores Into Nature

LESSON 7:

THREE TREASURES & THE CIRCULATION OF WATER AND FIRE

三 寶
San Bao

Lesson Seven: The Three Treasures & the Circulation of Water and Fire

The Three Treasures: Jing, Qi & Shen

The concept of *Jing* was introduced in Lesson Two. It might be a good idea to go back and read about *Qi* and *Jing* again, as these concepts will be part of the current discussion. *Jing* is the material basis for the physical body, its physical infrastructure. Therefore it nourishes, moistens and fuels the body. *Jing* produces the bone marrow and is the foundation of the blood and fluids of the body. It is energetically related to semen in men and the uterus and ovum in women. *Jing* is the basal root of the body's energy according to Chinese Medicine. It is stored in the kidneys and the *Dantian*. The character for *Jing* contains the radical for a grain of rice on the left and then references the character for *Sheng* (life) over that of *Dan* as in *Dantian*.

$$米 \text{ mi (rice)} + \frac{\text{主 for 生 sheng (life)}}{\text{月 for 丹 for Dan (elixir/red)}} = \text{Jing 精}$$

This image is of an uncooked grain of rice as the seed of life being contained in the *Dantian*. As we saw earlier, the Chinese character for *Qi* also contains a grain of rice with vapors rising from it. The image is of rice cooking in a pot, producing steam. The vapor is seen as a kind of energy, or force, produced by a cooking or refining process.

Qi 氣

Qi is true breath permeating the whole body. It is the movement, change and transformation that permeates the body, and is directly connected to the movements and change in Heaven and Earth and in the universe around us. *Jing* and *Qi* are interdependent. Hence *Jing* is often referred to as *Jingqi*. The formation of the *Qi/Breath* is dependant on the *Jing*, and the *Jing* is in turn nourished by the transformative actions of the *Qi/Breath*. *Qi/Breath*, when it descends and gathers in *Dantian*, is transformed into *Jing*, just as Heaven's vapor becomes rain. When *Jing* rises, it is transformed into *Qi/Breath* (vapor), just as water evaporates to becomes clouds.

Jing and *Qi/Breath* must unite for there to be *Shen* (spirit/divine essence). *Shen* is an essential part of our vitality. It is our connection to the numinous, but at the same time it is both a product and a part of the ongoing bodily change and transformation that is rooted in the material body. The character for *Shen* references the radicals representing an altar and cultivated fields:

Shen 神

Shen combines 礻(示 *shi*) "altar" and 申 (*shen*), a phonetic related to 田 (*tian*) or cultivated field.[1] Stuart Alve Olsen believes that the vertical line running through 申, symbolizes the connection of heaven and earth.[2]

Jing, *Qi* and *Shen* are referred to collectively as the Three Treasures (*San Bao*). The three treasures are interdependent, hence they are often referred to together: *Jingqi* (Essence-Qi/Breath: Qi that is derived from or is a manifestation of Essence), *Jingshen* 精神 (Essence-Spirit: Spirit that is derived from or is a manifestation of Essence) or *Shenqi* 神氣 (that is dervived from or a manifestation of *Qi/Breath*).

Jing and *Qi/Breath* must unite for there to be *Shen*. The embrace of the two essences creates spirit. In nature this is called the coupling of Heaven and Earth – the essences of Heaven uniting with essences of Earth.[3] In human beings, it is the union of the essences of the parents creating a new being: *When two seminal essences strike against each other, it is spoken of as spirit.*[4] Through the spirit (*Shen*) human beings are capable of perceiving their own experiences and all transformation and change occurring both within and without. Through the spirit human beings are capable of perceiving the numinous.

Shen is stored in the heart and radiates out through the whole body. The radiance of the *Shen* manifests through the light, the brightness (*Shenming* 神明: "spirit brightness") shining out of a person's eyes. The mind-intention (*Yi*), associated with the heart, enables us to make and carry out plans, but we need the will (*Zhi*), associated with the kidneys to carry them through. In Chinese medicine the *Qi*/Breath and *Jing* of the kidneys provide the staying power to follow through to completion. Hence the statement in the *Ling Shu* (Spiritual Pivot):

> *When the heart applies itself we speak of intent;*
> *When Intent becomes permanent we speak of will.*[5]

Inter-Penetration and Inter-Transformation of *Jing*, *Qi* and *Shen*

Jing is converted into *Qi*/Breath, which is refined and raised up to the brain. During this process *Shen* is nurtured. *Shen* manifests itself through the intent. Intent in turn leads the *Qi*/Breath. Just as water can be transformed into steam, *Shen* and intention can transform the *Qi*/Breath and the *Jing*. At conception, the meeting of the essences of the father and mother produces the *Shen*, which enters into the fetus, giving rise to the *Qi*/Breath, which then in turn engenders *Jing*. As one grows older, Daoist practices aim at reversing this order: refining *Jing* and transforming it into *Qi*/Breath which then fills, animates and stimulates the body, becoming *Shen*. This process nourishes life, revitalizing one's consciousness and very existence.[6]

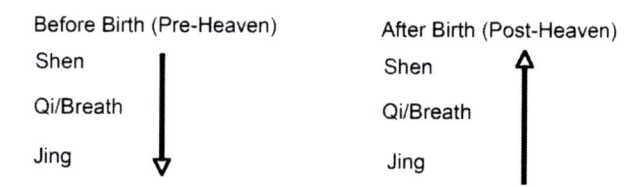

Before Birth (Pre-Heaven)	After Birth (Post-Heaven)
Shen	Shen
Qi/Breath ↓	Qi/Breath ↑
Jing	Jing

In Daoist meditation, for practical purposes, we can say that there is a lower, middle and upper *Dantian*. Employing this model:

1) *Jing* is associated with the sacrum, the *Lower Dantian* and *Mingmen*.
2) *Qi/Breath* is associated with the *Middle Dantian*, the breath, and the pulse. The *Middle Dantian* is just above the solar plexus between the breasts.
3) *Shen* resides in place behind center of the eyebrows, the *Niwan* (mudball) or brain: the *Upper Dantian*

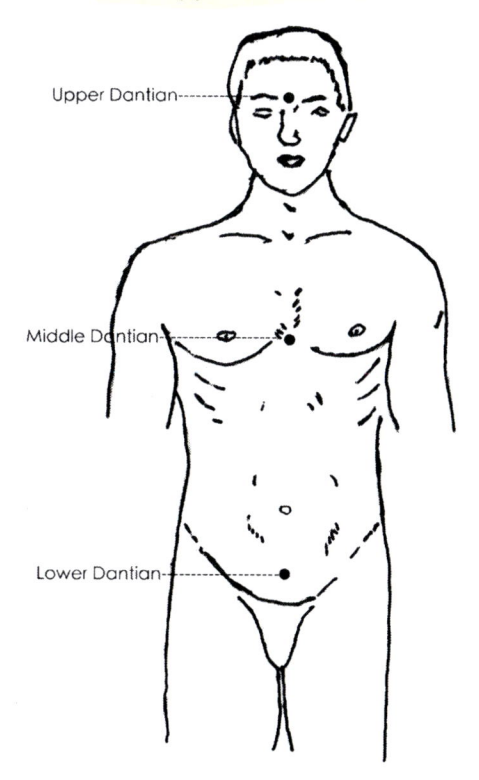

The inter-transformation of the Three Treasures and their relationship to the three *Dantian* is clearly illustrated in the diagram below adapted from *Qi Gong Essentials for Health Promotion* by Jiao Guorui.[7] It is easy to see that the *Qi-Breath* is the connecting link or the pivot between *Jing* and *Shen*.

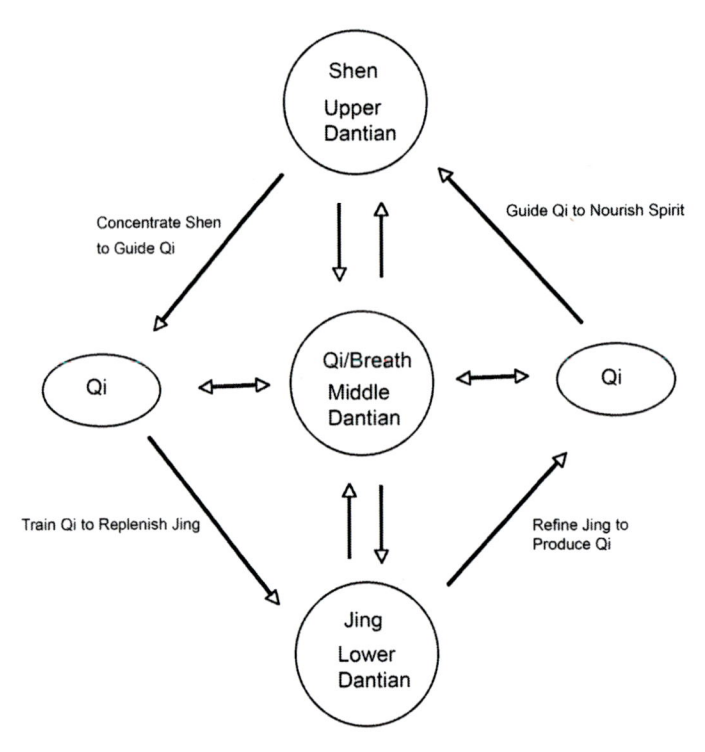

```
                    Shen
                    Upper
                    Dantian

Concentrate Shen                    Guide Qi to Nourish Spirit
to Guide Qi

                    Qi/Breath
    Qi   ←→         Middle        ←→    Qi
                    Dantian

Train Qi to Replenish Jing              Refine Jing to
                                        Produce Qi

                    Jing
                    Lower
                    Dantian
```

Interrelationship of Jing, Qi and Shen

The Inseparability of the Three Treasures

Jing, Qi/Breath and *Shen* are inseparable from each other. They are less individual entities than an indivisible process of transmutation. *Qi/Breath* lies at the very center of this process. It is the middle connecting element, the pivot, the ceaseless movement and transformation, the energetic breath that fills everything between Heaven and Earth. Therefore the *Qi/Breath* is the crucial tool that we harness and employ in Daoist meditation and Inner Alchemical practices. In the *Huang Di Nei Jing* (Inner Cannon of The Yellow Emperor) it says:

The wise observe their sameness, the foolish observe their differences. "The wise observe their sameness" means that Essence, Breath and Spirit are a single entity and operate with each other. The transformation of the three is achieved by the transformation of Breath within the human body.[8]

This close interlinking of the three treasures is illustrated in a the drawing below which is adapted from the *Hsing Ming Kuei Chih*.[9]

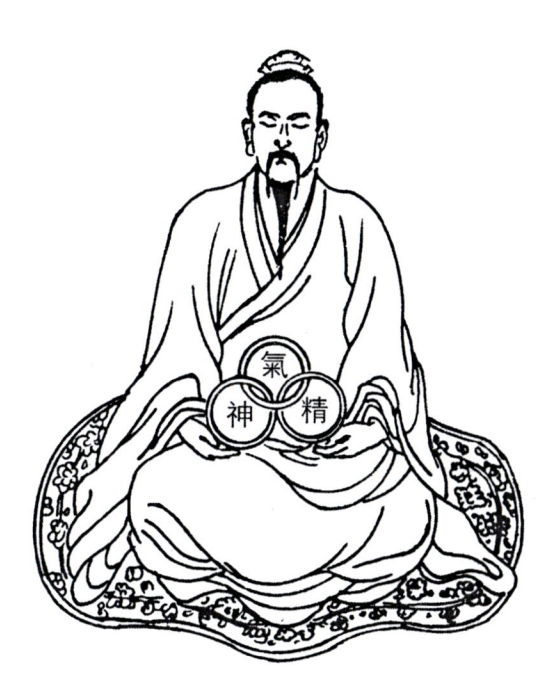

Jing Qi and Shen Interlinked
(Adapted From the Hsing Ming Kuei Chih)

Kan-Water & Li-Fire

Movement produces Yang-*Qi*. Stillness produces Yin-*Qi*. The yang breath descends from the heart or the brain, and the yin breath rises upwards from the kidneys. The heart is associated with Fire and is represented by the trigram *Li*. The kidneys are associated with Water and are represented by the trigram *Kan*.

Li–Fire: is related to the Heart

Kan–Water: is related to the Kidneys

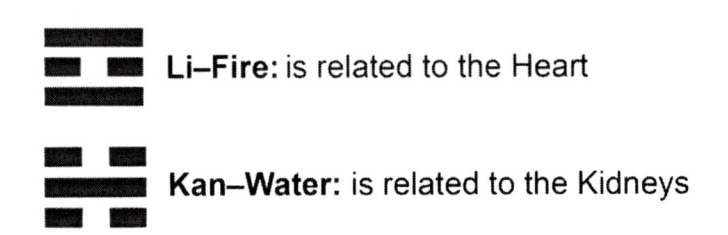

The trigrams of the *Yi Jing* (*I Ching*: Classic of Change or Book of Changes), are a way of diagramming the flux of Heaven and Earth and yin and yang. The solid lines are yang: active, full. Strong. initiating, creating. The broken lines are yin: quiescent, empty, weak, receptive, completing.

In Daoist meditation the trigram Kan-Water represents the kidneys and *Dantian*. Kan-Water is full in the middle (it has a solid yang line in the middle). The yang line in the center indicates that there is a yang-fire hidden within yin-water. It also means that the kidneys are replete, full and abundant. This fire within yin-water is also called the "moving qi between the kidneys" or the *Mingmen* (life-gate) fire.

Li-Fire represents the heart and chest. Li is empty in the middle (it has a broken yin line in the middle). This symbolizes the hidden yin-water within yang-fire. Normally, fire is light and rises to the chest and water is heavy and sinks to the *Dantian*. The broken line in the center of Li-Fire represents a relative emptiness inside the heart. The heart is relatively empty, in comparison to the lower abdomen where Kan-Water has a solid (full) line in the middle. This means there is space inside the heart and that the spirit can reside comfortably inside the heart.

The spirit is said to be "housed" by the heart. The spirit can only be undisturbed, be clear in its perception, by having space in the heart. This means the heart cannot be overflowing with emotions and desires. When the heart is relatively empty, as illustrated by the empty yin line in the center of the Li trigram, then the blood and breath can move smoothly and without impediment through the heart and chest. When the blood and breath move without impediment through this space, then intention and perception are clear. The heart and intention can then reflect and exhibit wisdom (a "knowing how"). Then it is possible to nourish life (*Yang Sheng*).[10]

The abdomen and the *Dantian* are relatively full in comparison to the heart and chest. The *Qi/Breath* sinks to *Dantian*, so that the lower abdomen and the *Mingmen* are full. This consolidates and replenishes the *Jing*, which in turn generates the *Qi/Breath*. If unimpeded, the *Qi/Breath* then nourishes the *Shen*. This transformation of the body's vital energies is sometimes referred to as "internal alchemy." In particular this involves replenishing the *Jing* (essence) and transforming essence into *Qi/Breath* and *Qi/Breath* into *Shen* (spirit). This transformative process, symbolized by the trigrams Li-Fire and Kan-Water, is achieved through quieting the mind and guiding the *Qi* with the breath and the intention.

The Circulation and Inter-Transformation of Kan and Li

Normally fire is light and rises to the chest, and water is heavy and sinks to *Dantian*. This is the "post-heaven" or "after-birth" state whose trigram configuration moves temporally from birth to death. This configuration is represented by hexagram #64: *Wei Ji* (Not Yet Fulfilled; Before Completion; Incomplete); fire above and water below. Because water sinks and fire rises, the two trigrams move in opposite directions; they do not integrate and harmonize.

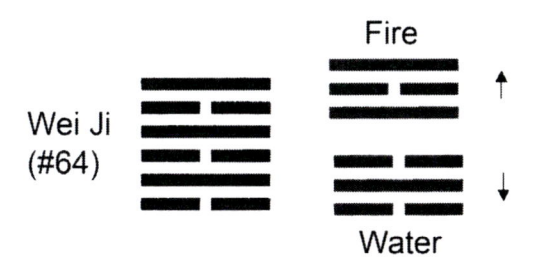

However, if fire is beneath water, it creates steam and condensation which is a rarefied energy. This process can be likened to water heated on a stove, creating a vapor which rises upward only to coalesce and descend again. The two elements must act in relation to each other and in balance with one another. If the heat is too great, the water will all evaporate. If the water boils over, the fire will be extinguished. This state of balance is represented by hexagram #63: Ji Ji (Completion), in which the trigram for water is above and the trigram for fire below. Here, water and fire interact and inter-transform.

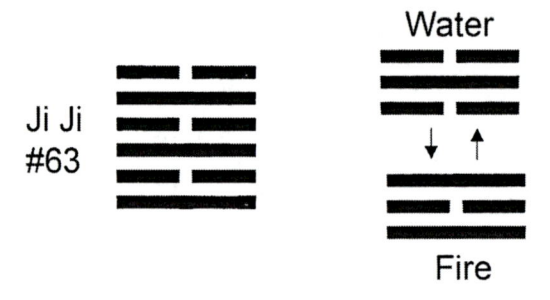

Ji Ji #63

Water

Fire

By employing proper posture, breathing and stillness of the mind, the *Dantian* acts like a stove that heats water, so that water transforms into a vapor that rises up to the chest and heart, where it coalesces to become water and then sinks back to the *Dantian*. Daoist meditation acts as a kind of inner alchemy, plucking the yang-solid line from the center of Kan-Water to fill the yin-broken line in the center of Li-Fire, thereby producing Qian-Heaven, represented by three solid-yang lines. The yin-broken line in the center of Li-Fire then moves to the center of Kan-Water, thereby producing Kun-Earth, represented by three broken-yin lines. When the middle lines of the trigrams switch places and form the Qian-Heaven and Kun-Earth trigrams there is a return to the original pre-heaven (before-birth) state, which in Daoist beliefs leads to stopping of the temporal movement and therefore "immortality" (or more practically speaking: peace and tranquility). This alchemical transformation is represented by Hexagram #11: Peace. In this hexagram, yin is ascendant, invoking prosperity, peace and upward progress, *bearing even in its character-structure evidence of the fertilizing living waters flowing down from the sacred mountain Tai Shan.*[11]

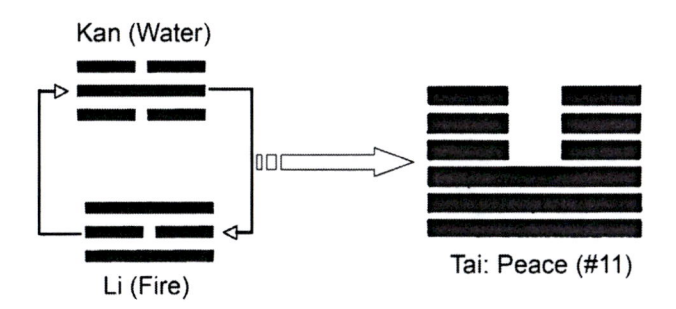

Qian-Heaven and Kan-Earth are respectively firm and yielding. Qian envelops and Kun is enveloped. The dynamic between them is one of opening and closing. As you breathe, the firm and the yielding rub against each other - they form the image of Qian and Kun, yin and yang, opening and closing.[12]

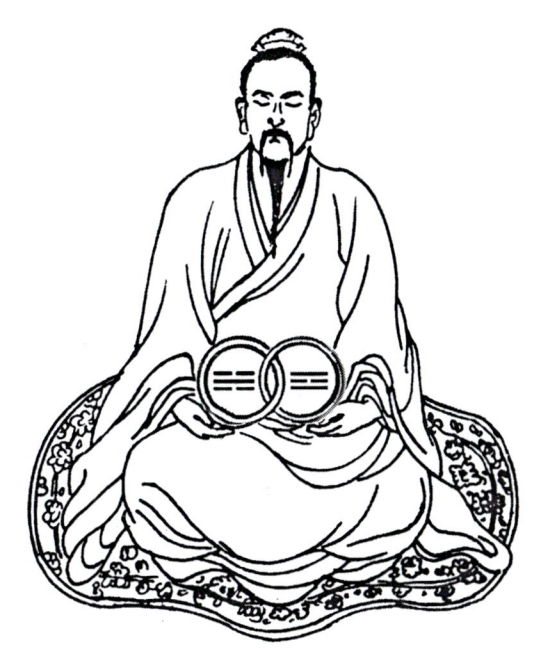

Inter-Transformation of Kan & Li
(Adapted from the Xing Ming Gui Zhi: Directions for Endowment and Vitality)

The Story of the Weaving Maiden and the Cowherd as a Metaphor for the Circulation of Water and Fire

One day the cowherd comes across maidens bathing in a lake. He takes the clothes of one of them. When the others fly up to the sky clothed in feathers, this maiden is left behind. The cowherd marries her and eventually they have a child. The cloak of feathers is hidden and the maiden contributes to the household by weaving. The child later finds the hidden cloak of feathers and the maiden puts it on and flies back to the sky. The cowherd is sad without the maiden. One of the cows, moved by master's sadness, has him slaughter her, and he uses her hide to ascend to the sky. The couple is reunited and are so happy that they forget to do their work. The King of Heaven decides that thereafter, they can only meet once a month. A magpie is entrusted to deliver this decree to the couple, but the magpie makes a mistake and tells them that they can rejoin each other only once a year. So once a year, on the 7th day of the 7th lunar month (the annual feast of young girls), they reunite. On this day it is supposed to rain so that no one will see them (ie: their associated constellations) meeting in the sky.[13]

The maiden is yin, associated with water and the kidneys, but she also represents the true yang (hidden yang) within yin - the fire within Kan-Water. She weaves, spinning the *Qi/Breath* and the true yang qi upward. The cowherd is yang, but he also represents the true yin within yang or the water within Li-Fire. Therefore he is associated with the heart and Fire. This is the true yin that flows downward to reunite with the Kan-Water.

On the one night a year that the lovers meet, the magpie makes a bridge across the sky to join them together. Likewise the heart-fire and the kidney-water are separate, but can reunite through the practice of Daoist meditation. The "upper magpie bridge" relates to the tongue touching the upper palate which connects the *Ren* and *Du* vessels above, and the lifting of the anus is the "lower magpie bridge" which connects the *Ren* and *Du* meridians below. These two "bridges" connect the circuit so that circulation in these two principle meridians can flow freely.

Chen Tuan's Diagram Revisited

In Lesson Four we looked at Chen Tuan's *Wu Ji* diagram in order to understand the progression from *Wu Ji* to *Tai Ji* and back to *Wu Ji*. At that time we read the diagram from top to bottom. However, Chen Tuan's diagram can also be read from bottom to top. Originally carved into the face of a cliff in the Hua Shan Mountain, the diagram had explanatory labels carved next to each tier. These labels, placed below have been adapted from Da Liu's book *Tai Chi Ch'uan and Meditation*.[14]

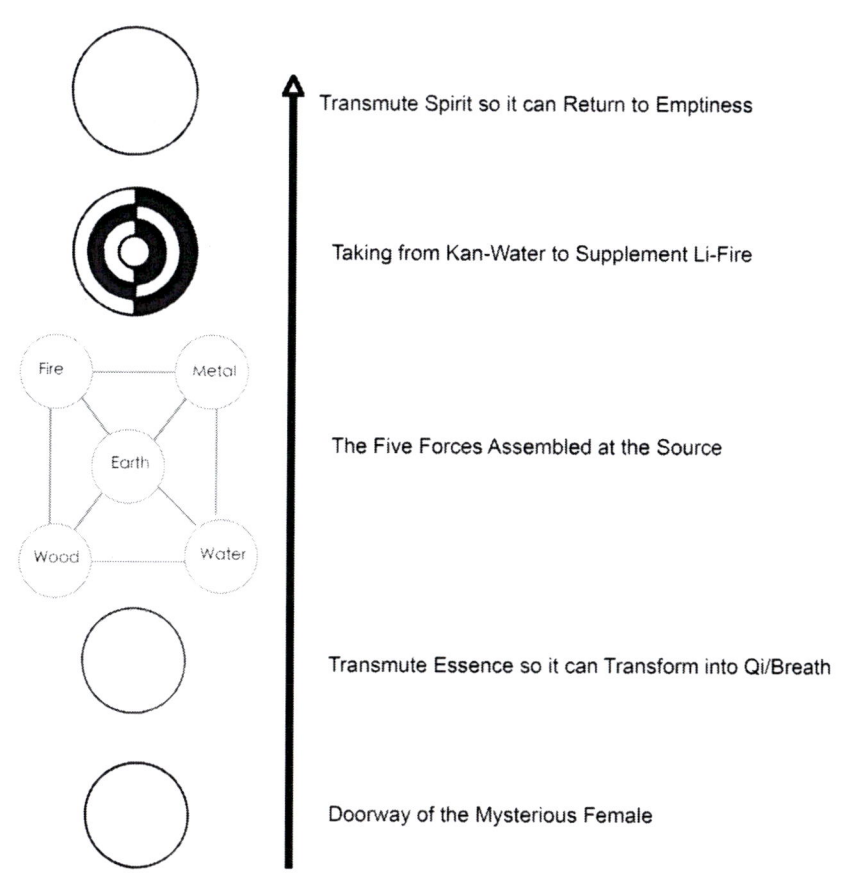

Transmute Spirit so it can Return to Emptiness

Taking from Kan-Water to Supplement Li-Fire

The Five Forces Assembled at the Source

Transmute Essence so it can Transform into Qi/Breath

Doorway of the Mysterious Female

This way of looking at Chen Tuan's diagram illustrates a reversion of the temporal sequence through an alchemical transformation involving the Three Treasures, *Kan*-Water and *Li*-Fire. This reversal is a return to the pre-Heaven State, to the origrinal "knowing" mind of the Dao.

The label, "Doorway of the Mysterious Female" is a reference to a passage in the *Dao De Jing*:

> *The Valley Spirit never dies.*
>
> *It is named the Mysterious Female.*
>
> *And the doorway of the Mysterious Female*
>
> *Is the base from which Heaven and Earth sprang.*
>
> *It is there within us all the while;*
>
> *Draw upon it as you will, it never runs dry.*[15]

The low ground represented by the "Valley Spirit," or "Water Spirit," as it is known in other texts, is the place where water collects. Through absorbing the "water spirit," plants, trees and other living things flourish and grow. The low ground, the valley, is considered to be *nearer to the Dao than the hills; and in the whole of creation, it is the negative, passive, "female" element alone that has access to the Dao, which can be mirrored in a still pool.*[16] A key element in all methods of Daoist meditation is the cultivation of inner stillness, which creates the proper internal environment for the transmutation of the essences of the body, so the heart and spirit can return to emptiness.

Reverse Breathing: Connecting the Kidney and the Heart

Reverse Breathing is not really different than Kidney Breathing (see Lesson Two). It is merely a natural extension of Kidney Breathing which occurs as *Qi/Breath* sinks to the Lower *Dantian* and moves back toward the *Mingmen*. On the inhale the *Qi/Breath* sinks into the *Dantian*, and then moves back toward the sacrum and the *Mingmen*. From the sacrum and *Mingmen*, the *Qi/Breath* then **naturally** moves upward to reach the chest in the area just above the solar plexus (the middle *Dantian*), or to reach the Upper *Dantian* in the brain. The lower abdomen may "feel" like it contracts slightly during this process, but generally there is no visible contraction. On the exhale, the *Qi/Breath* sinks, moving down the front portion of the body to return to the Lower *Dantian*. The lower abdomen may "feel" like it expands slightly with the return of the *Qi/Breath*, yet again there may be no visible expansion.

Because this is merely a natural development of Kidney Breathing, the *Qi/Breath* rises and sinks without physical effort, just as water becomes vapor and rises to form the clouds that bring gentle rain. Therefore the circulation of the *Qi/Breath* should be natural, slow, smooth and even. In his excellent book, *The Way of Qigong*, Ken Cohen provides a very useful image that can make this method of breathing easier to visualize. During inhalation, as the abdomen feels as though it contracts, imagine the *Qi/Breath* being drawn back toward the sacrum and adhering to the *Mingmen* which is roughly opposite the navel. During exhalation, the *Qi/Breath* moves forward. It may be helpful to imagine a pearl in the abdomen that rolls backward and forward with each breath.[17]

Lesson 7: Practice - Connecting Heaven & Earth, Circulating Fire & Water

Exercise 1: Connecting Heaven and Earth

1) Begin in the Wu Ji Posture (Lesson 4):
- Stand with the feet facing forward and parallel.
- The feet are directly underneath the hips.
- Make sure the whole foot is on the floor - that you are not standing more on one part of the sole, such as the heels or the outside of the foot.
- Bend the knees slightly but keep them relaxed.
- The knees are in line with the front of the hip and the space between the first and second toes.
- Bend slightly at the hip fold.
- Relax the hip: keep the *kua* open. *Kua* refers to the inguinal area in the front of the pelvis going up to the top of the ilium including both the internal and external structures.
- Round the crotch.
- Relax the waist.
- Sink the tail like a plumb line.
- Gently lift the perineum and anus (this is more an idea and less a physical action).
- Raise the upper back and soften and relax the chest but don't collapse it.
- Let the shoulders hang and relax.
- Let the elbows sink and drop.
- Keep space under the armpits, as though there is a ball under each armpit.
- Relax the wrists and fingers.
- The head lifts as though suspended by the vertex and the chin is slightly pulled in.

- The eyes look down and forward with a soft gaze.
- The tongue is on the upper palate and the mouth is closed.
- Bring your attention to the *Dantian*. Breathe naturally and deeply feeling the lower abdomen expand with each inhalation.

Remember each component of the body alignment is part of a whole and works synergistically with the others.

1) Draw the *Qi/Breath* of Earth up to the *Dantian*

As you stand in *Wu Ji*, imagine the *Qi/Breath* of the Earth coming upward through the *Yong Quan* (Kidney 1: "Bubbling Well") acu-point on the bottom of the foot. Each time you inhale you gently pull the *Qi/Breath*. At first it may be difficult and the *Qi/Breath* may only reach the top of the foot or the ankle. Anchor it there as you exhale. As you inhale again, pull the *Qi/Breath* of the Earth upward a little higher, perhaps to the ankle or shin. Each time you inhale, you raise the *Qi/Breath* of Earth a little higher, stretch it upward a little bit more, each time anchoring it as you exhale. It is like stretching something elastic, anchoring it and stretching it again. When the *Qi/Breath* reaches *Dantian*, anchor it there and continue to breathe. With each inhale you strengthen the feeling of the *Qi/Breath* reaching upward from the Earth and connecting to *Dantian*.

2) Draw the *Qi/Breath* of Heaven Down to the *Dantian*

With the Qi/Breath anchored in *Dantian*, direct your attention to the top of your head and imagine the *Qi/Breath* of Heaven pouring downward through the top of the head. With each inhale draw it through the *Bai Hui* (DU 20: "Hundred Meetings") acu-point. Just as you did in Step One above, pull the *Qi/Breath* downward a little more each time you inhale, anchoring it so that it does not pull back on the exhale. At first it may be difficult to get past the head, but as you continue to breathe you will gradually pull the *Qi/Breath* of Heaven down through the head and into the torso until it reaches the *Dantian*.

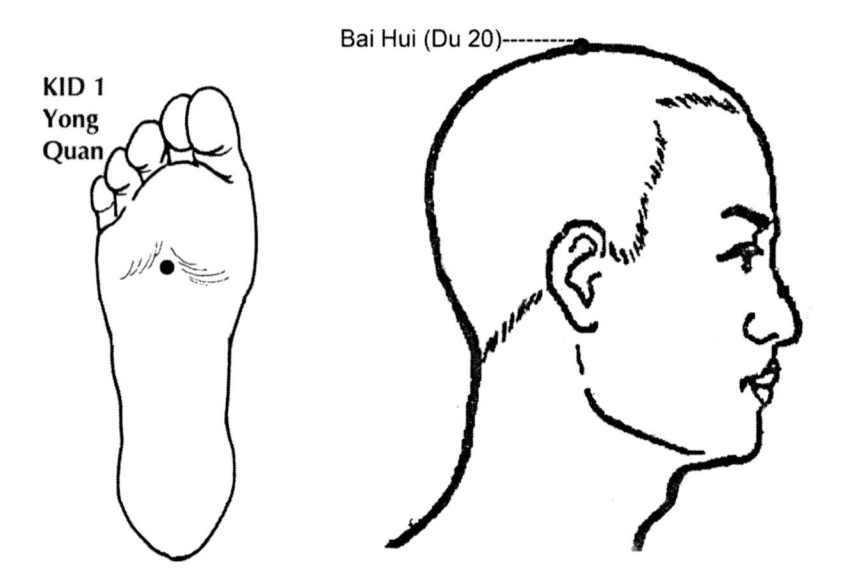

3) Connect the Breaths of Heaven and Earth

Now imagine that these two lines of *Qi/Breath* are like rods with hooks. Hook them together in the *Dantian* and let them become one. Once hooked together they become one line, one rod, that goes through the body connecting it to heaven and earth. Continue to breathe in the *Dantian*. Each time you inhale, you experience the *Qi/Breaths* of Heaven and Earth meeting in the *Dantian*. With each breath they become more and more one line, one breath. Feel the vibration of this line through the body. It is like a tuned string on a musical instrument that vibrates when plucked or strummed. Tune-in to the vibration. You may feel a vibration or swelling in your hands, or a faint sensation of the whole body vibrating. Stand this way for several minutes.

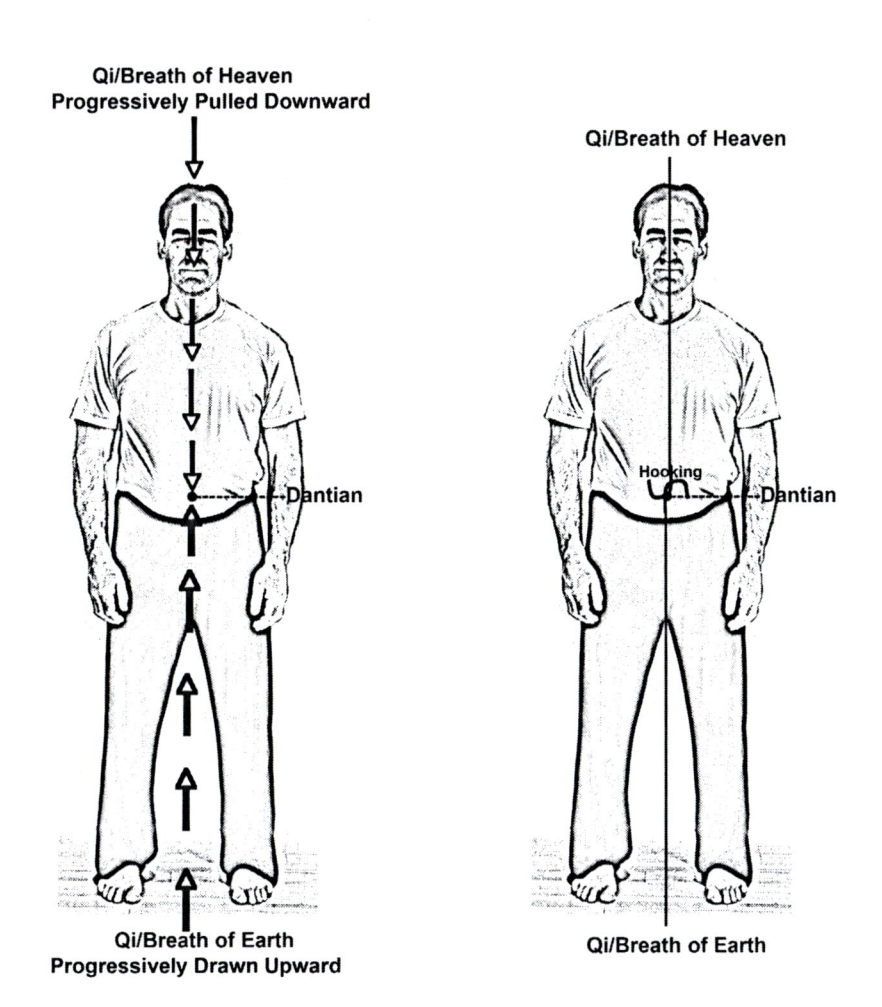

Exercise 2: Circulating Water and Fire

Water and Fire are the yin and yang corollaries of Heaven and Earth in our bodies. Water is associated with the kidneys, the storehouse of the *Jing* (essence), and Fire is associated with the heart the storehouse of the *Shen* (spirit).

1) In This Exercise We Will Return to Using a Sitting Position for Meditation.

Since you have been practicing standing meditation the last few lessons, it may be useful to review the alignments for seated meditation.

Sitting in a Chair
- The feet are flat on the floor with the knees over the ankles.
- Ideally choose a chair height that allows the knees to be bent 90 degrees and the thighs to line up with the hips.
- The hips , knees and feet are lined up.
- Ideally sit towards the front of the chair, so that your buttocks are on the seat of the chair, but your thighs are for the most part, not touching the chair.
- If you feel your back needs support, then sit farther back in the chair with a small pillow supporting your low back area.

Sitting on a Cushion
- Make sure the cushion is sufficiently high that the *kua* (inguinal area) is open and the back is straight rather than slumped.
- The hips must be relaxed and open.

General Alignments (Chair or Cushion)
- The back is relatively straight from the tail to the vertex. The lumbar area is relatively flat, not arched.
- The head and upper thoracic spine are lifted while the shoulders drop.
- The head is suspended from the vertex, but draw the chin in slightly in order to lengthen the neck.
- The hands are palm down on the knees with the elbows bent.
- Alternatively the hands can be palm up on the knees or enclosed within each other in a yin-yang configuration.
- Keep space under the armpits as though there is a ball under each armpit.
- Lift the ribs of upper back without raising the shoulders and drop and soften the chest muscles.
- Relax and loosen the shoulders.
- Sink the tail down and slightly under.
- Open the *kua*.

- The vertebrae are stacked one upon the other.
- Relax your face and jaw.

<u>Connect the Ren and Du Channels Internally</u>
- Touch the tip of the tongue to the roof of the mouth behind the upper teeth. This connects the *Ren* and *Du* meridians above (the "Upper Magpie Bridge").
- Gently have a sensation of lifting the perineum upward. This connects the *Ren* and the *Du* meridians below (the "Lower Magpie Bridge"). Remember, it is not necessary to tense or forcibly contract your anus to do this. Instead, use the synergy of the other alignments (suspending the head, sinking the tail and keeping the back straight, with the vertebrae stacked one upon the other) and gentle application of the mind-intention to "lift" the perineum.

2) Practice "Reverse Breathing"
- Now that you are seated and aligned, begin to practice this variation of Kidney Breathing. As you inhale, let the *Qi/Breath* sink to the *Dantian* and then move back toward the sacrum and *Mingmen*. Remember that *Mingmen* is roughly opposite the navel. As you continue to inhale, the *Qi/Breath* naturally moves upward from *Dantian* and *Mingmen* to the chest, just above the solar plexus. The lower abdomen may feel like it "contracts" as this happens.
- On the exhale, the *Qi/Breath* sinks, moving down the front portion of the body to return to the lower *Dantian* below the navel. During this process the *Dantian* area may feel like it expands slightly.

Remember, Reverse Breathing is really just a natural development of Kidney Breathing that often arises spontaneously on its own. It may be helpful to imagine a pearl in the abdomen that rolls backward and forward with each breath.

3) The Circulation of Water and Fire

As you inhale, the *Qi/Breath* moves to *Mingmen* and then upward toward the chest and heart. You may notice that there is a simultaneous and subtle complementary downward movement going from the chest to the *Dantian* and the kidneys. Simply observe this movement. As you exhale, the *Qi/Breath* sinks downward to the *Dantian* and kidneys. You may notice that there is a subtle and complementary movement upward toward the chest and heart. The *Qi/Breath* permeates the entire body. Movement of the *Qi/Breath* in one direction is always accompanied by counter-movement in the opposite direction, creating balance.

As *Qi/Breath* rises up, it also sinks downward; as yang *Qi* moves upward and outward, yin *Qi* moves downward and inward. The movement of the *Qi/Breath* is like an endlessly turning wheel. As a wheel turns, the spoke at the top becomes the bottom spoke and the spoke that was at the bottom moves to the top position. The sun heats water so that it turns to vapor which then rises upward. In the sky, vapor coalesces into water droplets and rain falls back to earth. Similarly, inside us, we can imagine that the trigrams Kan and Li move upward and downward in a continuous cycle that rises and falls and spirals upwards and downwards simultaneously.

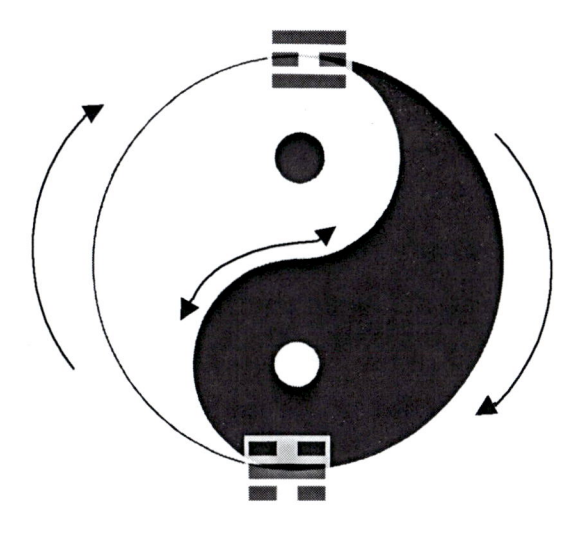

The Inter-Transformation of Kan and Li

Important Points :

At first it may be difficult to perceive the circulation of the *Qi/Breath* between the heart and the kidneys. Be careful not to use either muscular contraction or the mind-intention to force the *Qi/Breath* to circulate. Overexertion of this kind will cause the *Qi/Breath* to block. The key is to employ "Reverse Breathing" and to let the mind become still. In time, the *Qi/Breath* will circulate as described above, but this will occur without effort, almost as though one is observing, rather than directing this circulation. It can be helpful to visualize the Kan and Li trigrams - Kan in the lower abdomen and Li in the chest.

- **Kan-Water is Full in the Middle** - Therefore, relative to the chest, there is a sensation of fullness in the lower abdomen
- **Li-Fire is Empty in the Middle** - Therefore, relative to the lower abdomen, there is a sensation of emptiness in the chest.

These qualities attributed to Kan and Li are encapsulated in the following two statements which are used as a kind of mnemonic:

1) Solid (substantial; full) abdomen, unimpeded chest (*Shi Fu Chang Xiong*).
2) Contain the chest (like something held in one's mouth) and draw up the back (*Han Xiong Ba Bei*).

Gently focusing on the images of Kan and Li and their relative fullness and emptiness can aid your ability to perform Kidney Breathing and to quiet and calm the mind. Visualize the *Kan* trigram in the lower abdomen and feel how it is full in the middle. Simply by doing this, the *Qi/Breath* concentrates and moves into the *Dantian* and kidneys. Visualize the *Li* trigram with its empty center in the chest. This allows the heart to be quiet and empty. If the chest is relatively empty and the lower abdomen relatively full, then the circulation of Water and Fire and "Reverse Breathing" will manifest easily and spontaneously.

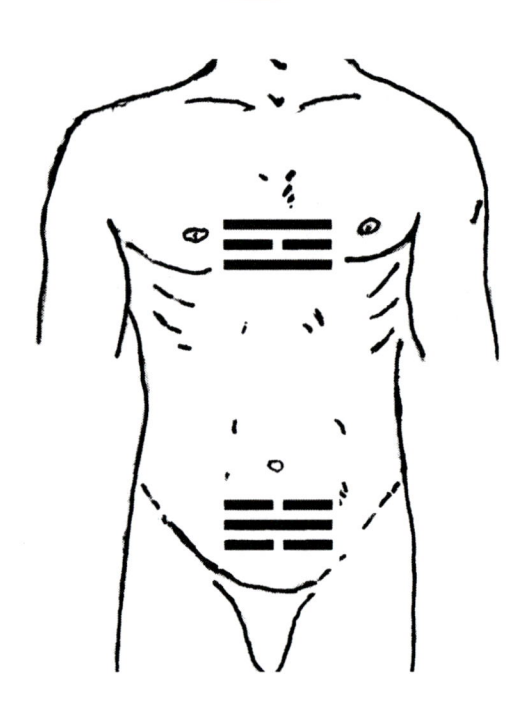

Supplementary Qi Gong Exercises to Assist the Circulation of Water and Fire:

Exercise 1: The Triple Heater Exercise

In Chinese Medicine the *San Jiao* (Triple Heater) is an internal pathway that oversees the transformation of *Qi/Breath* in the body. Emanating from the *Mingmen* and the kidneys, the *San Jiao* is the pathway through which *Mingmen* fire connects with the fire of the heart. The Triple Heater is the place where yin and yang are said to "meet and transform". Thus, it is a passageway for water and fire.

The Triple Heater Exercise is basic to many methods of Nei Gong because it aids in connecting the heart and kidneys and harmonizing fire and water. The movements can help us to feel the simultaneous upward and downward movement between the chest/heart and the *Dantian*, *Mingmen* and kidneys. The Triple Heater exercise can be performed as a stand-alone Qi Gong exercise that harmonizes and calms the body, and as a tool for perceiving the yin-yang interchange between the kidneys and the heart.

1) Stand in the *Wu Ji* Posture.
Remember to let the tongue tip touch the upper palate and to gently "lift" the perineum. Keep the head straight with the eyes looking straight ahead.

2) Inhale and curve the arms inward so that that they lift with the palms facing upward, until they reach chest level. As the arms raise and the *Qi/Breath* moves upward toward the chest, internally it feels as if the legs bend imperceptibly and there is a feeling of the whole body sinking and settling into the feet as though rooting into the ground.

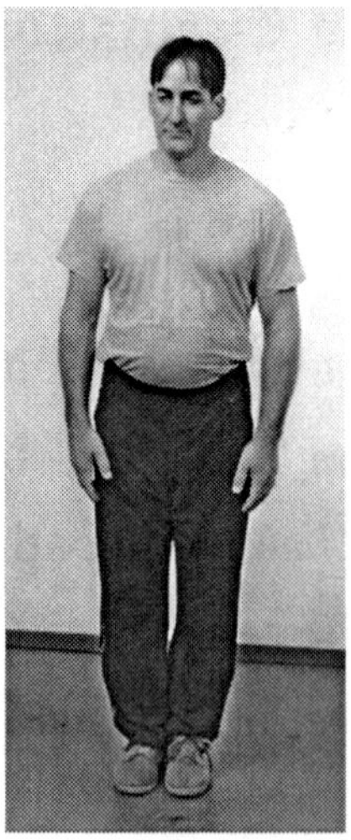
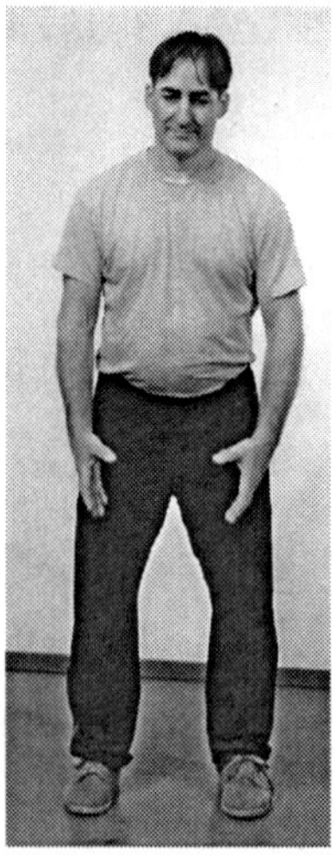
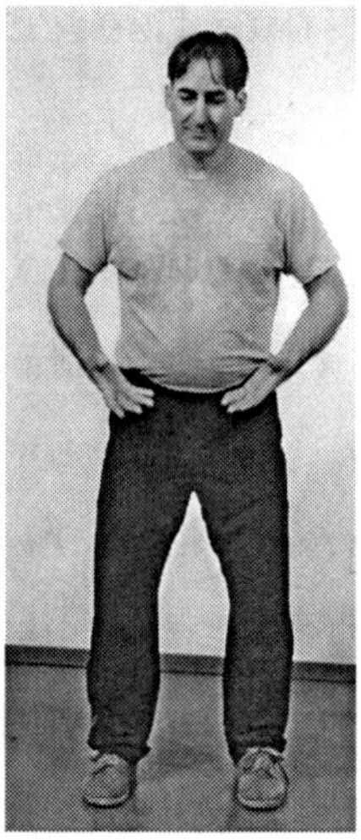
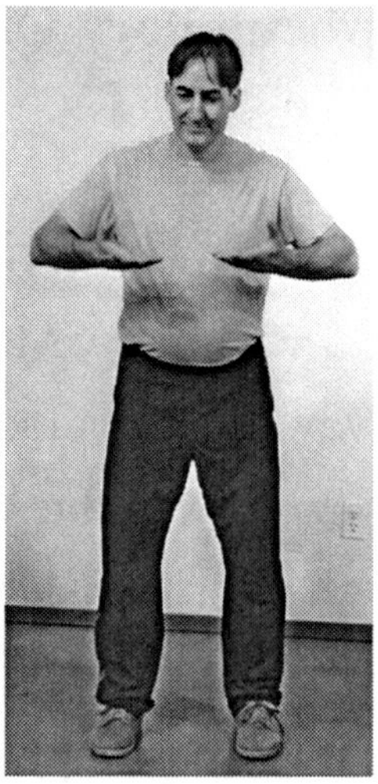
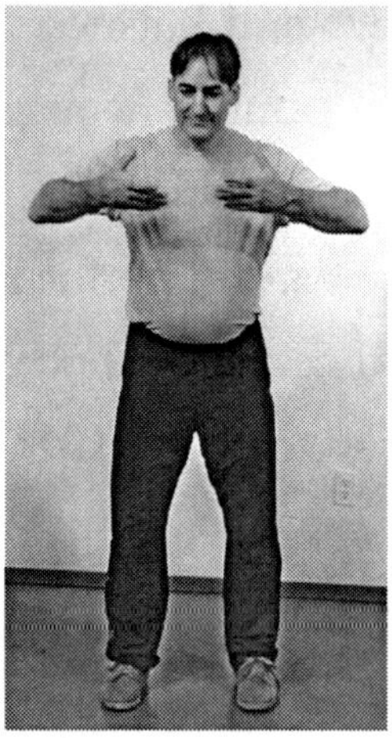
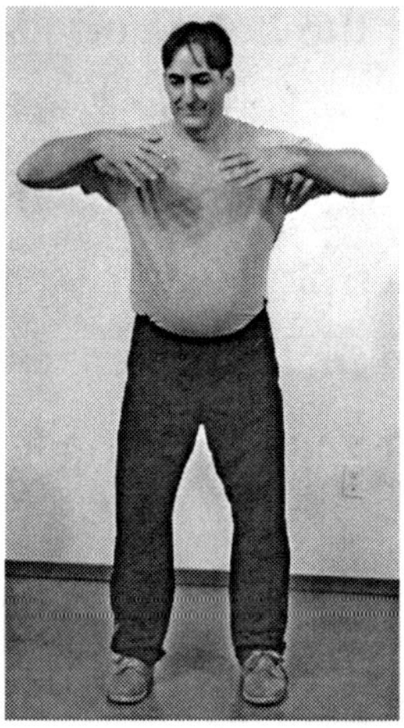
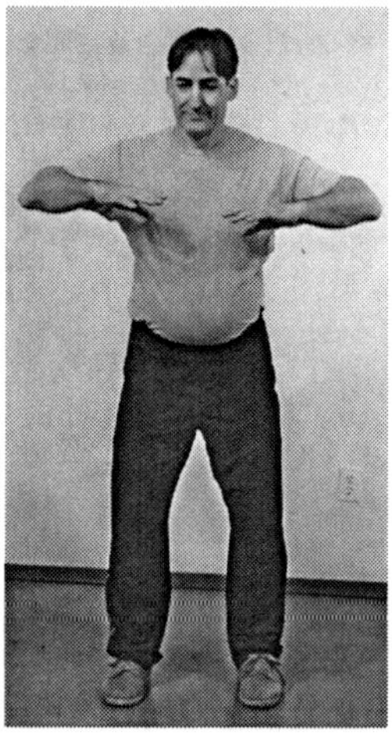
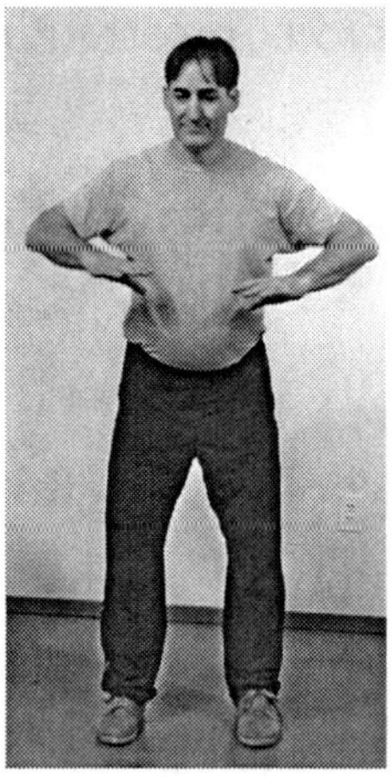
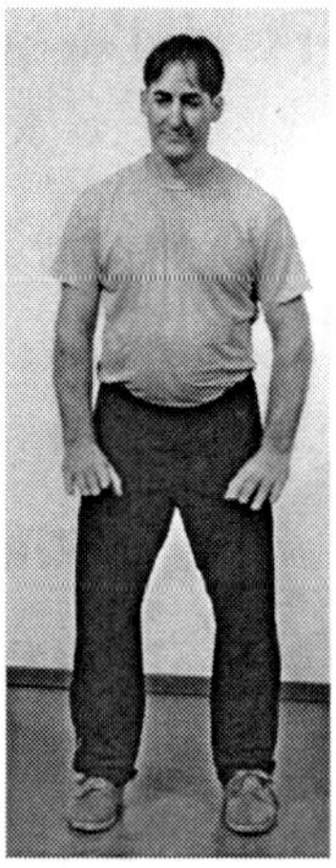
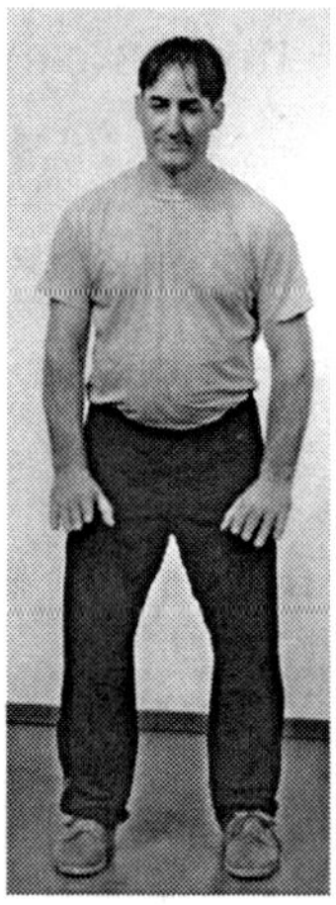
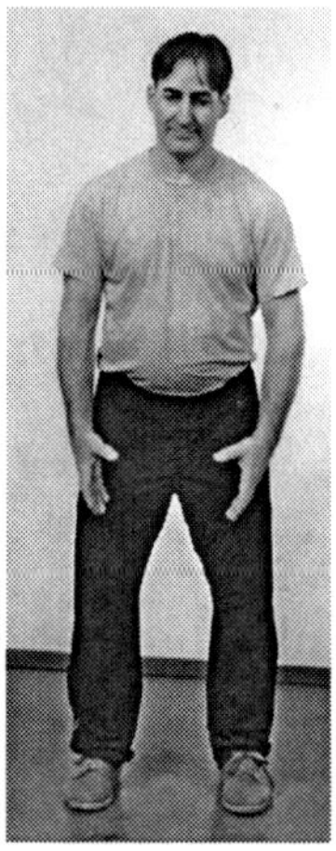

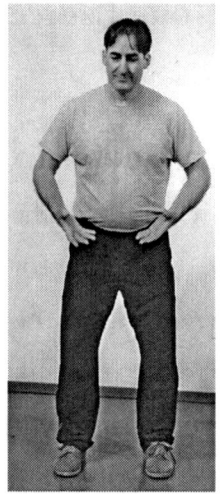

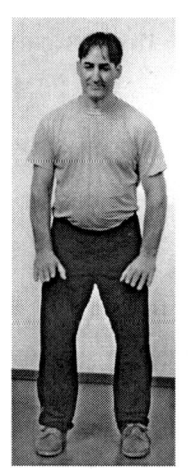

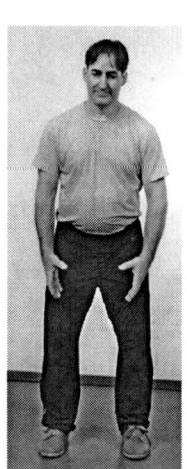

3) When the hands reach the chest, turn them palm down and exhale as you press the palms gently down until the hands reach the lower abdomen below the navel. As the hands and the *Qi/Breath* descend, the knees internally feel as though they straighten. Simultaneously, there is a feeling of erecting upward throughout the body.

4) Repeat these movements for 3-5 minutes.

Exercise 2: Connecting the Kidneys and the Heart

This exercise builds from the previous exercise and also works with the Triple Heater. Because it employs a circular movement of the hands, it can create a stronger sensation of the *Qi/Breath* spiraling between the *Dantian* and the heart.

Start: stand with your heels together. Let the tongue tip touch the upper palate and gently "lift" the perineum. Keep the head straight with the eyes looking foward. The knees are slightly bent and the toes turn slightly outward. The elbows and shoulders are relaxed.

Part 1: Winding Inward

1) Inhale and begin to lift the arms palm up in front of you with the elbows bent.

2) The arms bend inward as they rise past the chest. As you continue to inhale, the elbows bend and the hands curve inward toward the chin. The backs of the hands touch and the elbows swing outward. The *Qi/Breath* moves up and toward the heart and chest.

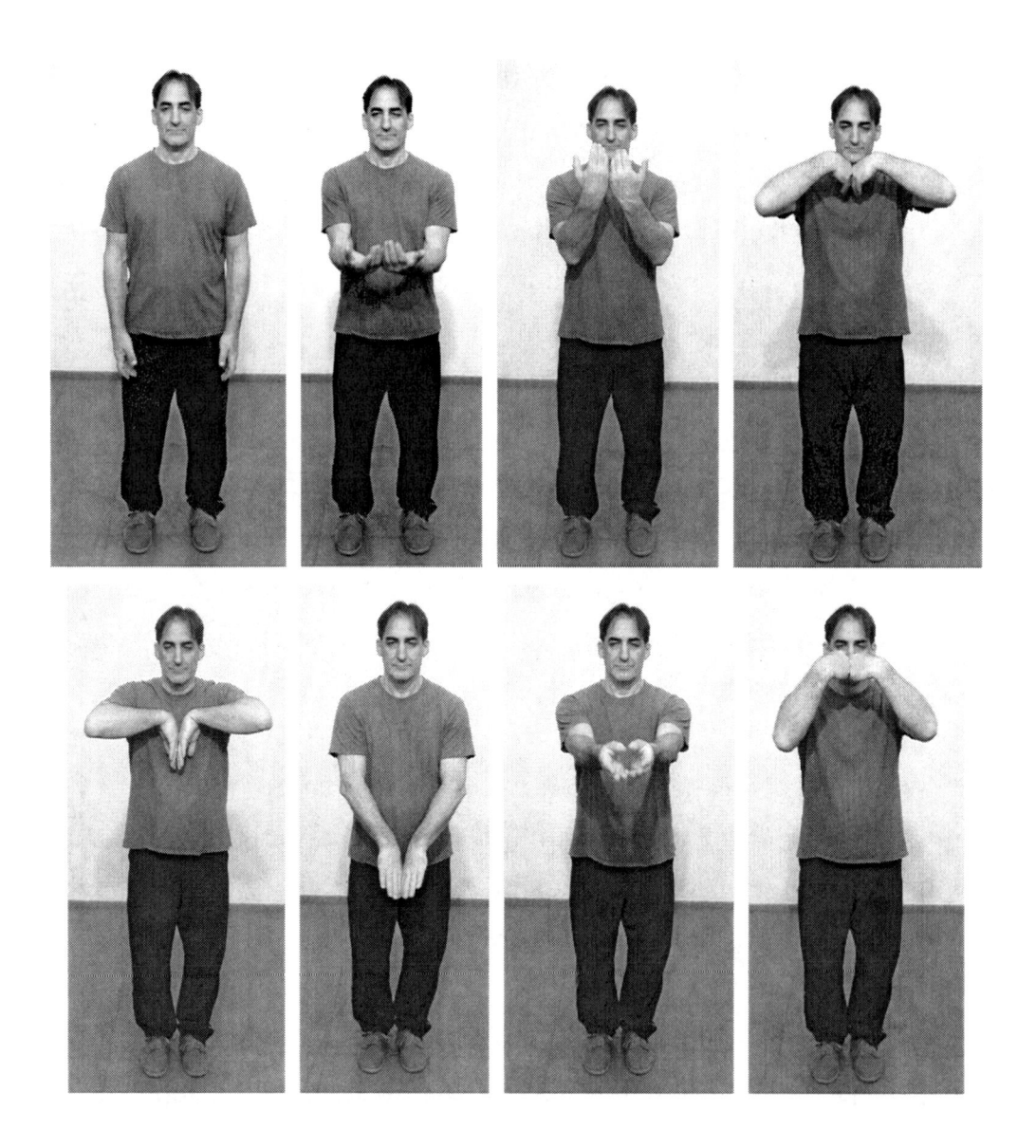

3) Exhale as the hands pass your chest and move down the body with the backs of the hands touching. As the fingers lead the downward motion, the elbows come towards each other naturally. Continue to exhale as the hands reach *Dantian*, the *Qi/Breath* following the movement of the arms. The palms begin to face down and out.

4) As the hands reach down toward the pubic bone, the arms extend outward and slightly rise. At this point, the palms face downward and the thumb and index fingers of the two hands connect with each other. As the

arms extend, the weight moves forward slightly on the feet with a faint sensation of the heels starting to lift.

5) As the arms rise past the navel, begin to inhale. At this point, the palms begin to turn so that they face upward. Continue to inhale and let the elbows bend as the hands curve slightly upward and inward towards your chin and then down to the center of the chest. The backs of the hands touch and the elbows swing outwards. The *Qi/Breath* moves up and toward the heart and chest.

6) Repeat these movements for 3-5 minutes.

Part 2: Winding Outward

From the start position, **reverse** the direction of the circle and the movements.

1) As you inhale, curve the hands inward leading with the fingers and begin to bring them upward along the front of the body. The hands can brush the front of the body.

2) Continue to inhale as you bring the hands upward along the body from the *Dantian* to the heart and chest and then under the chin. The elbows naturally swing inward as the backs of the hands come together and the fingertips lead the motion. The *Qi/Breath* follows the movements of the hands.

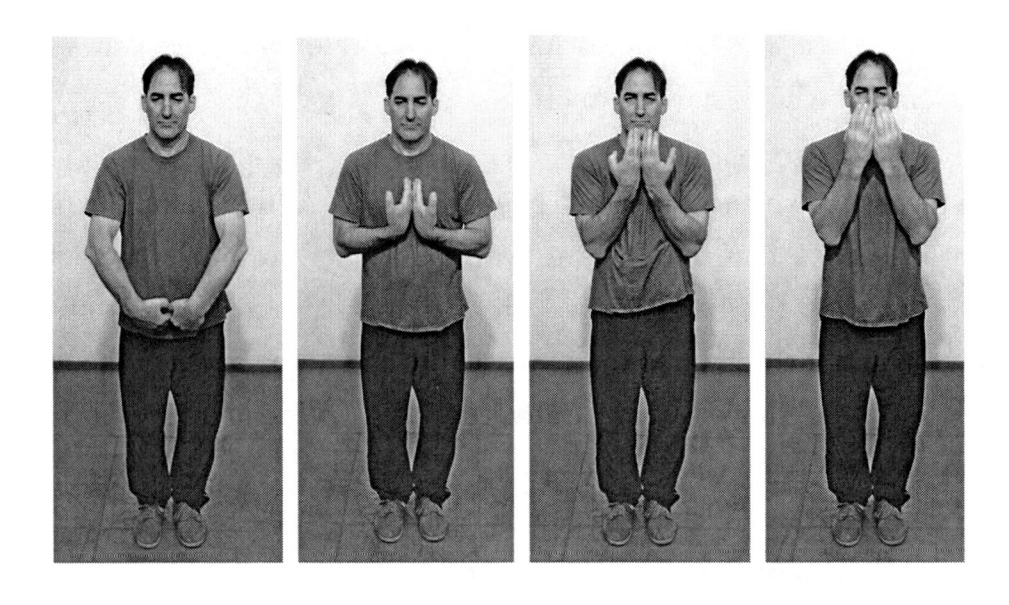

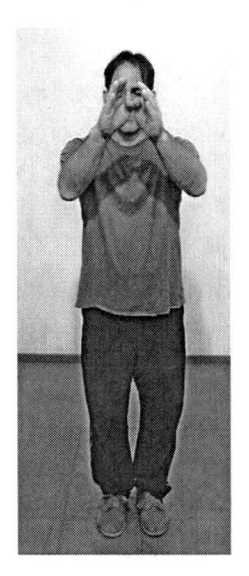

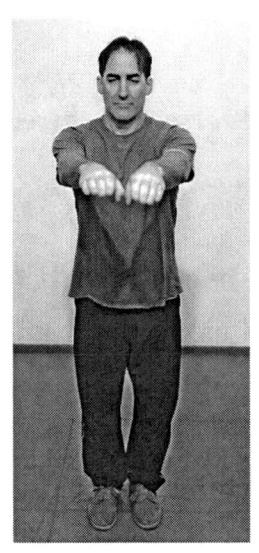

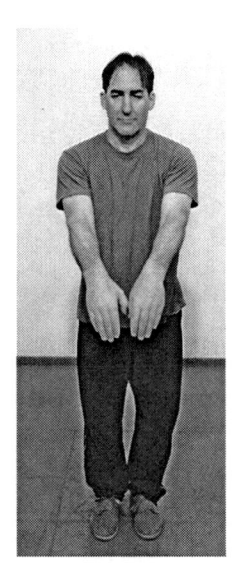

3) As the hands pass the chin, begin to exhale. The arms begin to extend, and rotate palm down. The elbows move outward as first the two pinkies touch and then, as rotation continues, the thumb and index fingers of the two hands connect with each other. As the arms extend, the weight moves forward slightly on the feet with a faint sensation of the heels starting to lift.

4) As you finish, continue to exhale; the hands reach forward and down. The *Qi/Breath* follows the movements of the hands.

5) When the hands reach the level of the pubic bone, they curve inward to rise along the front of the body as in Step Two above.

6) Repeat these movements for 3-5 minutes

Important Points:
- Feel how as the arms extend, the shoulders rotate and the muscles of the back are engaged.
- As the back engages, this action pulls you forward **slightly** towards the balls of your feet (not up onto your toes). As this occurs there is a very slight straightening of the legs. The knees do not lock.
- Keep the elbow and shoulder joints soft and relaxed.

Lesson 8:

Golden Fluid &

The Micro-Cosmic

Orbit

小 周 天
Xiao Zhou Tian

Lesson Eight: Golden Fluid & The Micro-Cosmic Orbit

Saliva: Elixir of Immortality

Saliva is a key element in Daoist meditation and internal alchemy. Swallowing saliva is a part of virtually every Daoist exercise, including many forms of *Qi Gong*. It is no surprise then that saliva is referred to by many nanes in different Daoist texts:

Golden Fluid	*jin ye*	金液
Golden Elixir	*jin yi*	金酏
Jade Dew	*yu lu*	玉露
Jade Fluid	*yu ye*	玉液
Jade Juice	*yu zhi*	玉汁
Jade Beverage	*yu yin*	玉飲
Divine Juice	*ling zhi*	靈汁
Heavenly Dew	*tian lu*	天露

As we shall see in this lesson, production of saliva is one sign that the meditation is being performed correctly. When *Jing* is concentrated in the lower abdomen, it transforms into *Qi/Breath* and moved upward, saliva is secreted and then descends to replenish *Jing*.

The tongue (known as the "red dragon") is sometimes used to further stimulate the production of saliva, as is the action of clicking the teeth. Isabelle Robinet tells us that the center of the mouth, where the saliva accumulates, called the "Jade Pool," is the upper-body equivalent of the lower *Dantian* where the sexual essence (*Jing*) accumulates.[1] According to Chinese medicine, saliva is made up of two basic parts. One part is more pure and refined. It is associated with the kidneys and therefore the *Jing*. This portion moistens and nourishes the teeth, themselves extensions of the kidneys, and the long-term cycles of growth and development associated with the kidneys. The other part is associated with the organs of digestion, particularly the stomach. This more turbid, less refined portion is related to digestive juices of the stomach and aids in breaking down food. Proper performance of "Reverse Breathing" and the Micro-Cosmic Orbit, which we cover in this lesson, promotes the production of a sweeter, thicker, more nourishing saliva, associated with the *Jing*. This "golden fluid" is then swallowed so that it can sink to *Dantian*.

Saliva flows from two channels under the tongue. If it is swallowed properly it can enter the *Ren Mo* ("conception vessel"), which runs down the center of the body to the *Dantian*, genitals and perineum, thereby returning to the *Dantian*. If not swallowed properly, saliva descends to the stomach. The proper method of swallowing the saliva is to have the tip of the tongue touching the upper palate. When the mouth fills with saliva (from correct practice of the micro-cosmic orbit), one must straighten the neck and swallow the saliva.[2]

Science & Saliva

Modern science has discovered that saliva has many important properties. Studies in Japan have shown that saliva contains various enzymes and hormones that help to aid digestion, maintain health and prevent disease. The digestive enzyme Ptyalin begins the process of breaking down carbohydrates. Other substances in saliva detoxify and protect against toxic substances in foods. There is some indication that saliva may even contain substances that fight cancer. Parotin, a hormone found in saliva, has been found to strengthen the activities of the muscles, maintain the blood elasticity of the vessels, maintain the elasticity of the skin and strengthen connective tissue, cartilage, bones and teeth.

Nutritionist Lino Stanchich tells the amazing story of his father who, during WWII, was taken prisoner in Greece and sent to a concentration camp in Germany. It was a work camp. His father was cold and hungry all the time and received only a slice of bread and coffee for breakfast and soup for lunch and dinner. He discovered that by chewing his food, and even his water, many times, it actually seemed to increase his energy. He showed two other prisoners what he had discovered, and they all felt warmer and more energized after chewing their food and water as much as 150 times before swallowing it. In the end only these three survived.[3]

Ren and Du & the Micro-Cosmic Orbit

The *Ren* and *Du* Vessels run along the midline of the body. The *Ren Mo* ("conception vessel") runs along the front midline of the body from the Perineum to the chin and mouth. *Du Mo* ("governing vessel") runs along the back midline of the body from the perineum to the top of head and then down through the forehead and nose to the inside of the upper lip and upper palate. Both vessels originate in the kidneys. When looking at the pictures of their pathways, it is important to keep in mind that *Du Mo* passes through the interior of the spine and *Ren Mo* passes through the interior of the abdomen. A number of points on these channels have alternative names or even several names. The names below are more specifically how they are referenced in Daoist meditation practices.

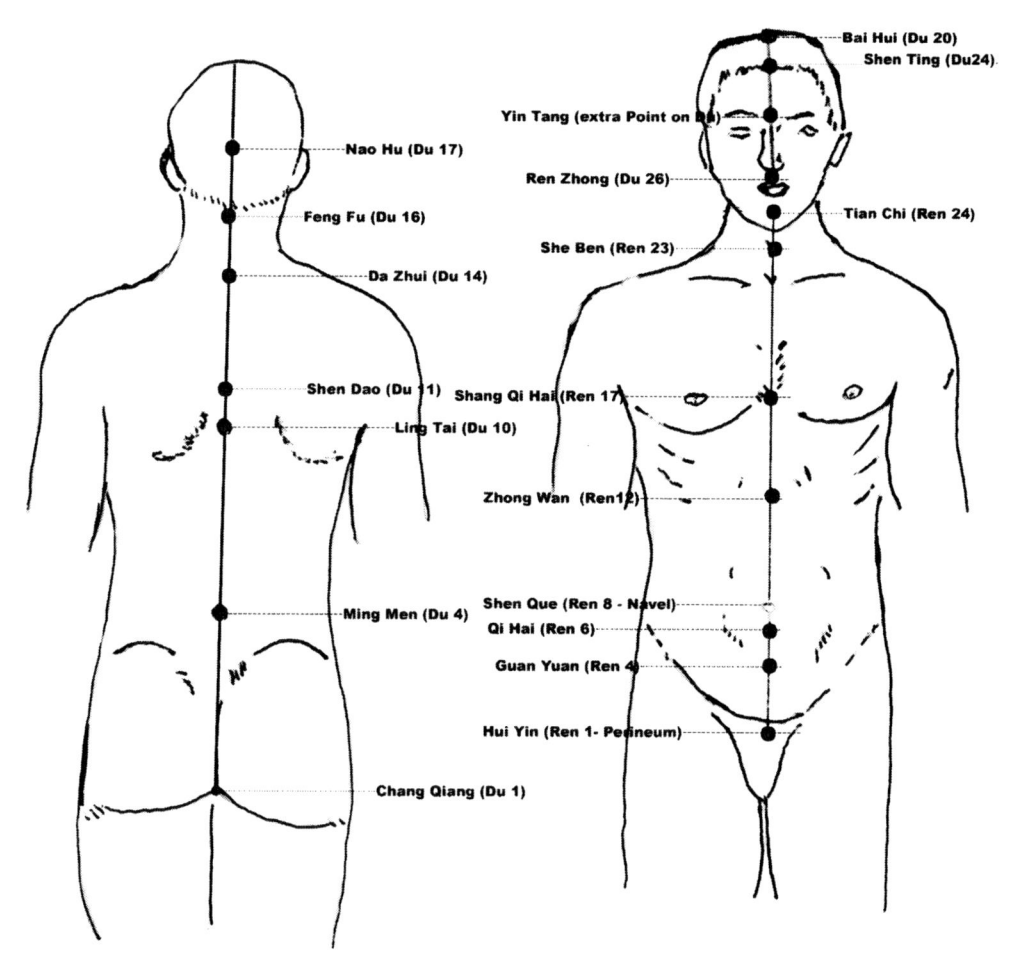

Pathways and Important Points on the Ren and Du Vessels

Important Du Channel Acu-Points

Du 1	*Chang Qiang (Wei Lu)*	Long Strong (Tail Gate)
Du 4	*Ming Men*	Life Gate
Du 10	*Ling Tai*	Spirit Tower
Du 11	*Shen Dao*	Spirit Path
Du 14	*Da Zhui*	Great Hammer
Du 16	*Feng Fu*	Wind Mansion
Du 17	*Nao Hu (Yu Zhen)*	Brain Door (Jade Pillow)
Du 20	*Bai Hui*	Hundred Meeting
Du 24	*Shen Ting*	Spirit Court

Extra	*Yin Tang (Zhu Qiao)*[4]	Seal Hall (Ancestral Aperture)
Du 26	*Ren Zhong*	Human Center

Important Ren Channel Points Acu-Points

Ren 24	*Tian Chi*	Celestial Pool
Ren 23	*She Ben*	Tongue Root
Ren 17	*Shang Qi Hai*	Upper Sea of Qi
Ren 12	*Zhong Wan*	Central Cavity
Ren 8	*Shen Que*	Spirit Gate
Ren 6	*Qi Hai*	Sea of Qi
Ren 4	*Guan Yuan*	Original Pass
Ren 1	*Hui Yin*	Meeting of Yin

Du Mo is the sea of all the yang vessels (meridians) in the body. It connects these vessels and ties them all together. *Ren Mo* is the sea of all the yin vessels. The true breath arises from the *Ren* and the *Du* and they are at the same time active expressions of the true breath.[5]

> *The two vessels of Ren and Du are but two branches with a single source. One travels along the front of the body and another travels along the back of the body. A person's body has the Ren and the Du, just as heaven and earth have midday (zi) and midnight (wu), which may be perceived as divided and united. Divide them and it is apparent that their yin and yang [aspects] cannot be separated. Unite them [and] it is apparent that they are coalesced without differentiation. The singular is plural and the plural is singular.*[6]

Ren Mo and *Du Mo* are where *Kan*-Water and *Li*-Fire intersect, where water and fire ascend and descend. Because of their relationships with the other meridians and their role in the transformation of water and fire, it is said that: *If a person can open these two vessels than all of the hundreds of vessels can all be open.*[7]

The Microcosmic Orbit, or Small Heavenly Circulation (*Xiao Zhou Tian*), is a method of Daoist meditation that attends to the circulation of the *Qi/Breath* through *Ren Mo* and *Du Mo*. In the *Treatise of Affirming the Breath and Making the Soul Return*, it is described as follows:

The jing transformed into qi rises up toward the heights;
If the qi is not strengthened, the jing becomes exhausted.
The qi which becomes the saliva, descends to the depths;
If the jing does not return, the qi is altered.
It is like water which one heats in a tripod;
If at first there is no qi,
How will qi be produced?
Because it descends and cannot escape.
By rising, water becomes qi,
Qi in turn becomes water when descending.
They rise and descend in endless rotation.[8]

By gently letting the breath sink to *Dantian*, it begins to flow up the *Du* channel to the top of the head. Apertures (acu-points) in the head allow the *Qi/Breath* to enter the brain and then descend down into the mouth, where saliva is produced and there is a connection with the *Ren* channel. From there the *Qi/Breath* (and the saliva) flow downward to the *Dantian* and the cycle is repeated. The *Qi/Breath* rises with inhalation and descends with exhalation. Through this process *Jing* is transformed into *Qi/Breath*, and *Qi/Breath* in turn nourishes the spirit (*Shen*). The *Shen* guides and harnesses the *Qi/Breath* to replenish the *Jing*. Through this process one is reconnected with the "true breath", the primordial yin-yang current that flows between Heaven and Earth. This not only invigorates the body by allowing the *Qi/Breath*, Blood and *Jing* to enter the bone marrow, tendons, ligaments, flesh and muscle, restoring the pliability of these structures, it also reconnects with our own innate wisdom, thereby re-inciting the life that is within us. Francois Jullien explains the importance of these channels as follows:

> *The principle artery or du, which irrigates the back from bottom to top and is the vessel through which energy flows. Why does our attention, once liberated from the endlessly spendthrift thirst for knowledge, focus on this artery as defining the line and rule of life? Because, as we have already discussed, this median artery has a regulative capacity that ensures respiratory constancy. And what is this respiration but a continual incitation not to dwell in either of two opposite positions – inhalation or exhalation? Respiration allows each to call upon the other in order to renew itself through it, thus establishing the great rhythm of the worlds evolution. Thus respiration is not only the symbol, the image or figure, but also the vector of vital nourishment.*[9]

Circulation of the Micro-Cosmic Orbit

As you inhale and the breath rises, the ribs in the back open. With the perineum (and anus) lifted, the tailbone sinking and the vertex lifting upward, the *Qi/Breath* is able to ascend through the spine. The chin is slightly held in, allowing the points at the base of the skull to open so that *Qi/Breath* does not get blocked at these points and thus enters the brain and rises to the top of the head.

With the exhale, the *Qi/Breath* is able to sink because the tongue tip touching the upper palate connects *Ren Mo* and *Du Mo*. The lifting of the head, the position of the neck and the open ribs allow the *Qi/Breath* to drop downward to return to the *Dantian*. As the *Qi/Breath* sinks, it seems to exhale not through the nose, but instead to exhale internally going down to *Dantian*. The *Dantian* then, naturally has a feeling of expanding as one exhales (the reverse breathing we practiced in the previous lesson). The flow of air is continuous, even and smooth like a thread being wound smoothly around a spindle.

As you inhale, visualize the *Qi/Breath* sinking to the *Dantian*. Then, by keeping the perineum lifted (the "lower magpie gate") and the tail sinking, the *Qi/Breath* rises through the tailbone to the *Mingmen* (Du 4: "life gate") and up through the center of the back to acu-point Du 16 (*Feng Fu*) where *Qi/Breath* enters the brain. *Qi/Breath* passes through Du 17 *Yu Zhen* ("Jade Pillow") at the occipital protuberance. From there it continues to rise to *Bai Hui* ("Hundred Meeting"; Du 20) point at the vertex and moves forward to *Shen Ting* ("Spirit Court"; Du 24) before beginning to descend with the exhalation.

As you exhale, the *Qi/Breath* moves into the mouth and connects to the Ren Channel via the tongue (the "upper magpie gate"), and then passes down the front of the body. Rather than passing out the nose or mouth, the *Qi/Breath* descends through the throat to enter the chest behind Ren 17 ("Upper Sea of Qi") and then down into the abdomen passing through Ren 12 ("Central Cavity"). From here, the breath returns to the navel (*Shen Que*; "Spirit Gate") and then to the *Dantian*.

Circulation of the *Qi/Breath* in *Ren Mo* and *Du Mo* is a bit like an electrical circuit. The two ends of the vessels must be connected for there to be an uninterrupted flow. The upper Magpie Bridge is the tongue, and the tongue touches the upper roof to link with *Ren Mo* and *Du Mo* in the upper part. The lower Magpie Bridge is in the perineum and links *Du Mo* and *Ren Mo* in the lower part. Thus, the *Ren* and *Du* are linked and the Heavenly Circle flows.

Waxing and Waning of Yin and Yang and the Micro-Cosmic Orbit

Yang *Qi* gathers as the *Qi/Breath* rises up the back and Yin *Qi* coalesces as the *Qi/Breath* sinks back to *Dantian*. Thus on the inhalation, yang waxes and yin wanes. On the exhalation, yin waxes and yang wanes. Similarly *Qian*-Heaven and *Kun*-Earth wax and wane just as day becomes night and night becomes day in endless cycles. In *Qian* there is opening, an opening of the gates for *Qi/Breath* to flow and change and transformation to occur. In *Kun* there is reception, closing and consolidation. Inhalation is opening and exhalation is closing, like bellows pumping. The changes and transformations, the opening and closing, are a product of Heaven and Earth's breaths, which also flow through us. The diagram below uses hexagrams from the *Yi Jing* (I Ching: the Book of Changes) to show this dynamic process. These twelve hexagrams are sometimes called: The Waxing and Waning Hexagrams, or the Twelve Sovereign Hexagrams. They are also used to describe the waxing and waning of yin and yang over the 12 months of the year.

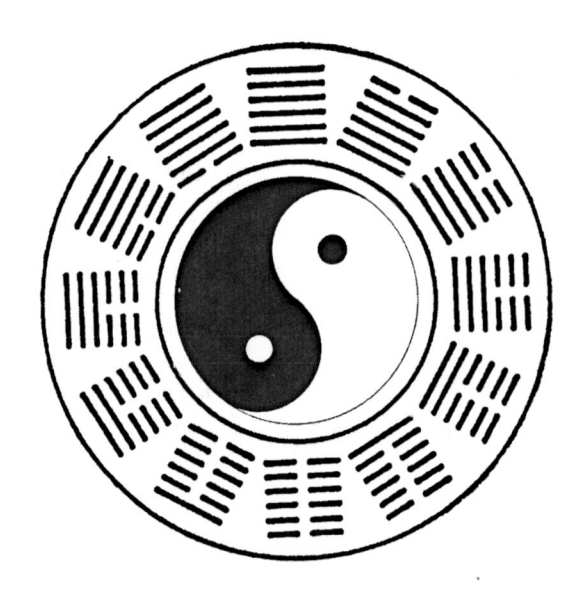

The hexagrams change from the bottom up, the yin lines pushing out the yang, beginning at the summer solstice, and the yang lines returning at the winter solstice.

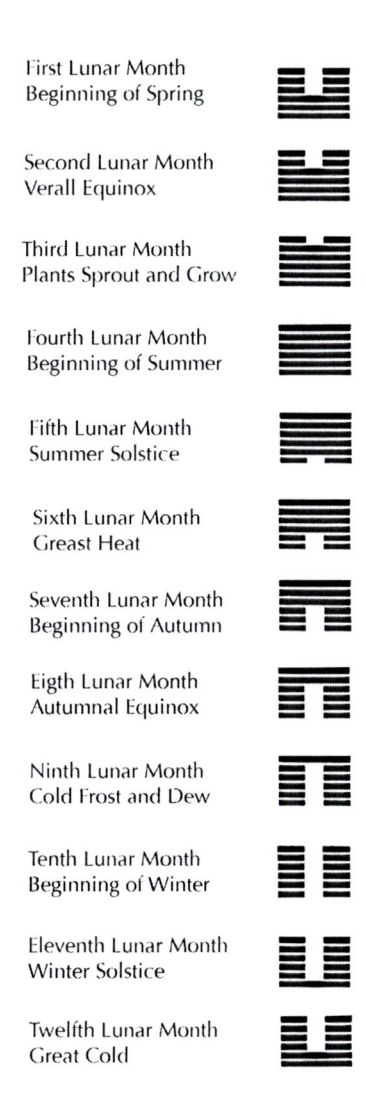

First Lunar Month Beginning of Spring	䷊
Second Lunar Month Verall Equinox	䷡
Third Lunar Month Plants Sprout and Grow	䷪
Fourth Lunar Month Beginning of Summer	䷀
Fifth Lunar Month Summer Solstice	䷫
Sixth Lunar Month Greast Heat	䷠
Seventh Lunar Month Beginning of Autumn	䷋
Eigth Lunar Month Autumnal Equinox	䷓
Ninth Lunar Month Cold Frost and Dew	䷖
Tenth Lunar Month Beginning of Winter	䷁
Eleventh Lunar Month Winter Solstice	䷗
Twelfth Lunar Month Great Cold	䷒

During Micro-Cosmic Orbit Meditation, these same yin-yang transformations occur inside us. As we inhale, yang begins to grow, rising from the kidneys and the perineum, and moving up the *Du* vessel until yang peaks just before reaching the top of the head. Then yin returns and begins to grow at *Bai Hui* (Du 20). Yin gathers until all the lines return to yin again at the perineum.

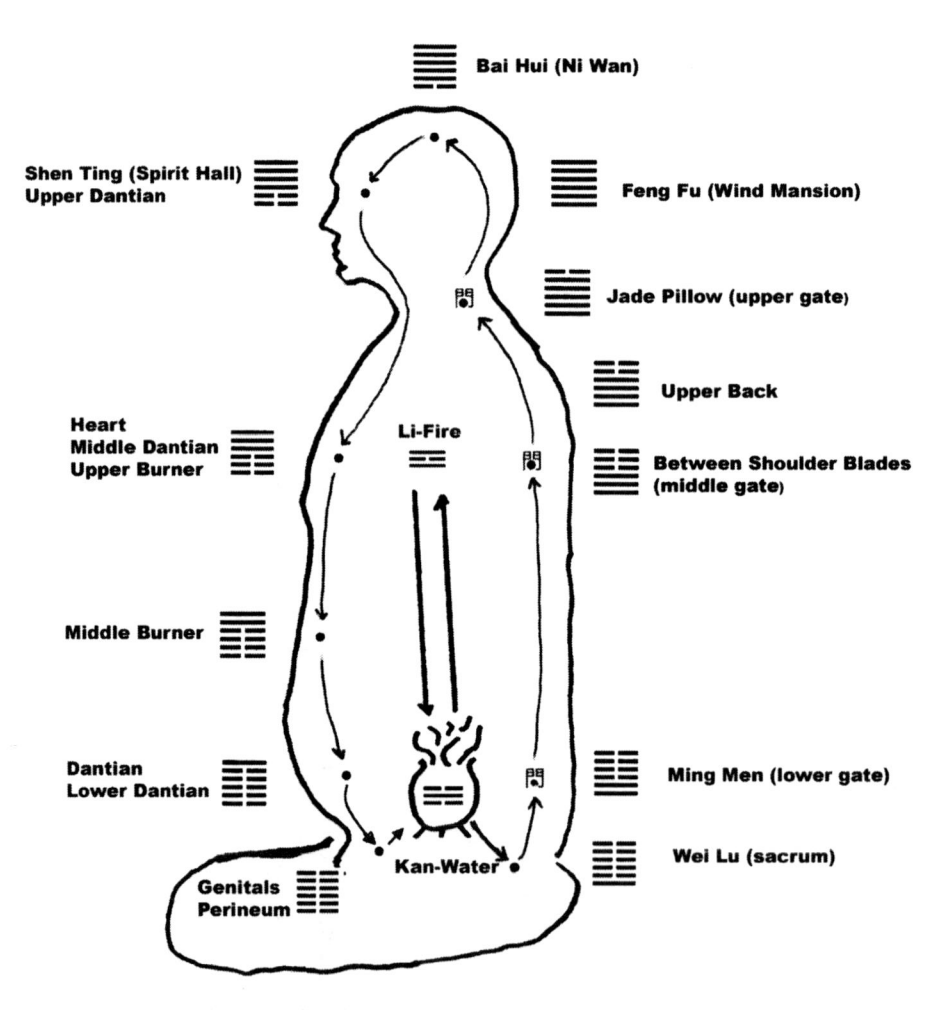

The Waxing and Waning of Qian and Kun (Yin and Yang)
Qian - The Opening of the Gates - Inhalation
Kun - The Closing of the Gates - Exhalation

Drawing adapted from The Complete System of Self Healing: Internal Exercise, by Dr. Stephen T. Chang. San Francisco: Tao Publishing 1986, p. 200.

Hormones, Jing, and the Endocrine System

Modern Chinese physicians sometimes relate *Jing* to hormones and the endocrine system, and some believe that microcosmic orbit breathing activates, stimulates and regulates the endocrine system. They theorize that when *Jingqi* from the kidneys moves upward to nourish the brain and the spirit, it may connect the adrenal glands with the hypothalamus which lies just above the brain stem. The hypothalamus has direct connections with the pituitary gland which is also located in the brain. The hypothalamus not only links the nervous system to the endocrine system, it regulates secretions from the pituitary and co-ordinates many hormonal and behavioral circadian rhythms. Endocrine glands that signal each other in sequence to produce hormonal triggers are referred to as an "axis." One such axis is the hypothalamic-pituitary-adrenal axis which increases production and release of corticosteroids.[10] Dr. Tian He Lu of Shanxi province in mainland China points out that the hypothalamus and pituitary are in the *Upper Dantian* and the adrenal glands and gonads (whose hormonal secretion is also controlled by the pituitary) are in the *Lower Dantian*. Furthermore, Dr. Tian feels that practice of the microcosmic orbit directly effects the endocrine system, particularly the hypothalamic-pituitary-adrenal axis. He attributes the health benefits ascribed to the Micro-Cosmic Orbit to its stimulation and regulation of the endocrine system.[11]

- Pineal Gland
- Pituitary Gland
- Thyroid Gland
- Thymus
- Adrenal gland
- Pancreas
- Adrenal gland
- Ovaries
- Kidneys
- Testes

Endocrine System

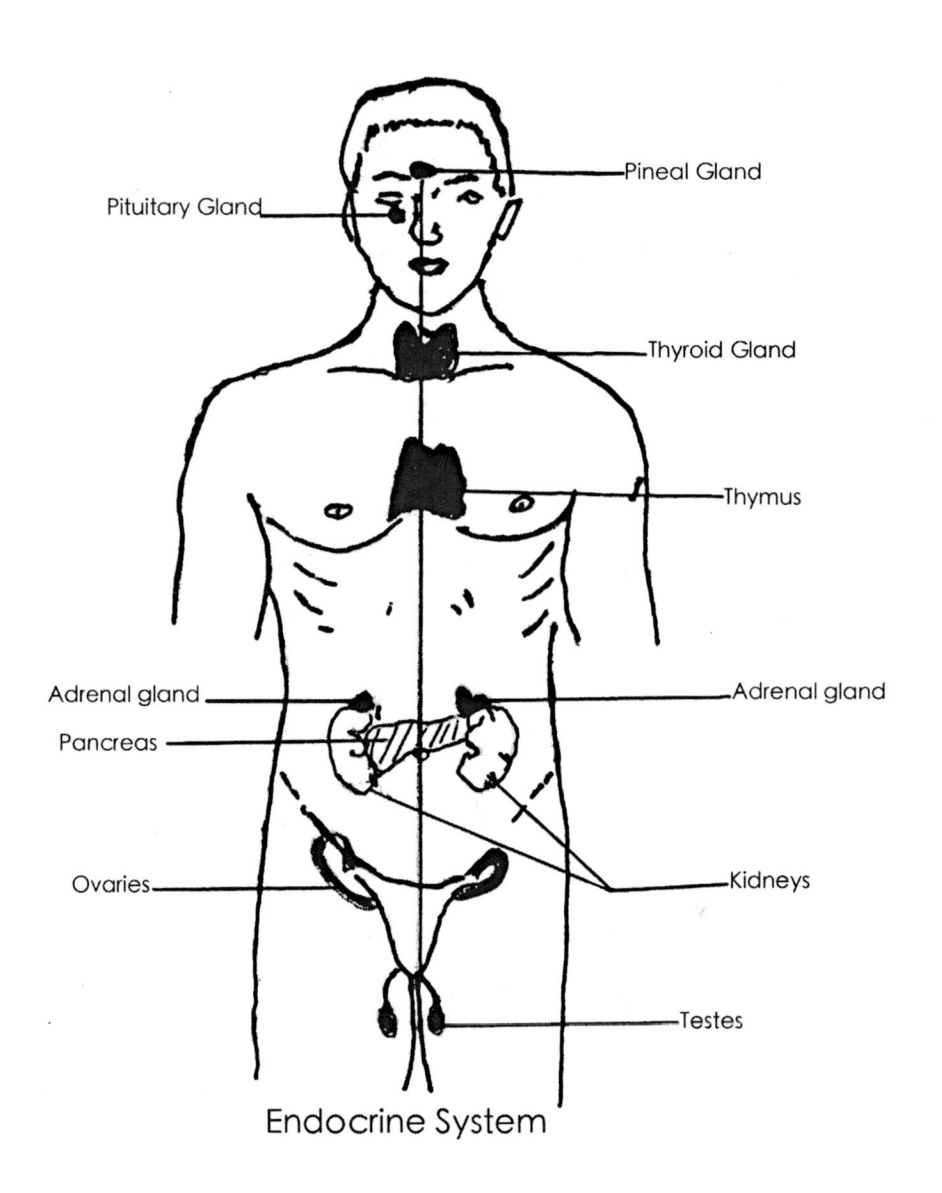

Lesson 8: Practice - The Micro-Cosmic Orbit

      Assume the seated meditation posture you used in Lesson Seven. Remember to connect the Ren and Du channels internally through the upper and lower magpie bridges: gently lift the perineum and touch the tip of the tongue to the upper palate. Do this without muscular effort by using the synergy of the various alignments that are built into the seated meditation posture.

1) Practice "Reverse Breathing" and Let *Qi/Breath* Flow Through the Micro-Cosmic Orbit.

Inhale softly, smoothly and evenly through the nose. Remember, on the inhale the *Qi/Breath* sinks into the *Dantian,* and then moves back toward the sacrum and the *Mingmen.* From the sacrum and the *Mingmen,* the *Qi/Breath* then **naturally** moves upward. The lower abdomen may "feel" like it contracts slightly during this process, but generally there is no visible contraction.

Continue to inhale, allowing the *Qi/Breath* to naturally move upward from the sacrum and *Mingmen,* so that it travels up the *Du Mo* toward the base of the skull and then *Bai Hui* (at the vertex). As the *Qi/Breath* moves forward to *Shen Ting* (at the frontal hairline) and down into the mouth, the exhale begins.

As you exhale, rather then passing out through the nose, the *Qi/Breath* feels as though it follows *Ren Mo*, moving from the mouth, down through the throat, and into the chest, then going backwards toward the spine; flowing smoothly, evenly and continuously. The *Qi/Breath* continues to sink until it reaches *Dantian*. During this process the *Dantian* area feels like it expands slightly.

Throughout this process, the movement of the *Qi/Breath* is slow, even and unforced as it moves through the *Ren* and *Du* vessels.

The Chinese liken this movement to a silkworm winding thread: pull too hard or force the motion, and the thread breaks or tangles; pull slowly, smoothly and evenly and it winds effortlessly and seamlessly. The mind-intention should not force the breath. It initiates, but does not make the breath happen; it participates, but also observes. It takes daily practice to achieve this. If you do not feel the *Qi/Breath* making the complete circuit, imagine that it does and in time you will observe the *Qi/Breath* flowing seamlessly and easily through the *Ren* and *Du*.

As you inhale and the breath rises, the ribs in the back open. The postural alignments of sitting meditation - lifting the perineum, sinking the tailbone, the tongue lifting to the roof of the mouth and the vertex lifting upward - all assist the *Qi/Breath* to ascend through the *Du* vessel. Withdrawing the chin slightly opens the acu-points at the base of the skull so that *Qi/Breath* does not block at these points, and thus is able to rise to the top of the head.

With the exhale the breath is able to sink because the lifting of the head, the position of the neck and the open ribs allow the breath to drop downward to return to the *Dantian*. As the *Qi/Breath* sinks, it seems as though it does not leave the body through the nose, but returns to the *Dantian*. The *Dantian* feels as though it expands and fills with the *Qi/Breath* as one exhales.

2) Count Nine Breaths Attending to the *Qi/Breath* Flowing Through the Micro-Cosmic Orbit.

Continue to perform Micro-Cosmic Orbit Breathing for nine breaths. Count each breath on the exhale. If you lose count, simply begin again starting at "one." Don't worry if you lose count or even if you find it impossible to get to nine – simply return to the exercise, bringing the attention back to the movement of the *Qi/Breath* through the *Ren* and *Du* vessels. It may be useful to review Lesson Three in which we practiced quieting the mind and counting the breaths.

3) Upon Reaching Nine Breaths Swallow the Saliva.

With correct practice of the Micro-Cosmic Orbit, and the stimulation of the tongue tip on the upper palate, the mouth fills with saliva that is sweeter and thicker than normal. In the beginning, and even after more extensive practice, if the mouth does not fill with saliva, one can circle the tongue around the inside and outside of the upper and lower teeth to gather saliva. When the mouth is full of saliva, gather it together, straighten the neck, lift the head and swallow the saliva. Observe the saliva passing down *Ren Mo* to the *Dantian*. Upon reaching *Dantian*, imagine the saliva vaporizes (like water hitting a fire) into a mist which fills the *Dantian*. When gathered and swallowed in this manner, the saliva is sometimes referred to as the "Golden Pill." It may be useful to use an image mentioned earlier in Chapter Two, in which the center of the *Dantian* is visualized as a rock that radiates heat. Water, or in this case the gathered "pill" of saliva that comes into contact with the rock, turns to vapor immediately.

Another method of swallowing the saliva is to swallow the mouthful of liquid in thirds. Once the first part reaches the *Dantian* and becomes vapor, swallow the second part, let it vaporize and then swallow the third portion. This sometimes referred to as "stringing pearls" – each portion following the next like pearls on a string.[12]

4) Continue for 36 Breaths, Pausing to Swallow the Saliva After Every Nine Breaths.

Important: The *Qi/Breath* cannot be forced to move through the *Ren* and *Du* vessels. If you are patient and focus on the three key points listed below, over time you will feel the *Qi/Breath* move naturally and without effort through the Micro-Cosmic Orbit:
1. Align the body correctly so that it is open and relaxed.
2. Practice Kidney Breathing.
3. Turn the attention inward to observe the thoughts and quiet the mind.

Chapter XI of the *Nei Yeh* (Inward Training) gives us similar advice in a clear and pithy manner:

> *When the body is not aligned,*
> *The inner power will not come.*
> *When you are not tranquil within,*
> *Your mind will not be well ordered.*
> *Align your body, assist the inner power,*
> *Then it will gradually come on its own.*[13]

Assisting the Micro-Cosmic Orbit: Deer, Crane and Tortoise Breathing

There are three breathing exercises that are traditionally used to assist the Micro-Cosmic Orbit. They can be used both to assist the movement of *Qi/Breath* through the *Du* channel, and to promote the inter-transformation of *Jing*, *Qi/Breath* and *Shen*. The deer, crane and tortoise are all symbols of longevity in China, and each corresponds to one of the three treasures in *Nei Gong* and *Qi Gong* practices.

Deer	*Lu*	鹿	Essence (*Jing*)
Crane	*He*	鶴	Qi/Breath
Tortoise	*Gui*	龜	Spirit (*Shen*)

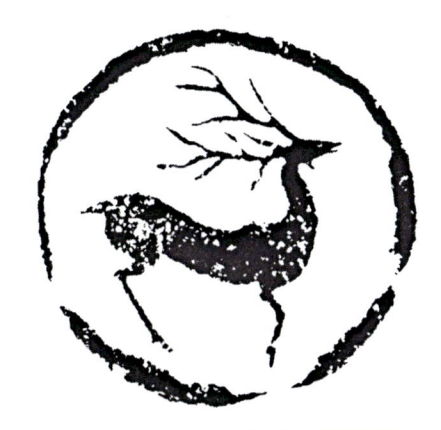

The deer is associated with endurance, speed and long life. The deer was also considered to have strong sexual and reproductive abilities. The word deer (*lu*) is the phonetic equivalent of another *lu*, which literally means "good income" or "prosperity. The antlers of the deer are prized by the Chinese as a longevity tonic and velvet deer horn is a traditional medicinal that supplements the kidney yang, strengthens tendons, ligaments and marrow and nourishes the blood, hence it is often employed to treat depletion of the *Jing*. As a medicinal, velvet deer horn is also said to fortify yang and tonify *Du Mo*.

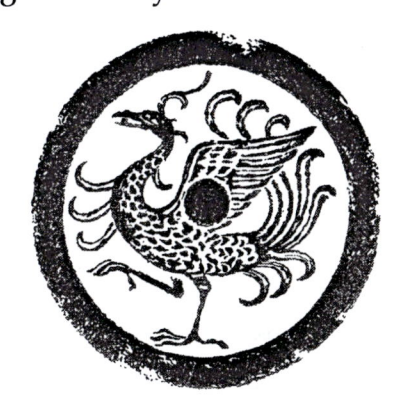

The bird is one of the four celestial animals, associated with the south, the heart and Fire. Sometimes the crane takes the place of the bird as a celestial animal. The crane is a symbol of longevity and wisdom. The crane is often pictured with a deer, standing on the back of the tortoise, or with pine trees (another symbol of health and longevity). Daoist immortals are often pictured as riding on the back of cranes. Similarly those who attain immortality are sometimes said to be carried off by cranes.

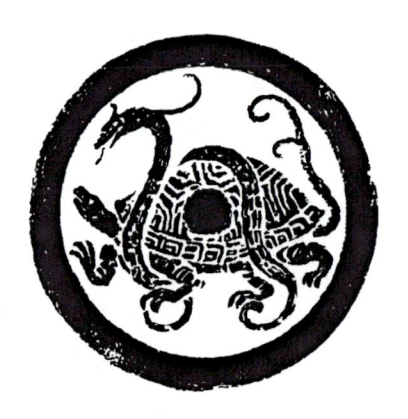

The tortoise is also one of the four celestial creatures, and is associated with the north, the kidneys and Water. The tortoise symbolizes immutability and steadfastness as well as immortality. Partially this is because tortoises live a long time relative to other animals. It was originally believed that there were no male tortoises and that female tortoises mated with snakes. Hence the tortoise is often depicted with a snake as the emblematic animal of the north. This representation appears on grave stone tablets supporting the inscription tablets of Emperors.[14] As a traditional medicinal, tortoise shell is said to enrich yin and regulate *Ren Mo*.

The Deer Exercise enables opening of the *Du* vessel, and through a lifting action of the inguinal area and pelvic floor, the exercise acts like a pump to lift the *Qi/Breath* up the *Du* channel. The ability of birds to expand their bodies, literally puffing up with *Qi/Breath*, is mimicked in the

Crane (Bird) Exercise which aids in promoting the movement and transformation of Qi/Breath. The Tortoise Exercise opens *Ren Mo* by lengthening its neck as it exhales:

> *The deer wags its tail and moves yang through the spine, hence it is associated with the du vessel. The deer refers to the genitals, perineum and sacrum that are part of the alchemical process. The tortoise cannot be separated from its shell. It raises its head to breathe in through the nose and is associated with the ren. The deer and tortoise refer to specific exercises to open the du and the ren. Of course the association of the deer and the tortoise with the ren and the du, respectively, also finds its expression in herbal medicine.*[15]

Deer Exercise: **Activating *Du Mo***

- Inhale as you gently lift the *kua* and the pelvic floor. This is similar to the lifting of the perineum you learned earlier and although direct force is not applied, there is a more specific and direct application of mind-intention in this lifting action.
- Let the pelvic floor and the *kua* sink as you exhale. The perineum is still slightly lifted at the end of this action.
- Repeat this exercise seven times.
- To Finish: Rub your palms together to warm them and then place one hand over the other and rub around the navel 36 times clockwise and 36 times counter-clockwise (traditionally women put their left hand on top of their right to rub and men did the opposite).

Note: Remember, the *kua* is considered to be the inguinal area in the front of the pelvis going up to the top of the hipbone (ilium) and includes both the internal and external structures.

Crane Exercise: Enabling the *Qi/Breath*
- Embrace your lower abdomen (*Dantian*) with your palms, placing the thumbs over the navel.
- Exhale through your nose and lightly press the *Dantian* in order to expel all of the breath.
- Inhale with a short half-breath and then **let** body continue to fill and expand with *Qi/Breath* like a bird puffing up its body. Feel the *Qi/Breath* move up and outward through the body, expanding effortlessly, but all without continuing to inhale. Do not force the breath, but **let** it expand and fill the body.
- Repeat seven times
- To Finish: Rub your palms together to warm them, and then place one hand over the other and rub around the navel 36 times clockwise and then 36 times counter-clockwise as in the Deer exercise.

Tortoise Exercise: Activating *Ren Mo*
- Inhale into the *Dantian*. As you inhale, slightly shorten the neck and *kua* internally. These movements should be subtle and unforced.
- Exhale as you simultaneously extend the neck and *kua* slightly. Again this movement is subtle and will not necessarily be visible.
- Repeat seven times.
- To Finish: Rub your palms together to warm them and then place one hand over the other and rub around the navel 36 times clockwise and then 36 times counter-clockwise as in the Deer Exercise.

The Story of the Tortoise Exercise

According to Stephen Chang, the ancient Daoist story associated with the Tortoise Exercise involves a family that escaped the war-torn countryside to live in a cave. At some point, a landslide sealed them in the cave and they could not escape. As their food ran out, they discovered a tortoise which had been in the cave with them all along. They noticed that the tortoise seemed to subsist on only a small amount of water dripping from the ceiling, and that the only movements it made were to extend its head in and out of its shell. They began to imitate the movements of the tortoise and, even after running out of food, survived. Many years later when the cave was rediscovered and the boulders from the landslide removed the family emerged alive and well. Like the tortoise, they had survived by only drinking water and extending and contracting their neck.[16] Many of the modern *Qi Gong* and *Nei Gong* routines that promote health and longevity involve bending, turning and/or flexing and extending the neck.

SPECIAL SECTION:
Women's Practice and The Deer Exercise

Women's practices of the Golden Fluid Returning to Dantian Meditation revolve around what Dr. Stephen Chang calls the "female deer exercise."[17] The original purpose of this exercise was to stop menstruation ("the red dragon"), because rather than losing their *Jing* and *Qi* through loss of semen, women lose *Jing* and *Qi* through menstrual blood. To stop menstruation was considered very important in ancient Daoist internal alchemy practices, but it is beyond the scope of the book and can involve health risks if performed improperly. However, for women, the addition of the following exercise can greatly enhance the practice of the Golden Fluid Meditation which folows in Lesson Nine.

The breasts are thought to be where the secretions of "perfect yin" originate. These secretions normally descend into the abdomen and transform into menstrual blood. These secretions, which are the foundations of breast milk, therefore transform into the menses.[18] The breasts then, are one of the key centers for physical and spiritual cultivation in women. Catherine Despeux explains the basic theory as follows:

> *Men guard their kidneys and stabilize their semen, refining it into qi by moving it up the spine into the niwan palace. This is called "return to the origin." Women guard their heart and nurture their spirit, refining it into fire by sitting motionless and making the qi descend from the nipples to the kidneys. From here they move it up along the spine to equally reach the niwan palace. This is called "transmutation to perfection."*[19]

The exercise begins by accumulating *Qi/Breath* at *Shang Qi Hai* (Ren 17: the "Upper Sea of Qi"). This acu-point lies between in the center of the chest between the breasts.

1. Sit cross-legged with your heels against the genitals. If possible, press one heel against the perineum.
2. First click the teeth 36 times and then swirl the tongue in the mouth, nine times in each direction outside the teeth and nine times in each direction inside the teeth in order to stimulate the production of saliva. This also stimulates breast secretions.
3. Concentrate the spirit at *Shang Qi Hai* as you practice Kidney Breathing, and then massage the breasts slowly between 36 and 360 times in an outward motion. If the chest is taken as the clock face the right hand moves clockwise and the left counter-clockwise (see picture below). This concentration and massage will cause the *Qi/Breath* to rise upward to the breasts and the *Qi/Breath* will move naturally between the *Dantian* and Ren 17.
4. Massage around the navel with the left hand over the right: 36 times clockwise and 36 times counter-clockwise.
5. Inhale as you gently lift the *kua* and the pelvic floor. Let the pelvic floor and the *kua* sink as you exhale. The Perineum is still slightly lifted at the end of this action. Repeat this exercise seven times.
6. Follow this exercise with Micro-Cosmic Orbit breathing for 9-36 breaths as explained above.

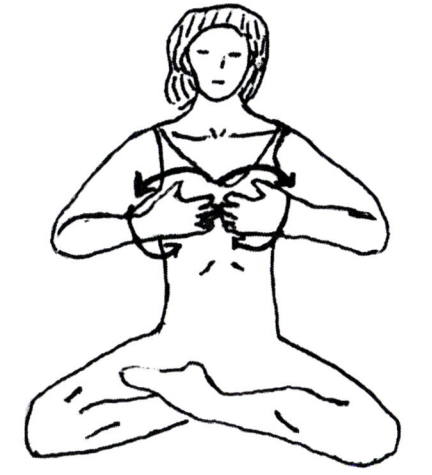

Adapted from the *Complete System of Self-Healing: Internal Exercises* by Stephen T. Chang

LESSON 9:

GOLDEN FLUID RETURNING TO DANTIAN MEDITATION

金 液
Golden Fluid

Lesson Nine: Golden Fluid Returning to Dantian Meditation - *Jin Ye Hai Dan Tian Nei Gong* 金液還丹田內功

In this lesson we will explore a method of Daoist meditation that combines many of the elements of the previous lessons into one exercise. The focus of this lesson is on the Golden Fluid Returning to Dantian Meditation (sometimes known as the seated Eight Brocade Qi Gong). It is one of the meditation practices through which *Jing, Qi/Breath* and *Shen* are inter-transformed and thus is considered a Daoist "alchemical practice." Golden Fluid Returning to Dantian Meditation builds on the previous lesson, in which we allowed *Qi/Breath* to circulate in *Ren Mo* and *Du Mo* in combination with swallowing the "Golden Fluid" (the saliva). Here, you will be employing the Micro-Cosmic Orbit practice in conjunction with various movements and self-massage techniques that facilitate the movement of the *Qi/Breath* through the *Du* and *Ren* vessels and the inter-transformation of the Three Treasures: *Jing, Qi/Breath,* and *Shen*.

Su Dong Po and the Golden Fluid Meditation

Su Dong Po (also known as Su Shi) was a famous poet of the Northern Song Dynasty. He was born into an illustrious family of officials and scholars. Both his father and brother were famous literati. Su Dung Po took the Imperial Exam in 1057, and in addition to his political career, he was an innovator and master of poetry, prose, calligraphy, and painting. He was one the founders of the Southern Song style of painting. His political career had many ups and downs. At different times he was imprisoned and exiled. Many of his poems are informed by Daoism and Chan Buddhism, and at various times he practiced both Daoist and Buddhist methods of meditation, including the Golden Fluid Returning to Dantian Meditation. He wrote of his personal experience in practicing this method:

Its effect is not sensed at the beginning, but after practicing for one hundred days, its effect cannot be measured and is a hundred times more effective than herbal drugs. Although the method is relatively simple and easy, real skill can only be obtained after long-term practice. After training for twenty days, I feel that my spirit is really different. I feel quite warm below the umbilicus, my low back and steps feel light. A shine remains on my face for a long time. I feel I am not far from being immortal.[1]

Su's fluid poetry reflects a spontaneity and fluidity that stem from his practice of Chan and Daoism, and his personal experiences with the poignancy of life; its pleasures, disappointments and vicissitudes. Two examples are below.

<u>Remembrance</u>
To what can our life on earth be likened?
To a flock of geese,
Alighting on the snow.
Sometimes leaving a trace of their passage.[2]

<u>Written on Abbot Lun's Wall at Mount Chiao (1074)</u>
The Master stays on Mount Chiao,
(though in fact he's never "stayed" anywhere).
No sooner had I arrived than I asked him about the Way,
But the Master never said a word.
Not that he was lost for words –
He saw no reason for replying.
Then I thought, Look at your head and feet –
Comfortable enough in hat and shoes, aren't they?
It's like the man with the long beard
Who never worried how long it was.

But one day someone asked him,
"What do you do with it when you sleep?"
That night, pulling up the covers,
He couldn't decide if it went on top or under.
All night he tossed and turned wondering where to put it,
Till he felt like yanking it out by its roots.
These words might seem trite and shallow
But in fact they have deep meaning.
When I asked the Master what he thought,
The Master smiled his approval.[3]

Li Ching Yun: "Immortal" of the Modern Era

In the modern era, the Golden Fluid method was made famous in mainland China, Taiwan and Hong Kong by Li Qing Yun (Li Ching-yun) who was purportedly born in Sichuan province in 1678 and died at age 256 in 1933. Some say that he buried 22 wives and had numerous children.[4] He joined the army at age 71, but was also an herbalist and perhaps a practitioner of martial arts. In 1927, General Yang Shen, impressed with Li Qing Yun's health, strength and youthfulness at an advanced age, investigated his life. He interviewed adults from Li's hometown who said he looked much the same now as he had when they were children. According to a Time Magazine article written in 1933, in 1930 Professor Wu Chung Chieh of Chengdu University found records indicating that *the Imperial Chinese Government had congratulated one Li Ching-yun in 1827 on his birthday. The birthday was his 150th, making the man who died last week - if it was the same Li Ching Yun, and respectful Chinese preferred to think so - a 256-year-old.*[5]

Part of the Li Qing Yun's secret, according to some, was methodical practice of the Seated Eight Brocade Exercises (Golden Fluid Meditation) which he maintained for over 100 years.[6] When asked about the secret of his long life, he merely said: *Keep a quiet heart, sit like a tortoise, walk sprightly like a pigeon and sleep like a dog.*[7] Whether or not the story of Li Qing Yun is true, if it inspires one to practice Daoist meditation, it is worth hearing.

The Three Passes (三關)

San Guan ("Three Passes" or "Three Gates") refers to three important places on the Du Channel. These three areas are the places where it is most difficult for the *Qi/Breath* to circulate, where it can become impeded. *Guan* (關) can mean a "mountain pass," a "barrier" or "bottleneck," "to close" or to "shut off." The ideogram contains the gate radical (門) with numerous strokes inside like threads being woven.

The first pass is the *Wei Lu Guan* (Tailbone Pass). The second is the *Jia Ji Guan,* located along the sides of the spine at the area around *Mingmen,* and proceeding upward on either side of the spine along the thorax (mid-back). *Jia Ji* means to "squeeze the spine" and is also sometimes a name for the area around the 6th thoracic vertebra, which lies just behind the diaphragm.[8] The third is the *Yu Zhen Guan* (Jade Pillow Pass) at the occipital region.[9]

Wei Lu Guan 尾閭關

Jia Ji Guan 夾脊關

Yu Zhen Guan 枕玉關

If *Qi/Breath* becomes stuck at the tailbone, there may be heavy aching pain in the sacrum. Focusing on the gentle lifting of the perineum without forcing the breath, will aid in smoothing the flow of the *Qi/Breath*. Blockage at the *Mingmen* area in the low back can result in aching across the low back. Often this occurs because of prior injury or tightness of the low back. Focusing on the *Qi/Breath* filling the *Dantian* and moving backward to the *Mingmen* as you attend to the tongue touching the upper palate will help move the *Qi/Breath* through this gate. It is most common for the *Qi/Breath* to become stuck at the occipital gate, resulting in stiffness of the neck and aching pain at the back of the head. Closing the eyes, and looking upward and inward as you subtly raise the head will help move the *Qi/Breath* through this gate. Practicing the deer exercise can help prevent blockage at the sacrum, the crane exercise can help prevent blockage at the *Mingmen* and *Jia Ji Guan,* and practice of the tortoise exercise can help prevent blockage at the occiput and neck.

The diagram below illustrating the waxing and waning of yin and yang during the Micro-Cosmic Orbit, uses the traditional Chinese character: 門 *Men* (gate-door), to show the location of the Three Passes:

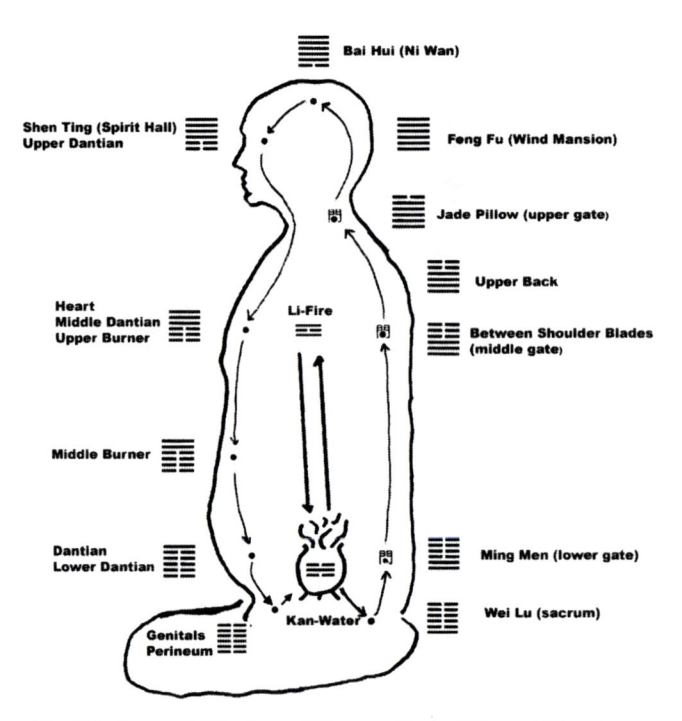

The Waxing and Waning of Qian and Kun (Yin and Yang)
Qian - The Opening of the Gates - Inhalation
Kun - The Closing of the Gates - Exhalation

Drawing adapted from The Complete System of Self Healing: Internal Exercise, by Dr. Stephen T. Chang. San Francisco: Tao Publishing 1986, p. 200.

The Image of the Waterwheel

A waterwheel turning along a millrace is a common image in Daoist meditation and is often used to describe the dynamic of the Micro-Cosmic Orbit. The waterwheel contains a hub at its center. The hub is still and empty relative to the buckets or paddles, which are full and move up and down at the periphery. As one bucket or paddle goes up from the bottom to the top, another moves downward from top to bottom. The hub represents the stillness of the spirit and heart inside. The turning buckets represent the movement of the *Qi/Breath,* the transformation of yin and yang in the *Du* and *Ren* Vessels. In the Nei Gong classic it says:

> *In front is the Ren and in the back is the Du.*
> *Between these the qi turns constantly.*[10]

In this passage, repetition of the character *gun,* "turn" (ie: *gungun* 滚滚) conveys the idea that the *Qi/Breath* literally turns, rolls, boils or spirals though the *Ren* and *Du* vessels, much like the action of water in a moving stream.

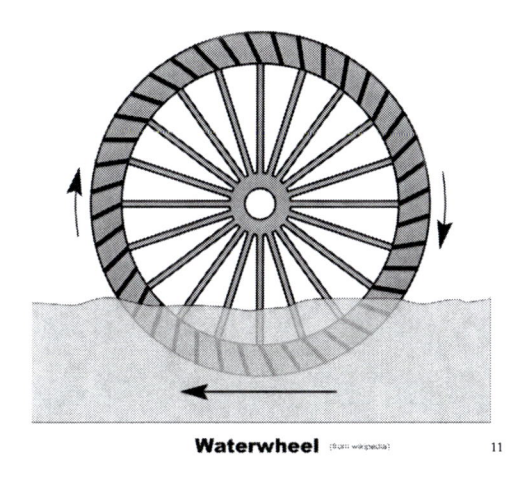

Waterwheel (from wikipedia) [11]

The circuit created by the *Ren* and the *Du* vessels transports substances that have water-like nature: the *Jing* (generative energy), the *Qi/Breath* (vapor), and the Golden Fluid (saliva). The upward movement of the waterwheel transmutes *Jing* into *Qi/Breath* and *Qi/Breath* into *Shen*.

The downward movement is concerned with the nourishing of the *Qi/Breath* by *Shen,* and the replenishment of *Jing* by *Qi/Breath*. With time, as the circulation becomes smooth, the movement travels in both directions simultaneously.[12]

> *First, the three gates along the Du meridian must be open. To open these gates, generative energy must be plentiful. When the generative energy is plentiful, it can be transmuted into vapor. When there is sufficient vapor, the vapor can thrust through the Du meridian and open the three gates. Second, the mind must be empty and still of thoughts. It is when stillness had reached its height that movement will begin.*[13]

Eva Wong tells us that two conditions must be met for the waterwheel to turn:

Lesson 9: Practice - Golden Fluid Returning to Dantian Meditation

Generally this practice is performed in the morning upon arising, but it can also be practiced around midnight before going to bed. It is divided into fourteen sections for ease of learning, but should be performed as an unbroken sequence. At the end of this lesson, there is a one page summary of the sequence. There are a number of spots in this meditation where you will massage the face and head, rub the back, tap the occiput, or stretch and move the body. These movements are important as they variously:

- Open up and unblock the sense organs in order to stimulate the spirit and the internal organs.
- Free up the Three Gates, so that the *Qi/Breath* can easily penetrate through them.
- Prevent the *Qi/Breath* from blocking by guiding or directing it.

Throughout this meditation, employ Micro-Cosmic Orbit breathing even during the transitional movements. At first this can be very difficult, especially when rubbing the face, combing the hair and performing the other movements that are part of the meditation. Like a martial artist learning a form, a dancer performing a piece of choreography or a musician playing a piece of music, it is at first difficult to coordinate all the different parts of the sequence, but in time, with daily practice, it becomes easier, automatic, and the breath and concentration become deeper and more subtle. The advantage of having a meditation "form" that one follows is that its outward structure gives the mind, consciousness and spirit a framework, a foundation that holds and leads the internal awareness and intention. This anchors, but also frees the conscious mind, aiding one's practice. The sequence is ultimately open-ended and can be expanded to become longer or it can be dissolved entirely as the *Qi/Breath* and the "mind within the mind" direct the practice.

1. Sit Upright and Concentrate the Mind

- Sit with the legs crossed (or in a chair with the back straight and thighs parallel to the floor) in tranquil relaxation.
- Half-close the eyes and place the hands on the knees (or below the navel, one hand nestled within the other) palms up. **The eyes will remain half-closed throughout this meditation.**

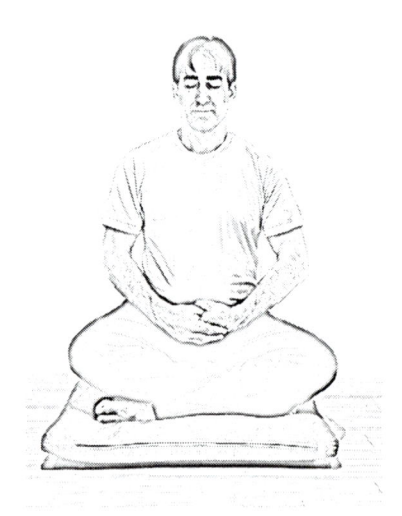

- Touch the upper palate with the tongue. **Concentrate the mind and regulate respiration naturally for nine breaths.**
- Inhaling and exhaling should be gentle and silent. Inhalation and exhalation are through the nose.
- **As you breathe, the *Qi/Breath* follows the Micro-Cosmic Orbit** (see Lesson Eight).
- **After nine breaths, rinse the mouth lightly with saliva and swallow it** as you straighten and extend the neck, imagining that the saliva passes down *Ren Mo* (the meridian running down the front midline of the body) to the *Dantian*. In the *Dantian*, imagine that the saliva vaporizes (like water hitting a fire) into a mist which fills the *Dantian*.

2. Knead the Ears

- Continue Micro-Cosmic Orbit breathing as you knead the right ear with the left hand eighteen times.
- Then knead the left ear with the right hand eighteen times.

Purpose: Acu-points in the ears connect with the whole body and the ear is dominated by the kidney. By massaging the ears, the kidney *Qi/Breath* and the whole body are strengthened.

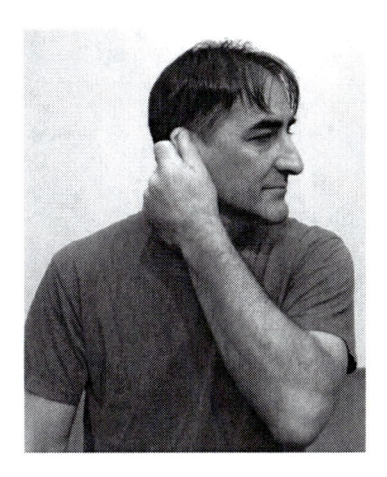

3. Press the Eyes with Warm Hands

- Continue Micro-Cosmic Orbit breathing as you **rub two hands** until they become warm.
- Gently press the eyes with the *Lao Gong* (palm center) point of the palm. Continue to perform Micro-Cosmic Orbit breathing as you feel/imagine the heat from your hands penetrating into the eyes and into the brain.

Purpose: The eyes link to the liver and brain, so this exercise brightens the eyes, stimulates the brain and regulates liver *Qi*.

4. Rub the Nose

- Rub the sides of the nose up and down with thumb portion of the palm (the thenar eminence) until a warm sensation is felt in and around the nose.
- Brace your forefinger with your middle finger and massage the *Ying Xiang* (LI 20: "Welcome Fragrance") acupoints, with the tip of the forefinger.

Purpose: The nose is linked to the lung. This exercise regulates the Qi/*Breath* of the lung and opens up the nose so that air can flow smoothly through it. This is especially effective for preventing the common cold and nasal obstruction.

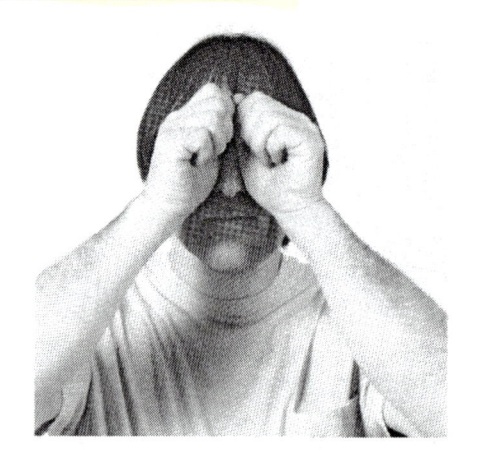

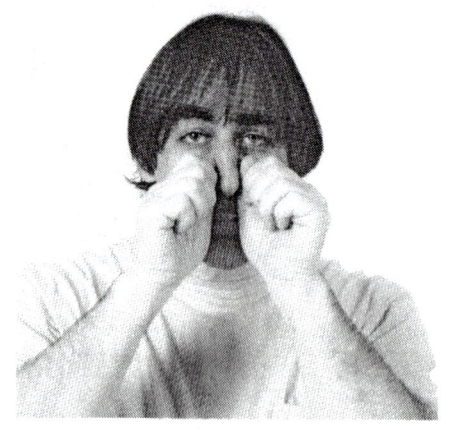

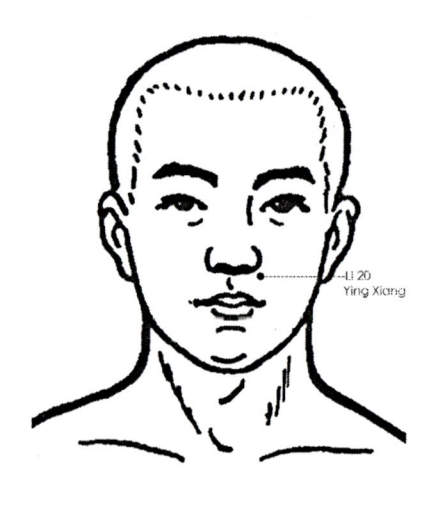

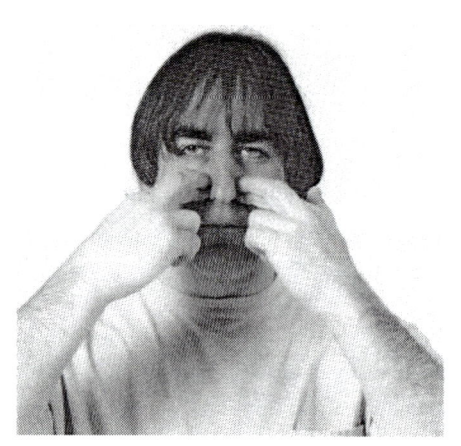

184

5. Wash the Face & Cultivate the Heavenly Palace, Comb the Hair with the Fingers

- *Tian Xin*, the "heavenly center" or "heavenly palace, is at the center of the forehead.
- Wash the face downward and upward nine times with the palms, gently pressing the face and forehead. Feel the warmth of the hands penetrate into the face.
- Comb the hair from the forehead to the occiput a minimum of nine times.

Purpose: This exercise regulates the meridians of the head and face, stimulates the brain and helps cultivate a radiant face and beautiful hair.

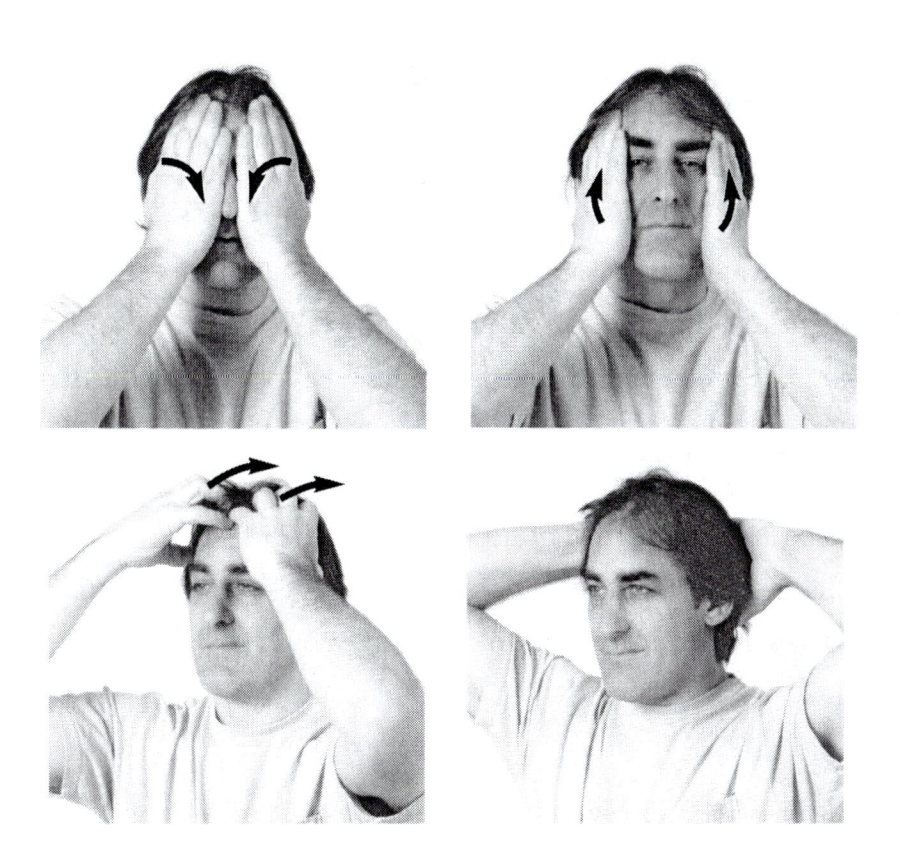

6. Knock the Teeth 36 times, Clench the Fists, Concentrate the Mind and Swallow the Saliva

- Repeat the first movement, "Sit Upright and Concentrate the Mind." Focus the mind-intention and perform Micro-Cosmic Orbit breathing for three breaths, as you clench the fists lightly with the thumb inside the four fingers. This helps to hold the *Qi/Breath* inside.

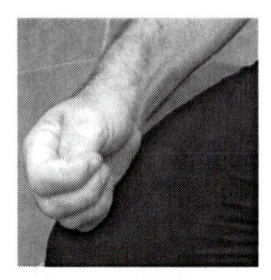

- Then with the hands still in fists, knock or tap the teeth lightly together 36 times, while listening to the sound of them clicking together. Do not click the teeth quickly or forcefully. Wait for the sound/internal vibration of each tap to dissipate before the next. Now swallow the saliva, as you straighten and extend the neck, imagining that the saliva passes down *Ren Mo* to the *Dantian*. In the *Dantian*, imagine that the saliva vaporizes into a mist which fills the *Dantian*.

Purpose: Clicking the teeth in this manner strengthens the bones and teeth. It also stimulates the brain, calms the heart and concentrates the spirit. Clicking the teeth stimulates the flow of saliva. Swallowing the saliva aids in the transformation of the Three Treasures and nourishes body fluids.

7. Regulate Respiration for Nine Breaths While Embracing Kun Lun with Two Hands

- *Kun Lun* here refers to the head. Embrace the head with two hands, but do not cover the ears. You can hold the head as shown

below or you can interweave the fingers. Make sure the lungs, neck and shoulders are relaxed and without strain.
- Use Micro-Cosmic Orbit Breathing.

Purpose: Stimulates the brain, opens the "Jade Pillow Gate" and helps the *Qi/Breath* to rise up the *Du* vessel.

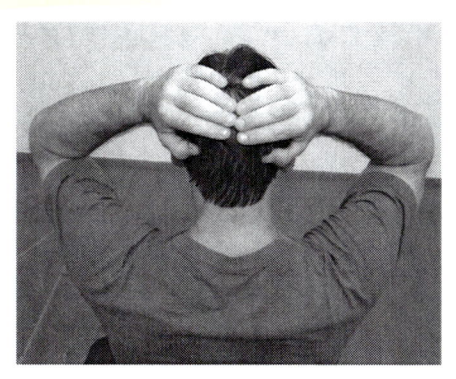

8. Strike the Heavenly Drum and Listen to the Sound 27 Times

- Cover the two ears with the palms. Press the forefinger with the middle finger to flick the forefinger against the occipital bone (the "Jade Pillow") 27 times, hearing the drum sound. Let the sound of each "drumbeat" fade before flicking the fingers again.
- Before removing the hands listen until the sound of the drumming fades away into silence.

Purpose: This exercise stimulates the brain, calms the mind, and concentrates the spirit. It aids in opening the "Jade Pillow Pass." This in turn allows *Qi/Breath* and blood to move freely up the *Du* vessel and nourish the brain.

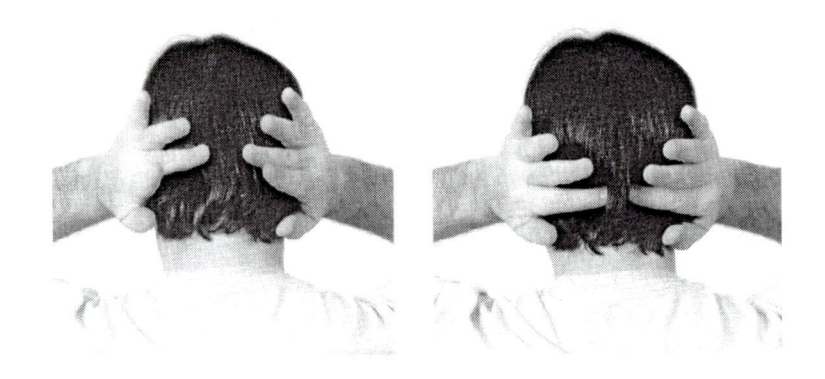

9. Shake the Heavenly Pillar Slightly and Stir the Golden Fluid with the Tongue

- Turn the head to the left as you inhale and then turn to face front as you exhale. Then turn the head to the right as you inhale and turn to face front as you exhale. Repeat three times.
- When turning the head make sure muscles of the neck and torso are relaxed. Do not force the head to turn to its limit. Instead, feel as though it turns smoothly and effortlessly. Feel as though the whole spine from the tip of the tailbone to the top of the head is subtly turning, almost as though the turning comes from the spine itself, rather than just the neck. Breathe slowly and evenly as the head turns.
- After turning the head, rotate the tongue in the mouth making nine complete circuits in each direction around the outside of the upper and lower teeth (between the cheek and the teeth), and then nine

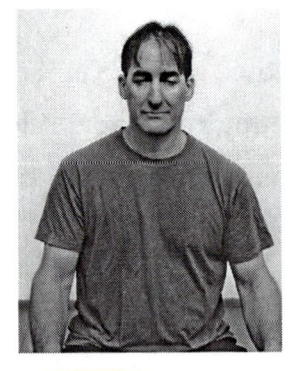

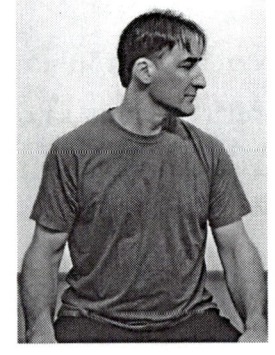

complete circuits in each direction around the inside of the upper and lower teeth in order to stimulate the secretion of saliva. .
- When saliva has accumulated, swirl and "rinse" the tongue and mouth with the saliva as you continue to use Micro-Cosmic Orbit breathing.
- Now swallow the saliva in three parts. As you swallow each third of this mouthful of saliva, straighten and extend the neck, imagining that it passes down *Ren Mo* to the *Dantian*. In the *Dantian*, imagine the saliva vaporizes into a mist which fills the *Dantian*. You can imagine that you are swallowing three pearls.

Purpose: Turning the head frees up the *Du* vessel and stimulates the flow of *Qi/Breath* through the *Du* Vessel. It particularly helps to open the Jade Pillow Pass at the occiput and neck. Stirring the saliva with the tongue cleans, stimulates and nourishes the teeth and gums. Swallowing the saliva aids in the transformation of the Three Treasures and nourishes body fluids.

10. Hold the Breath, Chafe the Hands, Exhale, and Rub the Back

- Inhale and then hold the breath while chafing the hands to warm the palms.
- Keep the palms together as you exhale and concentrate the mind on the *Dantian*.
- Then rub the region of the lower back and *Shen Shu* (the acu-point BL 23, which is on either side of the spine at L2-L3 over the kidneys) with the warm palms 36 times. After rubbing, keep your palms on the kidneys for a moment or two and imagine the heat from your hands penetrating into the kidneys and *Mingmen*.

Purpose: Rubbing the kidneys concentrates the *Qi/Breath* in the *Dantian* and *Mingmen*. It also warms and activates the kidneys and frees up the *Jia Ji* Pass and the *Wei Lu* (Tailbone Pass).

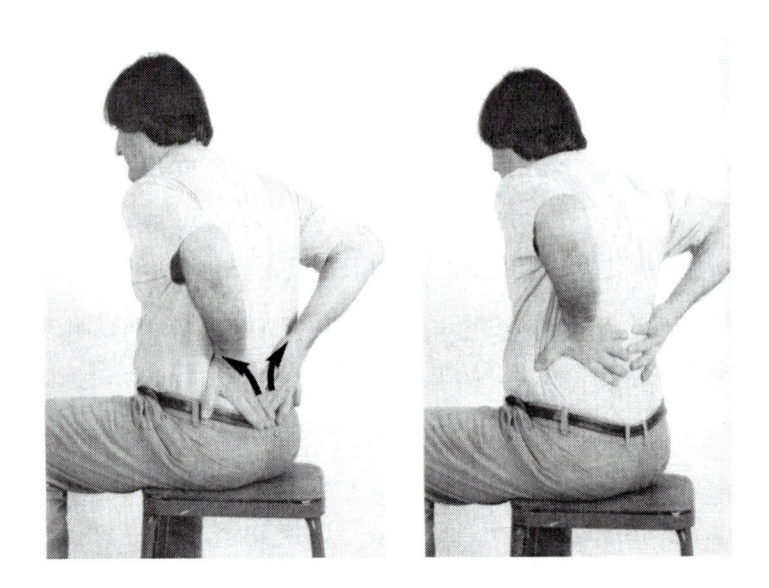

11. Regulate Respiration for Nine Breaths Focusing on Dantian

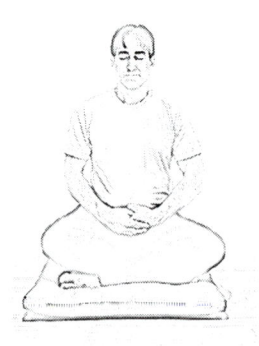

- This is essentially the same as the first exercise: "sit upright and concentrate the mind." Focus on feeling the warm sensation that penetrates *Dantian* as you perform Micro-Cosmic Orbit breathing. If you cannot feel the warmth, imagine that you feel it.

- At the end of the nine breaths, when saliva has accumulated swallow it by straightening and extending the neck as you visualize the saliva passing down *Ren Mo* to the *Dantian*. In the *Dantian*, imagine the saliva vaporizes into a mist which fills the *Dantian*.

12. Shake/Rotate the Two Shoulders in Order to Regulate the Ren and Du Channels

- With the hands resting lightly on the knees, continue to perform Micro-Cosmic Orbit breathing while rotating the shoulders in the shape of a figure 8 or infinity symbol nine times in each direction.
- Let the top of the head follow these movements so that it also makes a gentle figure eight shape.

Purpose: Frees up Ren Mo and Du Mo by literally shaking any restrictions loose. Opens up the ribs in the front and back of the body and opens the *Jia Ji* Gate.

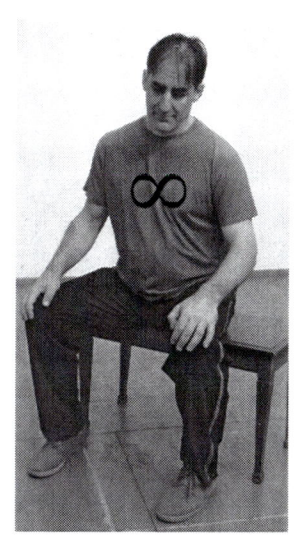

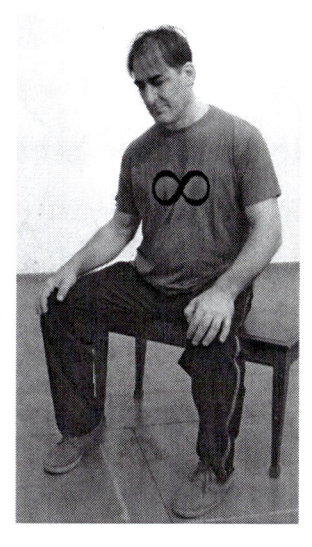

13. Extend the Two Legs, Bend the Body and Hook the Feet

- Extend the legs flat and flex the ankles back slightly.
- Stretch forward bending at the hips while the hands reach forward to "hook" the feet and knead the *Yong Quan* (KID 1 "Bubbling Well") acu-points at the center of balls of each foot with the tip of the middle fingers 36 times.

Purpose: Activates the kidneys and *Mingmen*. Frees up restrictions in the *Jia Ji* Pass and the Tailbone Pass. Unkinks the legs after sitting cross-legged.

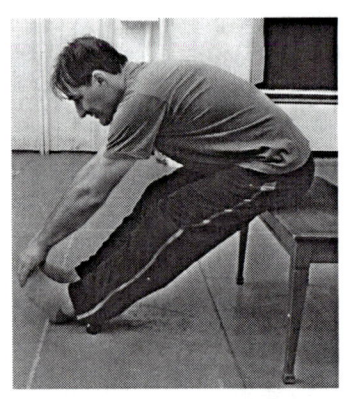

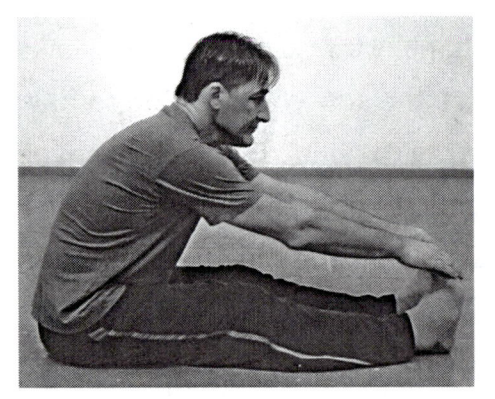

14. Count Nine Breaths, Wait for Heavenly Water, Rinse the Mouth and Swallow Saliva Again

- Return to the starting seated position to "sit upright and concentrate the mind" with Micro-Cosmic Orbit breathing. Count nine breaths.

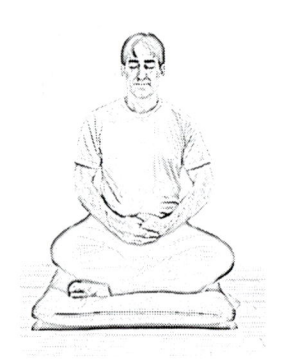

- Gather the saliva and swallow it by straightening and extending the neck, imagining that the saliva passes down *Ren Mo* to the *Dantian*. In the *Dantian*, imagine the saliva vaporizes into a mist which fills the *Dantian*.
- Continue to regulate respiration for another minute. This is the ending posture or, if you desire, you can extend the meditation by sitting longer - for 36 more breaths.

Cool-Down: Rubbing the Meridians

After completing the meditation, stand up and move around easily. It may be useful to rub the meridians as follows in order to help the *Qi/Breath* continue to circulate freely:

Arm Meridians:
- Turn the left arm palm up and stroke down the front of the left arm from the shoulders to the fingertips with the right palm.
- Then turn the left arm palm down and stroke up the back of the arm from the fingertips to the base of the neck with the right hand.
- Repeat nine times.
- Then repeat nine times on the other side.

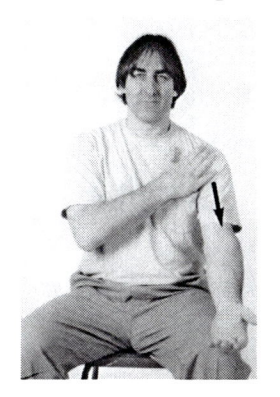

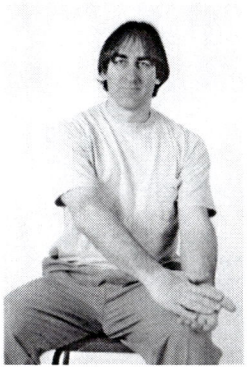

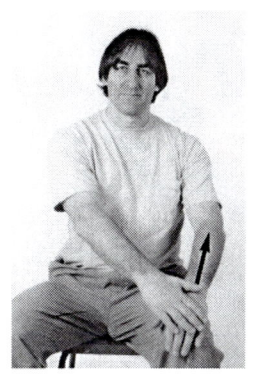

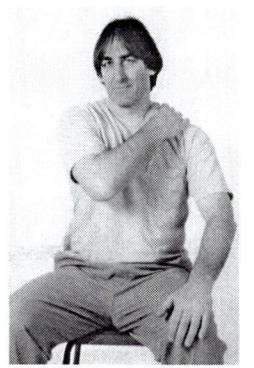

Leg Meridians:
- Massage with the palms down the back and side of the legs from the hips to the feet.
- Then massage up the inside of the legs from the feet to the abdomen.
- Repeat nine times.

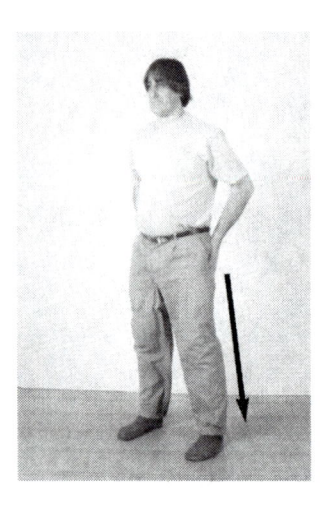

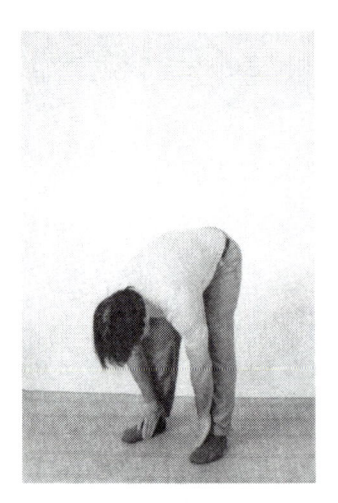

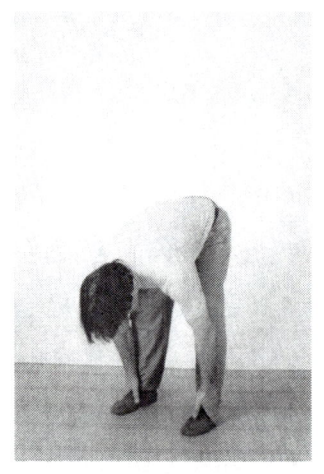

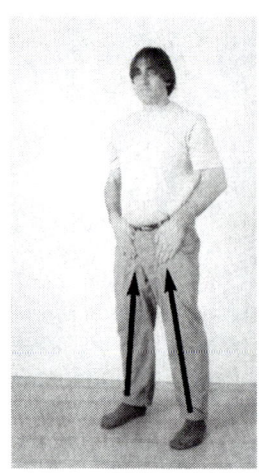

Golden Fluid Returning to Dantian – Summary

1. Sit Upright and Concentrate the Mind - Count Nine Breaths and then Swallow the Saliva

2. Knead the Ears

3. Warm the Hands and Press the Eyes Nine Times

4. Rub the Nose Up and down Until Warm. Press LI 20, Nine Times

5. Wash the Face with the Palms Nine Times & Comb the Hair with the Fingers Nine Times

6. Count Three Breaths as You Clench the Fists. Knock the Teeth 36 Times. Concentrate the Mind and Swallow the Saliva

7. Count Nine Breaths While Embracing Kun Lun with Two Hands

8. Strike the Heavenly Drum and Listen to the Sound 27 Times

9. Turn the Head Back and Forth Three Times, Stir Fluid with the Tongue Nine Times Inside and Outside the teeth) and Swallow the Saliva in Three Parts

10. Inhale, Hold the Breath and Chafe the Hands, then Exhale to *Dantian* and Rub the Back 36 Times

11. Count Nine Breaths Focusing on warmth in *Dantian* and then Swallow the Saliva

12. With Hands on the Knees, Shake the Shoulders in a Figure 8 Nine Times in Each direction while Regulating the Respiration

13. Extend the Two Legs, Bend Forward and Pull the Feet as you Massage Yong Quan (Kid 1) 36 Times

14. Count Nine Breaths Focusing on *Dantian*, and then Swallow the Saliva

BEYOND THE NINE LESSONS:

The Macro-Cosmic Orbit

大 周 天

Da　Zhou　Tian

Beyond the Nine Lessons – The Macro-Cosmic Orbit

In Daoist meditation our respiration as an individual human being is an expression of the primordial "breaths" moving between Heaven and Earth. Zhuang Zi tells us that that the respiration of the "True Man," the sage, is beyond deep:

> *The True Man of ancient times slept without dreaming and woke without care; he ate without savoring and his breath came from deep inside. The True Man breathes with his heels; the mass of men breathe with their throats. Crushed and bound down, they gasp out their words as though they are retching. Deep in their passions and desires, they are shallow in the workings of Heaven.*[1]

Another description of the breath of the "True Man" is found in another Daoist text, the *Cantong Qi*:

> *It will stream from the head to the toes;*
> *On reaching the end, it will rise once again.*
> *In its coming and its going, it will spread limitless,*
> *Pervading throughout and extending all around.*

This respiration of the "True Man" (the sage) emanates from the deepest reaches of his being and extends to the extremities, to the very limits of the body and beyond. In *Qi Gong* and meditation, "extremities" has a double meaning. It refers not only to the four limbs, but also to the end points of the body's innate energies:

> *The tongue is the extremity of the flesh,*
> *It should push upward against the upper teeth.*
> *The nails are the extremity of the tendons,*
> *They move slightly inwards so Qi/Breath can flow into the tendons.*
> *The teeth are the extremity of the bones,*
> *The teeth should touch lightly so Qi/Breath can reach the bones.*
> *The hair is the extremity of the blood,*

The hair should feel as though it stands on end to push up a hat.[2]

This deep and expansive breath is sometimes referred to as the Large Heavenly Circulation or the "Macro-Cosmic Orbit".

In this lesson, we will work with several exercises that explore Macro-Cosmic Orbit breathing. The Macro-Cosmic Orbit is an extension of the Micro-Cosmic Orbit. Rather than being a separate exercise it flows naturally from the Micro-Cosmic Orbit. For many people who practice the Micro-Cosmic Orbit, this larger circulation that moves through the whole body simply occurs spontaneously. Therefore, in the following exercises it is important to simply let the *Qi/Breath* move naturally and spontaneously.

Exercise 1: Combining Wu Ji and Tai Ji: Nezha Stirs the Sea

Nezha is a Daoist protection deity. The name of the exercise comes from a famous story. There was a severe drought brought on by a demon sent by Ao Guang, the Dragon King of the East Sea,. The demon is beaten by Nezha, who then stirs up the seas with his golden ring.

This exercise is an extension of the *Wu Ji* Posture. It is a somewhat advanced exercise which should only be practiced after working with the Wu Ji Meditation for a month or more. Nezha Stirs the Sea creates a powerful, spiraling (stirring) motion that moves through the whole body. This action leads to a powerful engagement with the spiraling movement of the *Tai Ji* and the *Qi/Breath* as they initiate movement between the poles of Heaven and Earth.

1) Stand in the *Wu Ji* Posture (see Lesson Four)
- Stand with the feet parallel and shoulder width apart and the knees slightly bent.
- The hands are at the sides of the body.

- With the eyes half closed, looking outward to the front and slightly down, focus the mind on the top of the head and the soles of the feet.

2) Rotate and Circle the Body

- Rotate the body gently, rocking it slightly left and forward and right and back. The body makes a circle moving on an axis that runs from the top of the head through the body to the ground between your feet.
- The body circles, but it stays in that middle place you discovered earlier in Lesson Four - the place where the leg muscles don't need to engage and contract to hold you up.
- Feel the axis of rotation not only as it passes through the body, but beyond the top of your head and down into the ground beneath you.
- Rotate nine times in one direction and then rotate nine times in the other direction. Repeat this for several minutes.

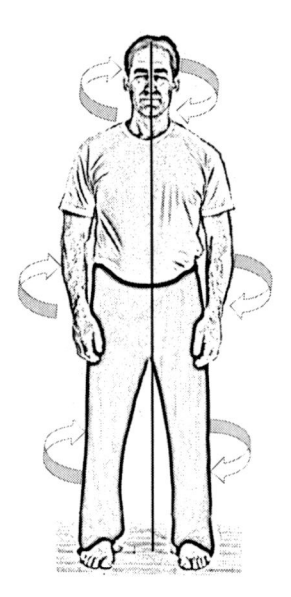

Nezha Stirs the Sea

3) End the Exercise by Standing in *Wu Ji* for a Minute or Two

<u>Important Points</u>:
- All the alignments are the same as in the *Wu Ji* posture.
- Employ Kidney Breathing throughout the exercise.
- If this exercise makes you dizzy, start with only nine times in each direction per practice session.

Exercise 2: Uniting the Original Qi

This exercise regulates the *Qi/Breath*. Kidney Breathing combined with the gentle circular movements of the arms create a global circulation of the "Original Qi" through the entire body, from the soles of the feet to the top of the head and the tips of the fingers.

1) Stand in the *Wu Ji* Posture
- The feet are parallel and the toes point straight ahead.
- Bend the knees slightly.
- Lift the head and upper back and sink the lower back.
- Place the tongue tip on the upper palate.
- Slacken the shoulders.
- Let the weight fall through the feet so that the whole sole is in contact with the floor.
- The eyes look straight ahead.
- The arms are relaxed and at your sides.

2) Inhale and Slowly Raise the Arms to the Left Side
- Inhale and raise the arms to the left side.
- As you continue to inhale, raise the arms until the wrists are just above the crown of the head and the palms turn to face forward.

3) Exhale and Slowly Lower the Arms to Right Side

- Continue to rotate the arms so that they descend to the right side, the palms slowly turning throughout the motion. As the hands reach the level of the groin and thighs, the palms are facing inward.

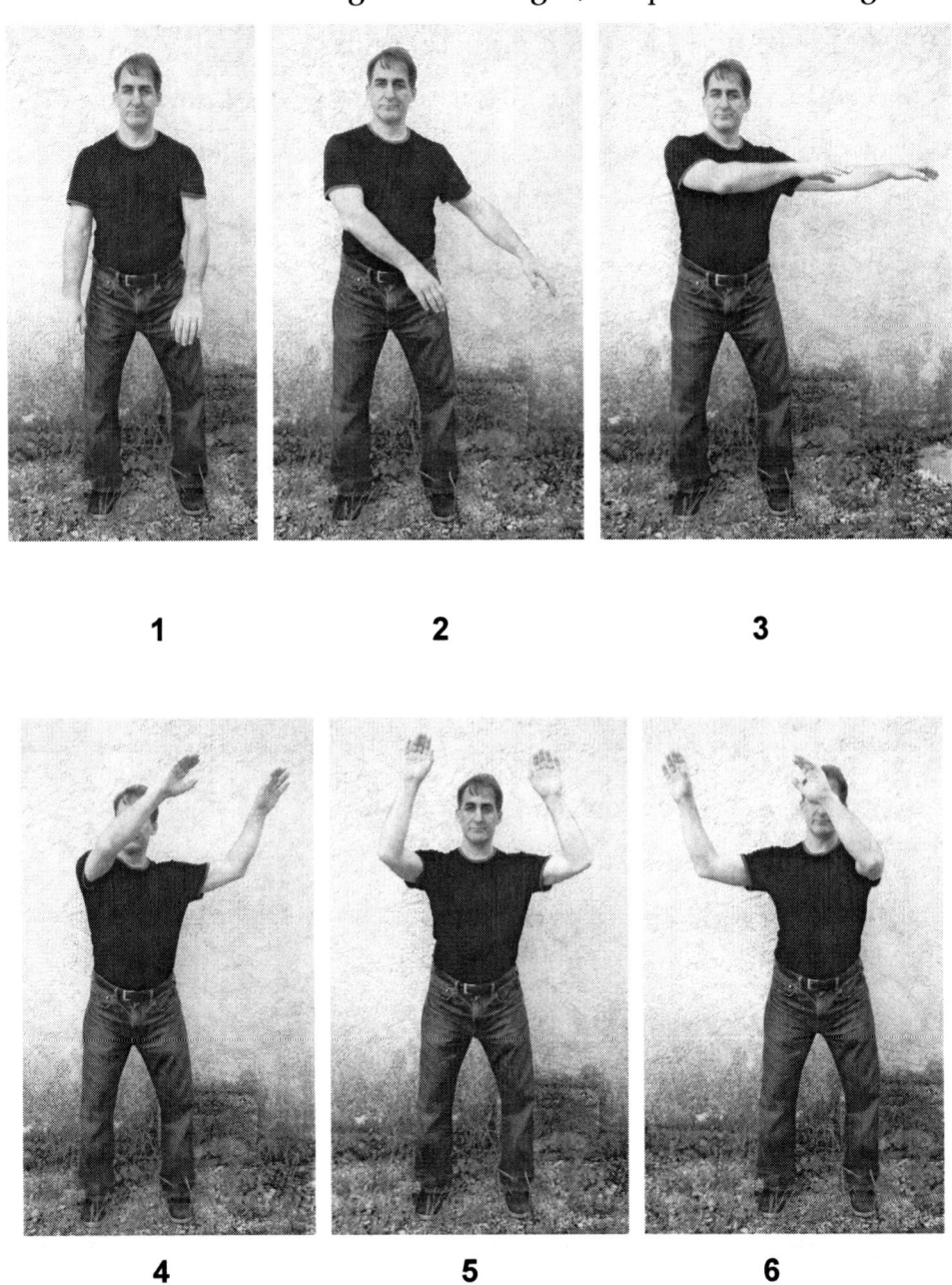

1

2

3

4

5

6

| 7 | 8 | 9 |

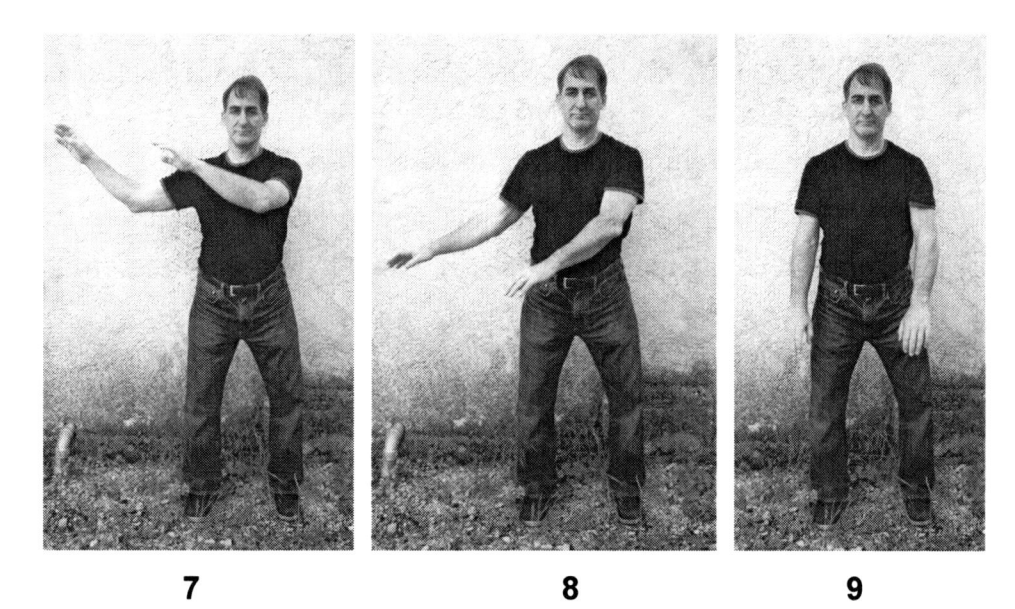

4) Perform 10-20 Repetitions. Then Repeat Rotating in the Other Direction.

Important Points:
- The arms should hold an open and relaxed shape.
- The shoulders slacken and the elbows sink.
- Keep space under the armpits.
- The fingers are spread slightly and the palm center slightly hollowed.
- Employ natural Kidney Breathing throughout. Coordinate the rising of the arms with the inhalation and the lowering of the arms with the exhalation.
- Move slowly and evenly, as though your hands are moving through water.
- Pay attention to the movement of the *Qi/Breath* as it moves through the entire body, rising from the soles of your feet to the top of the head and the tips of your fingers.

An excerpt from the "Song of Uniting the Original Qi" gives us insight into the movement of the *Qi/Breath* in this exercise:

At the top of the circle begin to exhale, at the bottom begin to inhale.
The energy comes from the Dantian, from the shoulder to the elbows.
The elbows push the palms and hands, the power reaches the four extremities.
The Qi and breath move in and out, the Dantian expands and contracts.
The Qi follows the movements of the palms, the palms move and the Qi goes.
Spirit and form unite as one, the intent first leads, it moves through a complete cycle and then returns in cycles without end.
Qi is full and the spirit concentrated, when the spirit is concentrated the heart is at peace, fire and water are united.
The kidneys are strengthened and the skill is refined.[3]

Exercise 3: Heel Breathing

Heel Breathing is more subtle than the exercise of Uniting the Original Qi. The movements of the body are very small, almost invisible.

1) Stand in the *Wu Ji* Posture with Your Arms Relaxed and at Your Sides. Inhale.

- As you inhale, attend to the *Qi/Breath* as it rises from the soles of your feet to the heel, and then up through the legs and torso, eventually reaching the top of your head.
- Simultaneously let the fingers curl into loose fists and feel as though the hands and shoulders rotate outward very slightly, and internally extend through the legs. The body internally extends, but this extension is not visible from the outside - it is an internal feeling. These movements "open" the body so that the *Qi/Breath* can flow upward more easily.

2) Exhale and Slowly Return the Body to the Start Position.

- As you exhale, attend to the *Qi/Breath* as it sinks back to the heels and soles of the feet.
- The bones feel as though they lift upward, but internally there is also a feeling of closing and sinking downward. This is almost invisible from the outside.

3) Repeat 5-7 Times Only.

Important Points:
- Breathe easily and naturally using Kidney Breathing.
- Do not force the *Qi/Breath* up to the top of the head or down to the soles.
- If the breath does not easily ascend or descend, just imagine that it does and in time it will.
- The movements of the arms and torso in opening and closing are subtle. They are relaxed without muscular tension.
- Thesensation of extending and sinking in the legs that accompanies inhalation and exhalation respectively are invisible – felt but not seen.
- The extension/opening and sinking/closing actions emanate from the *Qi/Breath* and the mind-intention rather than the bones, muscles, sinews and flesh.

The Macro-Cosmic Orbit and the Eight Extraordinary Vessels

The Macro-Cosmic Orbit is an extension of the Micro-Cosmic Orbit. In the Micro-Cosmic Orbit we worked primarily with the *Ren* and *Du* vessels, two of the Eight Extraordinary Vessels. The Eight Extraordinary Vessels and their interconnections have two important functions which are vitally important in meditation, *Nei Gong* practices, health preservation and martial arts. When they are free from obstruction, they:

1. Allow for the *Jingqi*, the vital generative force of the kidneys, to move and transform freely.
2. Allow the *Qi/Breath* to flow unimpeded through all the channels, meridians and interstices of the body.

Opening the Eight Extraordinary Vessels is therefore a key part of converting generative force to spirit in meditation, preserving the health of the body and resisting disease.

Four Vessels form the nucleus of the Eight Extraordinary Vessels. These four channels are interlinked and act in a unified fashion to circulate the *Jingqi*. They orient the vertical, horizontal, front and back and center lines of the body.

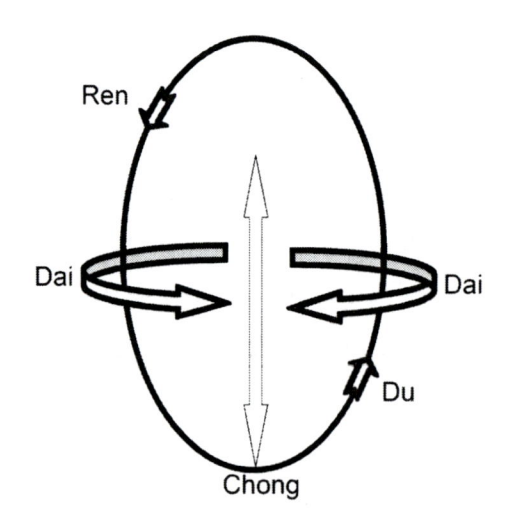

Orientation of the Four Central Extraordinary Vessels: the Ren, Du, Chong and Dai Vessels

1. **Du Mo** (Governing or Directing Vessel) rises from the perineum through the spine and enters the brain at the nape. Then it continues up and over the head and connects with *Ren Mo* in the mouth.
2. **Ren Mo** (Control or Conception Vessel) joins with *Du Mo* in the brain and mouth and descends down the front of the body to the

pubic bone and the genital organs, where it again connects with *Du Mo*, creating a circuit.

3. **Chong Mo** (Thrusting or Penetrating Vessel) runs up the center of the body. When connected and flowing freely, *Ren Mo*, *Du Mo* and *Chong Mo* are sometimes referred to as a single entity: The Central Channel.

4. **Dai Mo** (Belt or Girdle Vessel) is like a girdle around the area of the *Dantian* and kidneys that connects with and wraps the *Ren* and *Du* channels and all of the other meridians of the body. Unlike the other meridians which primarily run longitudinally through the body, *Dai Mo* runs horizontally around the body.

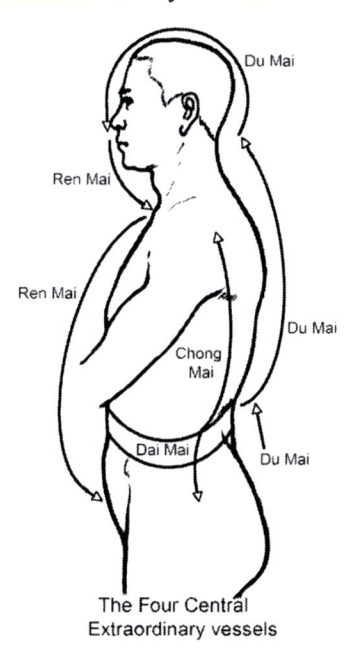

The Four Central Extraordinary vessels

The other four vessels act as an interlinked unit that serve to delineate and connect the sides of the body and the four limbs.

1. **Yang Qiao Mo** (Yang Heel Vessel) rises from the heel and ascends the outer portion of the leg and thigh to the rear rib sides. It continues upward to the scapula where it meets Yang Wei Mo.

2. **Yang Wei Mo** (Yang Linking Vessel) rises along the outer leg and then connects the ribs to the scapula and shoulder. Because it links all the yang vessels, it links the shoulders and outer sides of the arms with the fingers and the two palm centers.
3. **Yin Qiao Mo** (Yin Heel Vessel) rises from the heel, ascends the inner side of the leg and thigh. It connects to the genitals and rises along the front of the body to connect with Yin Wei Mo in the chest.
4. **Yin Wei Mo** (Yin Linking Vessel) rises along the inner leg and front of the torso under the breasts to link with the chest. Because it links all the yin vessels, it links the chest and inner side of the arms with the fingers and the two palm centers.

The pathways of the Eight Extraordinary Vessels are complex and the description above is merely an outline of their pathways. To make things more complicated, modern texts on traditional Chinese medicine are not always in agreement with older texts or with Daoist texts on the exact pathways of these channels – in particular the Linking Vessels. The description above is specifically to aid you in practicing the Macro-Cosmic Orbit Meditation, and is therefore based on the perceived internal movement of the *Qi/Breath* through these vessels during meditation. The most important thing to understand is that these eight vessels interlock, interconnect and ramify to form a network throughout the body. When the Eight Extra Vessels are unobstructed, the *Qi/Breath* and *Jingqi* can flow freely through this network.[4]

The Circulation of *Qi/Breath* in the Eight Extraordinary Vessels:

1. The *Qi/Breath* enters **Du Mo**, passing from the kidneys and sex organs through the coccyx, up the spine and into the brain, where it connects to **Ren Mo**.
2. The *Qi/Breath* passes down **Ren Mo** from the brain and mouth, down the front of the body to the *Dantian* where **Ren Mo** connects with **Dai Mo**.
3. **Dai Mo** circulates *Qi/Breath* around the body to the back, where it can then rise up the back to shoulder blades and connect to both shoulders.
4. From the shoulders, the **Yang Wei** (Yang Linking) vessels guide *Qi/Breath* down the outer yang side of the arms to the hands.
5. From the hands *Qi/Breath* circulates through the **Yin Wei** (Yin Linking) vessels, rising from the center of both palms, and traveling up the yin (inner) side of the arms to return to the chest.
6. *Qi/Breath* then falls to the *Dantian* and rises to the heart via **Chong Mo**.
7. *Qi/Breath* then descends to the *Dantian* and passes down the outer sides of the thighs and legs to the toes and sole of the foot via the **Yang Qiao** (Yang Heel) vessels.
8. From the KID 1 acu-point (*Yong Quan*: "bubbling well") at the bottom of the foot, *Qi/Breath* rises via the **Yin Qiao** (Yin Heel) vessels along the inner ankle and the inside of the leg and thigh retruning to *Dantian*.
9. From *Dantian* the cycle begins again.

Great Heavenly Circulation: Macro-Cosmic Orbit Meditation

The Macro-Cosmic Orbit circulation can most easily be performed either sitting in a chair or standing in the *Wu Ji* Posture.

To start, perform Kidney Breathing for several minutes. Continue to use this breathing pattern as you attend to the *Qi/Breath* moving through the body:

1. Observe the *Qi/Breath* moving up from *Dantian* to follow the Micro-Cosmic Orbit: ascending the *Du* vessel and returning down the *Ren* vessel to *Dantian*.
2. The *Qi/Breath* then flows smoothly down the outside of the legs to the feet and soles.
3. The *Qi/Breath* then moves up the inside of the legs to *Dantian* and then passes to the back via *Dai Mo* to proceed up the two sides of the back.
4. At the level of the shoulder blades, *Qi/Breath* splits into two streams passing through the shoulders, and then down the outside of the arms to the finger tips, before running up the inside of the arms to the chest, shoulders, mid-back and head.
5. From the head, the *Qi/Breath* moves downward along the front of the body to return to *Dantian*.
6. *Qi/Breath* then rises from *Dantian* to just below the heart and then sinks to return to *Dantian*.
7. From *Dantian*, the cycle begins again.

Important:

1) **The breath does not directly match with any particular part of this meditation.** You simply attend to the movement of the *Qi/Breath* using mind-intention. This will be difficult at first, but over time, with gentle application of the mind-intention, the sensation of the *Qi/Breath* flowing through this circuit will become stronger.

2) In the beginning, practice the Macro-Cosmic Orbit circulation as described above. However, after practicing the Macro-Cosmic Orbit Meditation regularly you will notice that **the movements described above are all happening simultaneously.** The *Qi/Breath* moves downward even as it moves upward; descends to the soles of the feet even as it rises up the back; goes out to the fingertips even as it returns to the mid-back, head and shoulders. **At this point it feels as though the movement of the *Qi/Breath* is spontaneous. You are not directing this movement, but observing it.** The *Nei Gong Zhen Chuan* describes this as follows:

> *This refers to the unified nature of Nei Gong. In one pathway the breath of Heaven and Earth, the Jingqi is accepted into the Dantian, while the Zhen Qi [True Qi] of the Dantian is transported from the armpits to the vertex. While this ascending occurs, the Zhen Qi is also descending from Yukou [area behind the diaphragm] to Dantian. This is one Qi arising from the origin. From the Dantian, Zhen Qi is transported downward from the inside of the crotch to Dantian at the sole of the foot [Yong Quan acupoint]. As Qi goes downward, there is a simultaneous rising of Qi from the sole, up the lateral side of the leg to the Dantian. Left and right together make two Qi arising form the origin. From the Dantian, Zhenqi is transported to the back, from whence the Qi again descends returning to Dantian. Left and right together make two Qi arising from the origin. All together five Qi arise from origin. One ascends and one descends; one falls, one rises; one goes out, one enters in; without contradiction, flowing constantly without stopping and without end.[5]*

Daoist Nourishing Life Longevity Methods

养 生

Yang   Sheng

Daoist Nourishing Life Longevity Methods

Yang Sheng or Nourishing Life Methods have always been a part of both Daoism and traditional Chinese medicine. Modifying and regulating one's lifestyle preserves health, aids the practice of meditation, and connects one's life with the changes of heaven and earth. Regulating your lifestyle includes:

- Living in harmony with the seasons
- Regulating the emotions
- Attending to diet
- Balancing activity and inactivity; work and rest
- Regulating sexual activity
- Practice of supplementary life nourishing exercises

The Inner Chapters of Ko Hung, an early text on Daoism from the Fourth Century tell us that in nurturing life, it is important not to be wounded:

> *Wounding occurs when our thought is troubled with things for which we lack talent; also when we force ourselves to do lifting without the requisite strength. Sadness, decrepitude, uneasiness and torment are wounds, as is also excessive joy. Constant covetousness wounds as do long conversations and the telling of pointless stories. Wasting time abed, archery contests, drunkenness and its vomitings, lying down after a heavy meal, getting breathless from running, shouts of joy and weepings, abstention from sexual intercourse – all these are wounds. When wounds have been accumulated to the point of exhaustion, death soon ensues.[1]*

The text goes on to tell us:

> *Therefore the prescription for nourishing life is this: Do not spit for distance [too much breath would be lost]. Do not walk too fast. Do not listen too intently. Do not look too long. Do not stay in bed until you get weak. Dress before you get chilled. Lighten your dress before you get*

overheated. Do not overeat when you have been starving. Eat only to satiety. Do not over-drink when you have been parched. Do not over-drink. Overeating begets congestions, and over-drinking produces accumulations of mucus. Don't overwork or take too much ease. Don't get up too early or too late. Don't perspire. Don't race your carriage or your horse. Don't strain your eyes to see too far. Don't chew your food so long that it gets cold. Don't drink wine when you are going out in the wind. Don't bathe your body or hair too frequently. Don't overextend your will or desires. Don't scheme to achieve something ingenious. Don't seek too much warmth in winter or too much cold in summer. Don't lie without covers under the stars. Don't expose your shoulders when sleeping. Don't undergo severe cold, severe heat, strong winds or heavy fogs. Don't overemphasize any of the five savors when eating, for too much acidity [sour] harms the spleen, too much bitterness harms the lungs, too much salt harms the heart, too much acridity [spicy] harms the liver; too much sugar harms the kidneys.[2]

Living in Harmony with the Seasons and Climate

In Chinese medicine, each season is described in terms of its energetic signature. As human beings we are part of the natural world, no matter how much central heating and modern conveniences insulate us from climate and weather. The cycles of yin and yang that we observe in the natural world also occur within us and effect our health and well-being. For this reason, changing our behavior and activities in accordance with these seasonal fluctuations of yin and yang helps preserve and harmonize our own energies with the energetic changes that are constantly occurring in the world around us.

In order to fully understand this discussion of the seasons we must look at the Chinese calendar. Unlike the Western solar calendar, the Chinese calendar is partly based on the lunar cycle. Therefore the days on which important holidays and seasonal markers occur can vary from year to year. However, the Chinese also divide their calendar into 24 "Solar Nodes" or "Solar Terms." These 24 fortnight periods, reflect the climactic changes that occur as the earth rotates around the sun. The 24 Solar Nodes can easily be converted to the Western solar calendar as they occur at roughly the same time each year. However, as China is in the Northern Hemisphere, the dates must be reversed for people living in the southern hemisphere. Eight of these nodes mark the beginning of each season, the spring and autumn equinoxes and the winter and summer solstices.

Looking at these eight nodes you may be surprised to see that the Beginning of Spring in the Northern Hemisphere occurs on February 4/5. In the West, we usually think of spring as beginning on the Vernal Equinox (March 20th or 21st). In the Chinese lunar calendar, the beginning of a season comes somewhat before that season appears on the Western solar calendar. This is because the start of a new season actually begins when the energies of that season begin to develop. This first "stirring" of the new season's energy happens several weeks before those energies actually manifest in an obvious way. For example the "Beginning of Spring" is in early February on the Chinese calendar. This corresponds with the first stirring of rebirth and growth associated with the energies of spring. Often at this time a warm spring breeze will be felt for a day before cold returns. It is at this time that sap begins to rise in trees, and similarly we feel the "sap" rise within us.

```
Beginning Of Spring
Feb. 4/5 to Feb. 19/20
        |
Vernal Equinox
Mar. 21/22 to April 4/5
        |
Beginning of Summer
May 5/6 to May 20/21
        |
Summer Solstice
June 20/21 to July 6/7
        |
Beginning of Autumn
Aug. 8/9 to Aug. 23/24
        |
Autumnal Equinox
Sep. 22/23 to Oct. 8/9
        |
Beginning of Winter
Nov. 7/8 to Nov. 22/23
        |
Winter Solstice
Dec. 21/22 to Jan. 5/6
```

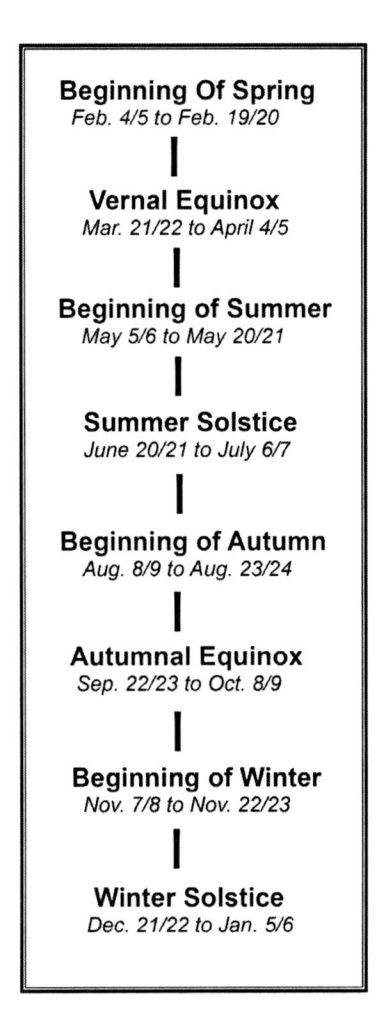

When yin and yang are discussed in the context of seasonal activity, the Chinese are referring to the cyclical transformation of yin and yang energies in the world that are a reflection of the climactic changes that occur in relation to the yang energy of the sun:

- **Beginning of Spring:** Yang *Qi* begins to dispel the cold. Plants and creatures begin to grow.
- **Vernal Equinox:** Day and night are equal in length. Yin and yang are equal. The days become warmer.
- **Beginning of Summer:** Yang continues to grow and living things flourish.

- **Summer Solstice:** Longest day of the year. Yang peaks and yin begins to grow.
- **Beginning of Autumn:** Yin *Qi* increases. Early fruits are harvested.
- **Autumn Equinox:** Yin and yang are again equal. Days grow cooler. Another time of balance in which we have an opportunity to harmonize yin and yang and collect vitality back to the center to strengthen health for winter.
- **Beginning of Winter:** Yin gains ascendancy and plants and flowers wither.
- **Winter Solstice:** Shortest day of the year. Yin peaks and yang is generated.

Spring

Spring brings the renewal of life and growth after the dormancy of winter. Living things are renewed and hibernating animals reappear. The world warms up and is full of life and energy.

The three months of Spring one calls "issuing and laying out".
Together Heaven and Earth give life,
The myriad creatures thereby blossom.
Sleep at night and rise early,
Stroll at ease around the yard,
Loose the hair and relax the body,
Allow intent to come to life.
Let it live, Don't kill it;
Give to it, don't steal from it;
Reward it, don't punish it.

This is the response to the Qi of Spring, the way to nourish the coming to life. If you go against it you harm the liver and in summer will suffer from chills; there will be too little provision for "the growing up".[3]

In the spring, getting up early and walking in nature allows the yang-*Qi* to circulate to the vertex (the Du 20 acu-point at the top of the head). This also helps the *Qi/Breath* of the liver to circulate smoothly and without obstruction to the tendons and ligaments. Therefore, stretching, and flexibility exercises will yield better results in the spring. Exercise early in the morning, when the sun comes up. More vigorous exercise is appropriate and healthy for the body in the spring.

In the spring the climate is changeable and can go from a bright sunny day to a cold windy day quite quickly. One should not switch to light clothing or shorts and t-shirts too soon. Wear a scarf if it is windy, and increase or reduce clothing according to the changes in temperature. In China people say: *Don't take off clothes in spring until the weather stays warm and don't put on clothes in autumn until the weather becomes really cool.*[4]

Summer

The Three months of Summer one calls "the thriving and fulfillment".
The Qi of Heaven and Earth mingle,
The myriad creatures flower and ripen.
Sleep at night and rise early,
Don't be too greedy for the sunshine,
Don't let intent get out of hand.
Let the flowering fulfill its growth,
Allow the Qi to seep out from you,
As though the not-to-be-wasted were outside.

This is the response to the Qi of Summer, the way to nourish the growing up. If you go against it you harm the heart and in autumn will suffer from fevers; there will be too little provision for "the gathering in".[5]

In the summer, life flourishes and plants reach their full flowering and bear fruits as the yang energy reaches its peak. The *Qi/Breath* of the heart is more active in the summer. At this time, the yang-fire of the heart circulates with the yang *Qi* in the exterior of the body.

Qi seeping outward refers to Qi moving outward through perspiration. The summer is a good time to rid the body of excess heat through exercise that causes perspiration. This both aids the *Qi/Breath* of the heart and protects the body against autumn illness. Stretching and strengthening exercises are appropriate and more effective, because the muscles are warm and adequately nourished by the blood, which circulates more easily in the summer. Yet these activities should be done early in the day, not in the sun's heat. Clothes for summer should have good ventilation, letting body heat out and allowing for evaporation. Lighter colors that reflect the light are better.

Fall

In autumn, yin begins to grow and yang wanes, as the world grows colder. This is the time of the harvest, when the earth and living things prepare for the winter. In autumn the balance of Yin and Yang is more equal.

The three months of autumn one calls "the contained and calm".
The Qi of heaven is then gusty.
The Qi of earth is then bright.
Sleep early, rise early,
Be up with the cock.
Keep intents firm and stable,
To ease the penalties of autumn.
Gather in the harvest of daimonic Qi
Keep the Qi of autumn calm.
Don't let the intent stray outside,
Keep the Qi in the lungs clear.

This is the response to the Qi of Autumn, the way to nourish "the gathering in". If you go against it you will harm the lungs and in winter will suffer from diarrhea; there will be too little provision for "the storing away".[6]

Because yin and cold begin to grow as yang and warmth diminish, exercise should be done later in the day and be more balanced between "motion" (vigorous movements) and "tranquility" (lighter, more inward directed exercises such as meditation, qi gong, yoga, etc).

The temperature becomes colder in autumn, and although the changes in weather are more steady and less unpredictable than in the spring, they are not stable. As the weather gets a little colder, delay putting heavier clothing until it is actually cold. This will help you adjust to the colder weather to come, and prevent the wind and cold from penetrating into the body through the perspiration. However, as an old saying about fall goes: *There are four seasons in a day and the weather changes even 5 miles away.*[7] Have layers prepared and add them gradually as the weather changes throughout the day.

Winter

Don't put strain on the yang.
Sleep early, rise late,
Be sure to wait for the sunshine.
Keep an intent as though lurking and hiding,
As though it were a private thought,
As though you had succeeded already.
Avoid the cold, stay near the warm,
Don't allow seeping through the skin,
Which lets the Qi be quickly stolen away.

This is the response to the Qi of Winter, the way to nourish the "storing away". If you go against it, you harm the kidneys and in the Spring will suffer from impotence; there will be too little provision for "the giving of life".[8]

In winter, the yang energy is hidden and the yin is shown on the exterior. The energy of living things should be stored and nourished for the coming spring. In winter, when the earth is cold and the yin prevails, it is important to avoid sweating too much in order to prevent wind and cold from penetrating the muscles and joints. One should also not overuse medicinal herbs that drive out pathogens through diaphoresis as this will deplete the yin and yang energies of the body at a time when these energies should be stored and nourished.

Exercise later in the day, when the sun is out and it is relatively warmer. During the winter, one should focus on storing and nourishing yin, while conserving yang. Therefore more dynamic exercise is reduced and stress is put on quiescent exercises.

In winter, it is important to wear clothing that is well insulated and warm, preventing loss of body heat. However, excessively warm clothing will cause sweating and make you prone to illness. Light wool undergarments are recommended because they are warm even if wet and wick perspiration away. Don't take clothes off when you are sweating, especially in drafts.

Gao Lian, a poet and medical scholar from the 16th century, adds several interesting seasonal considerations that expand on the above discussion. His treatise on *Promoting Health During the Four Seasons* is well worth reading. In relation to winter's cold, Gao gives the following advice:

Wear padded winter clothes during the coldest time, but add them gradually and not all at once; stop increasing the layers just when you have added enough to not feel cold anymore. Do not warm yourself in front of a roaring fire, since this winter habit may bring about particularly harmful consequences. The hands and feet, namely, have an affinity to the heart network, and should therefore never be toasted over a fire. The fire may otherwise be enticed into the heart and create symptoms of restlessness. For the same reasons, avoid grilling food over an open fire.[9]

Regulating the Emotions

Emotions are natural and part of what makes us human beings, but if the emotions tend too much in one direction, or teeter back and forth between extremes, they can cause illness and damage the *Qi/Breath* and *Shen*. Developing a positive and relaxed attitude to the vicissitudes of life can do a great deal to keep the body harmonious and healthy. Studies of healthy and active centenarians in China have shown that a large component of their longevity and vigor is due to a relaxed mental attitude and appreciation of natural beauty, painting, singing, music and art. A famous saying puts this simply: *Look forward, one thinks one possesses one thing, but lacks another, that he is short of this and that. Step back, one finds one can lead an easy life just by eating this bowl of porridge and wearing this garment.*[10]

It was mentioned in Lesson Two that the normal functioning of the body is achieved through the orderly motions of the *Qi/Breath* as it moves up, goes down, moves in and out, opens and closes, gathers and stores. These actions are collectively referred to as the "Qi Dynamic" (*Qi Ji* 氣機) in traditional Chinese medicine. When the Qi Dynamic becomes disordered or obstructed, it can result in congestion, stagnation, blockage, as well as excessive closure or opening, and excessive raising or lowering. This in turn can lead to a wide variety of somatic and/or psycho-spiritual symptoms.

The emotions are largely governed by the "Heart-Mind" (*Xin* 心). An exemplary person has a Heart-Mind that is broad and open, while a smaller person has a narrow Heart-Mind that is unhappy or sullen.[11] A famous passage from the *Ling Shu* (Spiritual Pivot) describes the Heart-Mind as a process that includes social, moral and psycho-spiritual elements:

> *When two seminal essences* 精 *[Jing] strike each other, it is spoken of as spirit* 神 *[Shen]. Following the spirit as it goes and comes is the animal spirit* 魄 *[Po]. Together with the seminal essence as it exits or enters is that which is spoken of as the human soul* 魂 *[Hun]. Those which are in accord with control of myriad things are the heart and mind. The mind has recall which is spoken of as thought* 意 *[Yi]. Thought is that which, when kept, is spoken of as will* 志 *[Zhi]. From will and that which is kept and changed is spoken of as consideration* 思 *[Si]. From consideration of distant longings comes planning* 慮 *[Lu]. From planning, to managing of myriad things, is that which is spoken of as wisdom* 智 *[Zhi].*[12]

In this context, *Po, Hun, Yi, Zhi, Si,* and *Lu* are not different things, but descriptions of different phases of the same continuous Heart-Mind - an unobstructed process of transformation which acts naturally in accordance with the context and the environment.[13] As long as emotions are moving and transforming in accordance with the movement and transformation occurring in the natural world, and in accordance with one's own immediate environment, then the Qi Dynamic, the movements of the *Qi/Breath*, will also move and transform without obstruction or blockage. Daoist meditation techniques like those discussed in Lesson Six can be used help us transform our emotions

Diet & Eating Habits

Correct eating habits and proper diet are complex subjects, but there are a few basic rules that have been part of nourishing life regimens for centuries.

Basic Eating Habits
- Don't fill up at dinner.
- Don't go to bed full.
- Drinking too much liquor disturbs the *Qi/Breath* and blood.
- Too many fluids damages the spleen and kidneys.
- Don't drink tea on an empty stomach.
- Eating more in the morning is better than eating more at night.
- Walk a hundred steps after a meal and knead and massage your abdomen with your hand.
- Don't eat too quickly, but don't over chew your food.

More Dietary Advice
1) The basis of proper nutrition is to eat whole, natural foods that are as fresh as possible.
2) Eat a diverse and balanced diet.
3) Eat primarily light and bland foods. Sun Si Miao, one of China's most famous physicians, advocated a diet that stressed natural light foods like cereals, grains, beans, vegetables and fruit. An excess of heavy, rich, greasy foods often result in a buildup of heat, dampness and phlegm.
4) Eat easy-to-digest food in order to nourish the stomach and spleen.
5) Excessive consumption of cold and raw foods like raw vegetables, salads and fruit can weaken the spleen and digestion.
6) Avoid refrigerated food and iced drinks and ice cream.

7) Eat meals that contain all of the five flavors. A diet that includes all of the five flavors, ensures that the *Qi/Breath* and blood are properly nourished and flowing, and that the functions of the internal organs are harmonious and balanced. Preference for one flavor over the others can lead to an imbalance.
   - Excessive Sour Flavor: damages the Sinews (Tendons and Ligaments)
   - Excessive Bitter Flavor: damages the *Qi/Breath*
   - Excessive Sweet Flavor: damages the Flesh
   - Excessive Spicy/Pungent Flavor: consumes the *Shen*
   - Excessive Salty Flavor: injures the Bone

The passage above reflects an idea basic to Chinese dietary therapy, in which foods are classified according to their tastes or flavors. These flavors indicate not only what something tastes like on your tongue, but the inherent qualities of foods which have certain traits and produce certain effects. In addition, each flavor "homes", or is drawn to, one of the viscera. Like our activities and emotions, the five flavors should also be regulated to conform to seasonal changes.

Eating with the Seasons

In spring, one should eat more mildly sweet food and less sour food. Because sour is associated with liver-wood, sour foods stimulate the liver. In the spring, when the liver is flourishing and active, it does not need to be stimulated. Instead, you should eat foods that nourish the spleen and stomach which aid in the building of blood and *Qi/Breath*. The nourishing quality of these foods helps one adjust to the harsh changeable climate of early spring.

Another way to think of this is in relation to the advice that in the spring, we should let down our hair and take long walks in nature. One should engage in more physical activity, particularly as the days become warmer. The sour nature of foods like vinegar, tones the viscera, muscles and sinews because the sour flavor tends to astringe the tissues. In excess, this astringent aspect of the sour flavor can cause muscles and sinews to tighten and cramp, causing pain and restriction. The spring is a time when the sap is rising, and plants and trees begin to grow again. The world is stretching and extending outward. We are also stretching and extending. Our *Qi/Breath* is reaching outward in harmony with the season - we want to exercise and move more after winter's retraction and withdrawal. The astringent nature of sour foods, if consumed to excess, interferes with this outward movement.

In summer, one should eat more pungent/spicy foods and less bitter foods. Eating spicy foods that heat us up in hot weather may seem counter-intuitive at first. Pungent foods home to the lung. They tend to warm the body, thereby accelerating the movement of the *Qi/Breath* and blood (the circulation). Therefore such foods tend to disperse stagnant moisture. Pungent foods also promote sweating which helps to release excess heat from the body. This is perhaps why a common feature of the traditional diet of peoples that live in warm damp climates includes spicy foods with hot peppers. If eaten in excess, pungent foods can exhaust the *Qi/Breath*, overheat the body and dry the tissues.

In summer the fire element and the heart energy peak. Bitter foods "home to" and stimulate the heart. They help the body eliminate heat and can disperse stagnant moisture and *Qi/Breath*. However in excess they can be drying, or can over-stimulate the heart whose energy is abundant at this time. It is natural to consume more cooling, yin foods such as fruits, juices and cooling drinks in the summer. However, too many cooling foods put out the digestive fires and damage the spleen and stomach leading to bloating, diarrhea and other digestive problems. Therefore one must balance cooling foods with some warming and pungent foods.

In autumn, the *Qi/Breath* of metal-lung flourishes. One should eat less pungent/spicy food and more sour food. This prevents metal-lung from interfering with the liver: *The acrid [pungent] taste acts on the lung. If the acrid taste is taken excessively, lung-metal will restrict liver-wood. As the liver determines the condition of the tendons, when the liver is restricted the tendons will become loose. Because the acrid taste also has the function of dispersing, the excessive taking of the acrid taste will consume spirit as well.*[14] In this season when yin grows and yang recedes, Qi/Breath and blood must be conserved and restrained from being pushed outward excessively. Exercise must be moderated and sweating contained so that Yang Qi/Breath is conserved and blood is not dispersed. In this way, the liver and tendons will be nourished and the spirit will be nurtured. The sour taste, through its astringing action, helps to restrain this outward movement of Qi/Breath and blood.

In winter, kidney-water flourishes. Salty foods are said to home to the kidneys. Salt has a powerful effect on the fluids of the body. Because the kidneys are the primary filter of body fluids, salty foods tend to concentrate Qi/Breath, blood and fluids and move them downward toward the lower body, aiding the kidney function. In excess, salty foods can cause stagnation and retention of fluids. *The salty taste can soften hardness and is superior to the blood, so when the salty taste is taken too much, it will damage bone and muscle.*[15] If the kidneys are over-stimulated, disharmony of the heart and spirit can also result. Therefore one should eat less salty food in winter and more bitter food which homes to the heart. This, in conjunction with more quiescent training and keeping the spirit calm and the mind without desire, protects and nourishes heart Qi/Breath. Although in winter it is natural to crave and consume more warming, stronger tasting and richer food, one must be careful to balance their consumption with yin moistening and cooling foods. Otherwise, it is possible to accumulate too much inner heat, which will overheat the heart and upset the spirit.

Work and Rest: Balancing Activity and Inactivity

It is important to have a balance between rest and quiescent activity and work and exercise. We expend *Qi/Breath* when we work and exercise and we restore and replenish it when we are at rest. When rest and work are balanced, *Qi/Breath* that has been expended is easily replenished. If we steadily overwork for months and years it cannot be replenished quickly enough and we draw on our *Jing* to keep going. As we have seen during the lessons on Daoist meditation, *Jing* is an essential component of the Micro-Cosmic Orbit breathing that needs to be preserved and replenished rather than expended. This is one reason why meditation can be an important counter-balance to an active life.

Excess of certain specific activities can imbalance or damage specific organs:

- Too much mental overwork damages the spleen and heart.
- Excessive use of the eyes injures the blood and the liver.
- Excessive lying down injures *Qi/Breath* and the lungs.
- Excessive sitting injures the muscles and the spleen.
- Excessive standing injures the bones and the kidneys.
- Excessive exercise/walking injures the sinews and the liver.

Other advice includes:

- Speaking less nourishes the *Qi/Breath*.
- Don't spit out saliva.
- Don't hurry or walk too quickly.
- Don't fatigue the eyes.

Li Dong Yuan on Economy of Speech[16]

Li Dong Yuan was one of the four great physicians of the Jin-Yuan Dynasties (1115-1386). In his essay called *Admonition on Economy of Speech*, he first reiterates the inter-relationships of the Three Treasures by reminding the reader that *Qi/Breath,* in its position at the center of the interaction of the Three Treasures, is the root of *Shen* and *Jing*. Li goes on to tell us that stillness and quiet are important in order to preserve the *Qi/Breath*, so that it can accumulate and produce *Jing* and foster *Shen*:

> Great is qi! When qi accumulates, it produces essence. When essence accumulates, it completes the spirit. Keep clear, keep still and abide by the Dao. A heavenly man can do all of these. He has the Dao and is able to follow it. But what am I? It will be ok for me just to practice economy of speech.

Sexual Activity

Sex is, in and of itself, neither good nor bad. It is our relationship to sex that can either enhance or harm our health. Too little sex can result in diseases of accumulation or stagnation, while too much can deplete and exhaust the body. In particular, ejaculation in men, and to some degree orgasm in women, is considered to exhaust the reproductive essence (*Jing*) stored in the kidneys, although for women the menses and multiple childbirths are more depleting than sex. The *Jing* is easily replaced by the young, but becomes harder to replace as we age and the vital energy declines. *Jing* forms the root of the body's energies. *Jing* nourishes the bones, which are associated with the kidneys and forms part of the blood which nourishes the internal organs and all of the tissues of the body, including the tendons and ligaments. Chinese medicine advocates less frequent ejaculations as a man ages. Because each of us is different, there are no hard and fast rules about sexual activity. If you are fatigued and experience a feeling of weakness for some time after sex then you may be having sex too frequently. There are two other caveats that the Chinese consider important.

- Don't have sex when full or drunk.
- Don't have sex when already very fatigued or exhausted.

Rejuvenating Sexual Energy

Da Liu, a well known teacher of *Tai Ji Quan* in New York City gives us the following exercise for restoring and increasing sexual potency and energy:

- Sit on a chair with the feet on the ground and cover your kneecaps with your hands.
- With the tongue on the upper palate, inhale through the nose while bending forward from the waist until the torso is at a 45 degree angle. As you bend, simultaneously feel the *Qi/Breath* flow upward from the soles of the feet, up the legs to the genital area.
- Then exhale and straighten the body while you feel the *Qi/Breath* flow down the legs and back to the to the soles. This exercise should be performed 10-20 times in the morning just after rising and again just before going to sleep in the evening.
- After several months the exercise can be further refined by directing the *Qi/Breath* up the legs to the perineum, and then slowly to the tip of the penis (for men). Women should direct *Qi/Breath* up the legs to the perineum, and then inward to the uterus.[17]

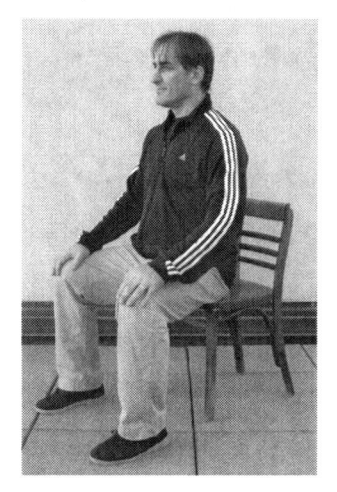

Start

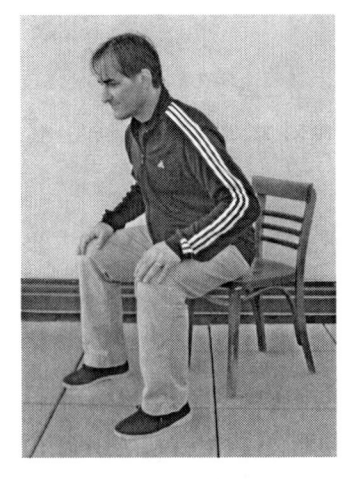

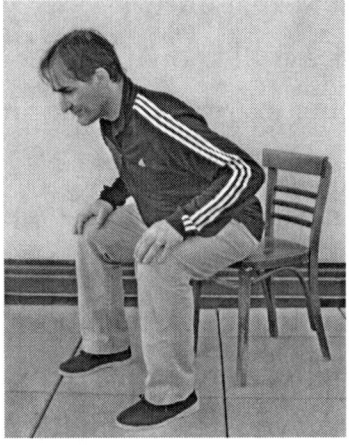

Inhale: *Qi/Breath* **flows from the soles of the feet, up to the genitals**

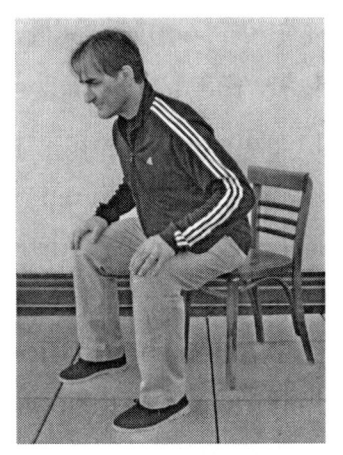

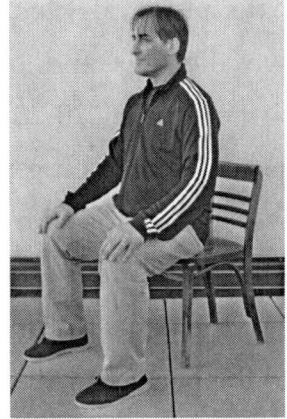

Exhale: *Qi/Breath* **returns to the soles of the feet**

Supplementary Life Nourishing Exercises

There are many life nourishing exercises that can aid and enhance the practice of Daoist meditation. Practicing active moving exercises such as the internal martial arts (*Tai Ji Quan; Xing Yi Quan* and *Ba Gua Zhang*), *Qi Gong* exercises and/or regularly walking two to three miles a day are an important balance to quiescent seated meditation, but there are some other fairly simple, yet surprisingly effective exercises that are not hard to integrate into your daily routine.

1. Cultivating the Kidneys Nourishes Life

1. Before sleep, sit on the bed. Gently lift the perineum and lift the tongue tip to the upper palate. Perform Kidney Breathing for one to two minutes.

2. Click the teeth together nine times. Then rotate the tongue in the mouth nine times in each direction around the outside of the upper and lower teeth and nine times in each direction around the inner part of the upper and lower teeth in order to stimulate the secretion of saliva. When saliva has accumulated, swallow it as you extend and straighten the neck, imagining that the saliva passes down *Ren Mo* (the meridian running down the front midline of the body) to the *Dantian*. In the *Dantian*, imagine the saliva vaporizes (like water hitting a fire) into a mist which fills the *Datian*.

3. While still performing Kidney Breathing, rub the kidney area, stimulating the Shen Shu (BL 23) acupoints 120 times until they are warm.

4. Then

For men: Lie on your back and continue to perform Kidney Breathing as you hold up the scrotum with one hand and rub the *Dantian* in a circle with the other hand 50 times. Switch hands and repeat. Then lightly knead the testicles.

For women: Lie on your back **and** perform the Deer Exercise (See Lesson Eight): Gently lift the *kua* and the pelvic floor as you inhale. This is similar to the lifting of the perineum you learned earlier and although direct force is not applied, there is a more specific and direct application of mind-intention in this lifting action. Then let the pelvic floor and the *kua* sink as you exhale. The perineum is still slightly lifted at the end of this action. Repeat this four times as you rub *Dantian* in a circle with the right hand,

and then four more times as you rub the *Dantian* in a circle with the left hand.

2. Rubbing the Abdomen Aids the Stomach and Intestines

This exercise is intended to mainly stimulate the blood circulation in the abdomen and organs of digestion by rubbing specific acu-points and massaging directly over the internal organs. This exercise can be done in the morning or after a meal.

1. Rub Zhong Wan (Ren 12): Put the pads of the three middle fingers of the right hand midway between the navel and the lower end of the sternum. Put the left hand on top and gently press and rub clockwise around this area.

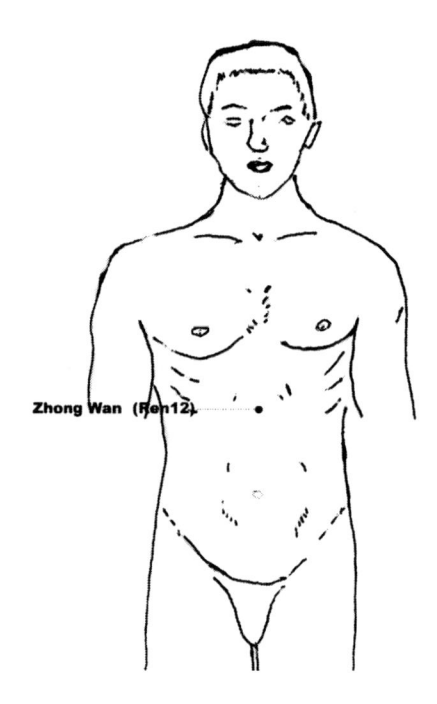

2. From the navel area use the palms to massage up along the sides of the ribcage until your palms are just below the breasts. Then bring the hands together and rub down the centerline to return to the navel. Repeat these movements nine times.

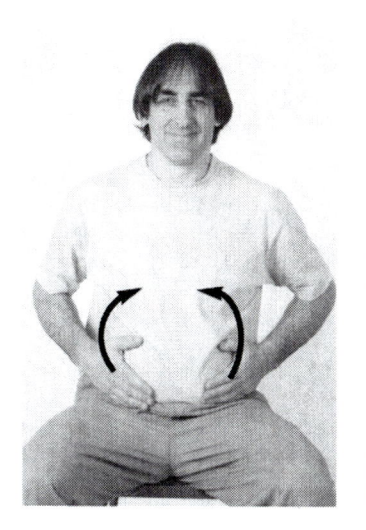

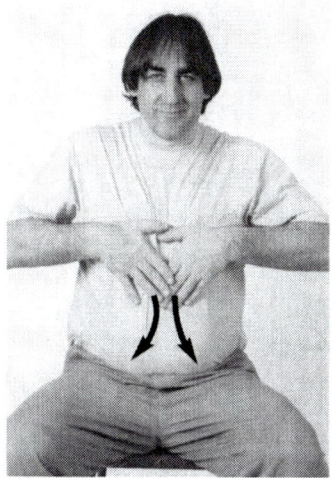

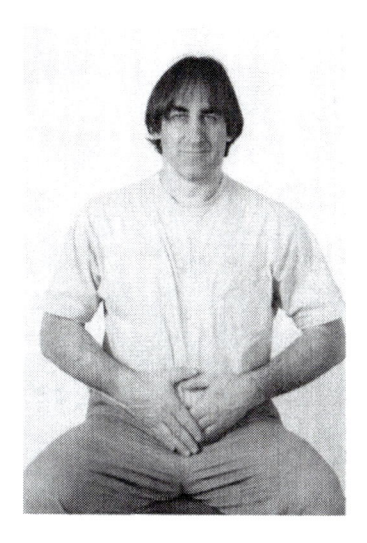

3. Use the palm to massage around the navel, making 36 circles clockwise and then 36 circles counter-clockwise.

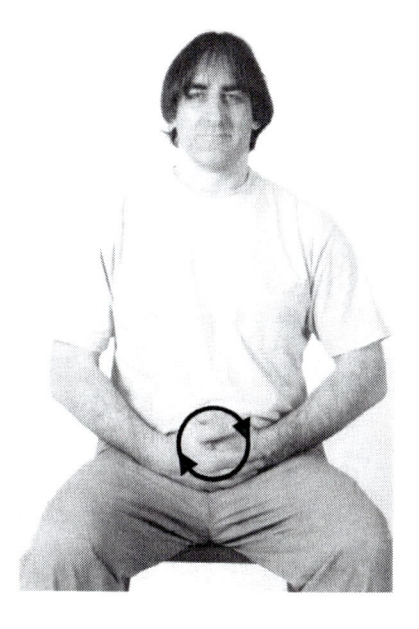

3. Combing the Hair Frequently Stimulates the Meridians and the Brain

All of the meridians in the body have either direct or indirect connections with the head, scalp and brain. Therefore stimulating the scalp by "combing the hair" can have global effects on the body's health by regulating the meridians. Combing the hair actually means to massage the scalp. This can be done by separating the five fingers and digging into the scalp as you comb backwards from the forehead to the occiput. Alternatively a wooden or horn comb can be used. The Chinese often use peach wood, sandalwood or buffalo horn combs to stimulate the scalp. These can be purchased online. Combing the scalp 100 times before bed calms the mind, producing peaceful sleep.

4. Other Exercises
- "Wash" the face frequently by rubbing your palms together until they are warm. Then massage downward from the forehead, down through the center of the face, and then upward along the sides of the face and cheeks, and back up to the sides of the forehead. Repeat from 9-27 times in a session.
- Click the teeth and swallow saliva frequently.
- Wash the feet in warm water before going to bed.

PART II

Cracking the Code: The Use of Symbolism and Imagery in Daoist Meditation

Cracking the Code: Daoist Imagery and Symbolism

Daoist texts are replete with imagery, symbolism and metaphor, offering a rich and multilayered tapestry of visual forms. Engagement with this aspect of Daoism is difficult, especially for Westerners who do not have the requisite cultural reference points. Where does one begin? And is it even necessary to delve into these sometimes fanastical, variegated images if one merely wants to learn meditation techniques?

This dense tapestry of symbol, image, metaphor and text does have a purpose and can greatly aid the practice of Daoist meditation if it is understood and used properly. I encourage you to engage with this aspect of Daoism. If you started the lessons, you have already encountered a number of images: Water, Fire, Kan, Li, Heaven and Earth, etc. You may have noticed that these images are helpful in practicing the different meditation methods and techniques.

Daoist imagery serves two primary purposes. First, to obscure the correct methods of practicing Daoist meditation by acting as a kind of code, within which these methods are hidden. In this way, only the initiated will understand the practice methods and they are thus empowered by this special and esoteric knowledge. As the goal hjere is to elucidate, rather than obfuscate, we will focus on the second purpose of Daoist imagery: to aid the meditator, giving him or her an alternative and imagery-rich language, a departure from ordinary language. Through this departure, the everyday mind is by-passed, allowing one to engage with another more subtle mode of perception, which in turn allows one to discern and engage with the almost imperceptable movements and changes taking place within the body.

Like a Zen Buddhist koan, one of the functions of the language of Daoist meditation is to destabilize habitual patterns of thought. To this end, different and multiple images are used to say the same thing in different or even inverse ways. The discourse of Daoist texts and images is repetitive and recursive, coming at the mind and spirit from multiple angles. It is always different, but always new.[1] This endless recursion continuously interweaves images and words so that our conscious, everyday mind is subverted and transformed. Some of the most important and symbolic devices in Daoist meditation are derived from the *Yi Jing*, one of the most important texts in the Daoist Canon, and perhaps in Chinese thought.

Susan Huang sums up Daoist visual imagery as representations pertaining to "true form" (*Zhen Xing* 真形): *The concept of true form is not static, but instead entails a vigorous quest, an active journey of seeing underlying and secret phenomena through a series of metamorphoses. This particular Daoist cultivating process of seeing the hidden and unknown parallels the cultivation of Dao through which practitioners integrate themselves with the cosmos.*[2]

In Daoism, the concepts of text and image are interwoven. Images **are** texts, and often maps, drawings, talismans, symbols, pictures, paintings and charts contain Chinese characters, themselves ideographic symbols, that interact with the imagery.

> *Numerous Daoist symbols exist in a gray zone between images and texts. An image can be a text not only because it imitates writing, but because Daoists see "viewing" as the faculty essential to decoding a text. From the Daoist perspective of sacred scriptures, moreover, an image is a text: any materialized form reflects the highest form of text – the writing from heaven, or heavenly writings (Tian Shu), condensed from graphic or picture-like patterns of the pure cosmic qi upon world creation.*[3]

In this context *Nei Dan* (inner alchemy) "texts" often take the form of maps, or charts. An example is the *Nei Jing Tu*, the Chart of the Inner Circulation of the *Qi/Breath* which depicts the inner landscape of the body. In the picture, a person is seated in meditation, their body configured like a Chinese landscape painting. This "text" represents an inner vison of the body and the macro-cosmic, micro-cosmic processes at work both inside the body and in the universe at large. There are characters interwoven with the image, and the images themselves represent stories and metaphors with multiple meanings and multiple layers of meaning. Other texts, like the *Dao De Jing,* do not contain images, but attempt to engage the reader's inner vision through words. For the Daoists, text and image are inextricably intertwined like the warp and weave of a tapestry.

In the sections that follow, we will look at a number of texts, symbols and images, and discuss their inter-relationships and their relation to Daoist meditation practices:

1. The *Dao De Jing* and its hidden meanings and images.
2. The *Nei Jing Tu* Chart of the Inner Circulation of the *Qi/Breath.*
3. Symbolism relating to Daoist meditation from the *Yi Jing,* the Five Phases or Powers, yin and yang, alchemical symbols such as the Dragon and Tiger and Lead and Mercury, Daoist numerology, the Nine Palaces and the dipper constellation.
4. The Gen Diagram from the *Yi Jing* and its relationship to Daoist meditation.

This will by no means be a thorough discussion of Daoist imagery, but will focus on decoding the imagery that helps flesh out, explicate and aid the meditation practices introduced in this book. The final chapter in this section, "The Message in the Code", will attempt to sum up the meaning of the images and their implications for the practice of meditation.

Dao De Jing on Daoist Meditation: The Hidden Message Within the Text

道 德 经

Dao　De　Jing

The Dao De Jing and Daoist Meditation: The Hidden Message Within the Text

The *Dao De Jing* (Tao Te Ching), attributed to Lao Zi, is often viewed as the central text of what is often erroneously called "Philosophical Daoism." The *Dao De Jing* (also called the *Laozi*) is a philosophical text, but it also addresses spiritual and religious issues of Daoist practice and therefore cannot be separated from these aspects of Daoism. In addition, the book has a veiled subtext that acts as an instruction manual for the practice of Daoist meditation. One of the oldest known commentaries on the *Dao De Jing* is attributed to He Shang Gong (Ho Shang Kung). In reading his commentary it is clear that He Shang Gong aims at enabling the reader to make practical use of the *Dao De Jing*, teaching him or her how to use the book as a guide to Daoist meditation. To this end, He Shang Gong gives chapter headings that serve as instructions or guideposts for the practice of Daoist meditation. Like a "how to" book, these headings attempt to instruct the reader. Some examples are "How to Embody the Dao", "How to Use Emptiness", and "How to Return to Purity". What follows is an introduction to the *Dao De Jing* as a guide to meditation. It is by no means a complete discussion.

Dao means 'way' or 'method' and by extension 'rule of life' or 'process'.[1] The *Dao De Jing* was originally divided into two halves, one called *Dao* (The Way) and the other *De* (power, potency, potential, charisma or virtue). Although both *Dao* and *De* are discussed in both sections of the book, the first half concerns itself largely with instruction in the *Dao* - in the context of our discussion, the way of practicing Daoist meditation and asceticism. The second half of the book concerns itself with *De*, the charisma and potency of the sage (one who has embraced the *Dao*) and the relationship of governance of oneself to the governance of others. The government of the "sage" rests on the fundamental point that the ruler himself must embody emptiness and non-action. Disorder stems from the dominance of desire, which reflects the unruly presence of confused and agitated *Qi/Breath*. In this way, self-cultivation and government are shown to form an integral whole.[2]

Chapter 1: How to Embody the Dao[3]

This is perhaps the most famous and most quoted passage of the *Dao De Jing*

> *The Dao that can be discussed,*
> *Is not the eternal Dao.*
> *The name that can be named,*
> *is not the eternal name.*
> *The nameless is the beginning of Heaven and Earth.*
> *The named is the mother of all things.*
> *Always without desire, thereby one beholds its secret.*
> *Always having desires, thereby one sees its return.*
> *The two are of the same origin but different in name.*
> *Together they are called the dark one.*
> *The one still darker than the dark one.*
> *The gate of every mystery.*[4]

The first chapter of the *Dao De Jing* tells us that both the man who has desires and he who has none, receive the same breath of Heaven - the "Dark One." According to He Shang Gong, the "One still darker then the Dark One," means that within heaven there is another heaven[5]; within the breath, there is another breath; within the mind, there is another mind. In the breath there is both fullness and emptiness, which allows us to cast aside feelings and desires and remain in the middle, in harmony.[6]

This first chapter also tells us that the *Dao* represents something subtle and difficult to grasp with the conscious, coneceptual mind. The *Dao* is a mysterious and numinous unity that underlies and sustains all things, and is therefore inaccessible to normal thought, language and perception.⁷

The parallel lines of the first chapter are juxtaposed in such a way that there both is and is not a constant *Dao* with a constant name. This juxtaposition of apparently contradictory statements forces us to seek connections where least expected. Like successive blows hitting the reader from opposite sides, they push him or her in an unexpected direction, a place somewhere in the middle. ⁸

Chapter 2: How to Cultivate the Personality⁹

The text tells us that opposites both generate and complete each other:

> *Existence and non-existence generate each other.*
> *Heaviness and lightness perfect each other.*
> *Longness and shortness form each other.*
> *By beholding shortness it becomes longness*
> *By beholding highness it becomes lowness.*¹⁰

> *He follows the doctrine of not speaking.*
> *All things rise,*
> *And they are not rejected.*
> *He acts and puts no stress on it.*¹¹

Already in these first two chapters there is an idea of putting no stress on anything, having no termination that defines and apprehends meaning. Rather then limiting definitions, these utterances serve as a kind of bridge.¹² Through non-differentiation one is then able to engage with the incessant ongoing transformation of things, *whose continuity 'cannot be named' but whose indistinction leads us beneficently toward the fundamental harmony which Daoists have called the 'Dao'.*¹³ He Shang Gong's commentary tells us that *acting, but putting no stress on anything, is what the Dao is* *doing.*[14] Allowing transformation to unfold, one "produces without owning" just as *the pristine breath produce all things without owning them.*[15]

Chapter 5: How to use Emptiness[16]

Heaven and Earth are not humane,
They regard all things as straw dogs.
The saint is not humane,
He regards people as straw dogs.
The space between heaven and earth,
Should it not be like a bellows?
Who talks much is soon emptied.
This is not equal to keeping to the center.

People are like straw dogs. Heaven and Earth follow their own natural interaction of which human beings are but a part, and therfore not subject to any special regard. The text of the *Lao Zi* tells us that the space between Heaven and Earth is like a bellows. The bellows is empty yet it possess a resounding breath.[17] It is empty yet it is inexhaustible and full. If the intake is too fast or too hard, the flow of air through the bellows will not be efficient. If too slow, little will be drawn in or expelled. The secret is to be gentle, consistent, steady and even.[18] The bellows represent the flow of the *Qi/Breath*, the flow of life, moving in a harmonious flow.

Similarly in meditation, one should keep strength inside, let the breath move and fill the emptiness and thereby cultivate the spirits of the five organs. Talking empties rather than fills this space, so save and cultivate the breath, and diminish idle talk. Words themselves often create a gap between the speaker and listener. Countless elements shape the meaning and quality of words, and both transmission and comprehension are often colored by one's internal conflicts, needs and emotions. A true understanding of one's moment-to-moment reality - the *Dao* - cannot be described with words. It can ony be hinted at:

The Dao that can be discussed, is not the eternal Dao.

Hence communication without words and understanding without words often facilitates a truer and deeper understanding.

Keeping to the center means not going too far in one direction or another. Then one is able to move in any direction as circumstances dictate, because one's potential for change and transformation remains full and potent. Francois Jullien points out that in Chinese thought, *the less evident a quality, the greater its capacity to grow; this is not remotely a question of humility. Rather, restraint is the very condition of non-exhaustion.*[19] Simplicity and plainness are the measure of authenticity - it is situated opposite in relation to the flavorful or colorful, *whose intensity and seductiveness are doomed to wear themselves out.*[20]

Chapter 6: How to Complete the Idea[21]

The spirit of the valley never dies
It is called the mysterious female.
The door of the mysterious is called the root of Heaven and Earth.
Flimsy and continuous, as if barely existing,
Yet use will never exhaust it.[22]

In He Shang Gong's commentary, he refers to the mysterious as the "dark" or the "dark one", sometimes differentiating it as yang or Heaven associated, as opposed to yin, associated with Earth:

The valley is what nourishes. Those able to nourish the spirit do not die. 'Spirit' means the spirits of the five organs. When these five are injured the five spirits leave. 'Dark' refers to Heaven. In a person this means the nose which links us with Heaven. The female refers to 'Earth'. In a person, this means the mouth which links us to Earth. The breath that passes through our nose and mouth should be finer than gossamer silk and barely noticeable, as if it weren't actually present. It should be relaxed and never strained or exhausted.[23]

The five spirits are rarefied essences of the five *Qi*/Breaths of the five viscera related to the internal organs. The five spirits produce the senses of the body. There are two key spirits. The *Hun* (spirit associated with the liver) is yang. It is connected to Heaven. Hence, it is mysterious and dark. The *Hun* relates to the liver and is in charge of what enters and leaves the body through the nose. The *Po* (associated with the lungs) is related to Earth and yin. The *Po* nourishes man with tastes which enter through the mouth. Relative to the rarified vapor of Heaven, foods and the tastes assciated with food, are turbid and dense. They "form" and provide nourishment for the frame of the body - the bones, muscles, flesh, etc.[24] The other spirits are the *Yi* (Intention) which is linked to the spleen and stomach, the *Shen* (Heart-Spirit) and the *Zhi* (Will), linked to the *Jing* (essence) which is stored in the kidneys.

When the *Hun* and the *Po*, the yin and yang manifestations of the spirits are harmonized, one connects or reconnects to an inner unity. This unity is itself a manifestation of the balanced and harmonious breaths of Heaven and Earth moving through us.

Breathing continuously, infinitesimally and smoothly is the door that connects us with the fundamental essences of Heaven and Earth, which in turn harmonizes and nourishes the spirits. The breath is described as being performed *uninterruptedly and in a mysterious way, as if one could flee and return, as if one did not exist.*[25]

The "Valley" is like the low ground where water collects without effort. This can be a metaphor for the *Dao*. It conjures up the image of a still pool, which can be likened to the cultivation of stillness in meditation - when the outward senses are withdrawn to look inward and the mind moves only within itself.[26]

Chapter 10: How to be Able To Act[27]

If one sustains the spiritual and animal souls,

And embraces unity, one may be without separation.

If one concentrates the breath, if one produces tenderness,

One may resemble a little child.

By purifying and cleansing, one gets the dark look.

Is one able to be without faults?

In loving the people, in governing the country,

Can one be without knowledge?

The gate of Heaven opens and shuts.

Can one not be a female bird?

If it resplendent penetrates the four quarters.

Can one be without knowledge?

It generates and nourishes.

It acts and does not possess.

It causes growth and does not rule.

This is called the mysterious Te.[28]

The spiritual and animal souls again refer to the *Hun* and *Po* respectively. There are two theories on the spirits. One is that the *Hun* and *Po* exist independently of the body and unite at conception. During life they are tied to the organic functioning of the body and the organs. At death the *Po* returns to Earth and the *Hun* to Heaven. In this way the *Hun*, the *Po* and their connection to the body are considered to be a microcosm of the Three Powers: Heaven, Earth and Human Beings. The alternative view is that the *Hun* and the *Po* are organically connected to the body and are part of its psycho-emotional functioning.[29] In its relationship with the physical body and earth, the *Po* is related to the Kidneys and essence (*Jing*).

Embracing Unity, or "Holding Fast to the One," is a method of Daoist meditation in which the practitioner seeks to still the mind so that no thoughts, emotions or desires arise. Both the body and mind are still, with the body aligned and the spine straight. Thsi gives one the potential to connect to the primordial, undivided state underlying consciousness. This state of Unity is sometimes called the "mind of the Dao."[30]

What the Laozi calls the "One," according to He Shang Gong, refers to the purest and most potent form of qi-energy that brings forth and continues to nourish all beings. This is the meaning of de, the "virtue" or power with which the "ten thousand things" - i.e., all beings - have been endowed and without which life would cease. The maintenance of "virtue," which the commentary also describes as "guarding the One," is thus crucial to self-cultivation. A careful diet, exercise, and some form of meditation are implied, but generally the commentary focuses on the diminishing of selfish desires.[31]

If in meditation one concentrates on securing and concentrating the original breath, so that the breath and consciousness are not confused or disturbed, then the body becomes supple, tender and pliant like an infant, without worrisome thoughts or politically motivated actions.[32] *If one is able to resemble a little child, inwardly without fear and outwardly without action, then the spirits do not flee*[33]. By thus purifying the mind and cleansing the heart, it becomes clear and tranquil, profound and silent. When it becomes clear, *the mind stays in the dark* (mysterious; profound) *places, the look knows all its doings. Therefore it is called the dark look.*[34] The "dark look" also refers to the inward directed gaze associated with meditation. Often it is fixed inside the body below the navel or on the tip of the nose. If one is tranquil and without lust and desires ("without faults") then the breath will be saved and concentrated.

Other passages in the *Dao De Jing* also refer to being like an infant. In Chapter 55: On the Charm of the Mystery,[35] we are told that in an infant:

Its bones are soft, its sinew are weak, but its grip is strong.
Not yet to have known the union of male and female,
but to be completely formed.
To be able to scream all day without getting hoarse.
Means that harmony is at its perfection.[36]

Although the infant seems soft and weak, its intention is fixed and does not change, so it can grip things firmly and hold onto them. It does not know of sex yet its essence (*Jing*) is abundant. In other translations of the text "completely formed" is translated as having an erect member.[37] *Jing* is associated with reproduction and sexual energy. In Daoist meditation, *Jing* transforms into *Qi/Breath* and *Qi/Breath* transforms into Spirit. Spirit in turn then transforms back into *Jing*, thereby replenishing it. Thus, abundant *Jing* is both a requirement for and a result of harmonizing the five spirits. Restraining one's sexual desires also helps to guard the essence.

The infant's heart is also pure and does no harm to others and so is not harmed by others - *poisonous insects do not sting it, nor fierce beasts seize it.*[38] The infant's heart does not force the *Qi/Breath*. Through a natural letting-go (rather than active interference) the infant lets the *Qi/Breath* circulate freely and unobstructed.[39] The heart and the emotions, if not still and focused, if not harmonious, pull on the reservoir of *Qi/Breath* and *Jing*, depleting them. This is considered to be going against the *Dao*.

To be "without knowledge" means that one should inhale and exhale without the ears hearing it.[40] The gate of heaven is the nostrils; opening and shutting means to inhale and exhale. A female bird is quiet and still. A bird's bones are hollow and its body soft and light. As it breathes, the bird expands and fills with the *Qi/Breath* (see the Crane Breathing Exercise in Lesson Eight).

Both generating and nourishing, the *Dao* bequeaths, but does not control. Generation and nourishing become tools and methods for use. Both *Dao* and *De,* when present in the heart, are mysterious and invisible.[41]

Chapter 11: How to Make Use of Non-Existence[42]

This chapter talks about the usefulness of non-existence, the importance of emptiness in functionality.

Thirty spokes unite in one nave,

Through what has not, the wheel can be used.[43]

The nave or hub is empty within, yet it unites all the spokes of the wheel. In meditation, one gets rid of feelings and desires, thereby allowing the five viscera (the interior of the body) to be empty. When the interior is empty, the spirits can return and reside inside the body.[44] Hans-Georg Moeller tells us that the image of a wheel and the hub are also an image of the *Dao:*

> *That the Dao is depicted as a wheel, as the wheel of a cart, shows right away that the Dao is not static, that it is not something that eternally stands still, but rather something that moves – even though it does not change its shape. The wheel is not merely a thing, it is a kind of event, it is rotation and motion. The wheel is a running, it is a "pro-ceeding," a "process" (i.e., literally a "going forwards").*[45]

The hub of the wheel stands still. The wheel turns, but the empty hub is unchanged, still, doing nothing, yet by doing nothing it unites the spokes and the rim and allows them to turn and move. Stillness in the center, having an empty space inside, allows movement and change to occur and allows the spirits to be receptive.

Chapter 12: How to Keep Off Desires[46]

The five colors confuse the eye,
The five sounds dull the ear,
The five tastes spoil the palate.
Excess of hunting and chasing
Makes men's hearts go mad.
Products that are hard to get,
Impede their owner's movements.
Therefore the Sage,
Considers the belly, not the eye.
Truly, he rejects that but takes this.[47]

Earlier, the text and commentary told us that when feelings and desires are diminished, the five organs and their spirits are quieted and one reaches a place of stillness and emptiness. Then the *Jing*, the *Qi/Breath* and the spirits are harmonious. For most people, the eyes are the dominant sense receptors. Therefore our visual senses have a powerful effect on us and easily distract us. Striving for beauty, emphasizing visual stimulation, damages the spirits. Craving sounds and music, prevents the heart from listening to the "sounds of soundlessness."[48] In order to nourish the spirits, one should look within (to *Dantian*) and at the powers within oneself, rather than be diverted by external pleasures and delights. This does not mean we should not look and hear and move and taste.

The eyes can't help seeing and the ears can't help hearing and the mouth can't help tasting and the mind can't help thinking and the body can't help acting. They can't stay still. But if we let them move without leaving stillness behind, nothing can harm us. Those who are buried by the dust of the senses or who crave sensory stimulation lose their way.[49]

This passage has much congruency with the teachings of Ma Dan Yang, a 12th century Daoist master who told his disciples that the most important practice is "nourishing qi."

> *Even if songs and lyrics sing about dragon and tiger, Child and Maiden, these are simply words. Therefore, if you long for the wondrousness of the Dao, nothing is better than nourishing qi. But people drift and drown in profit and reputation and in the process squander and ruin their qi. Those who study the Dao do not concern themselves with anything other than nourishing qi. Now, if the ye-fluids in the heart descend and the qi in the kidneys ascends, eventually reaching the spleen, and the enlivening influence of original qi is not dispersed, then the elixir will coalesce. The liver and lungs are pathways through which [the fluids and qi] come and go. If you practice stillness for a long time, you yourself will know this. If you do not nourish qi, even if you carry Mount Tai under your arm and leap beyond the Northern Sea, this is not the Dao."* [50]

Louis Komjathy comments on this passage as follows:

> *Nourishing qi is accomplished, first and foremost, by sealing oneself off from every source of dissipation. By sitting in silent meditation, emptying and stilling excess emotional and intellectual activity, one begins to return to one's original condition of energetic aliveness and integration. One is no longer swayed by concerns with profit and reputation. The above passage suggests that the cultivation of stillness and concentration on the lower elixir field initiates an inner alchemical process. It is unclear if there are specific neidan techniques being employed, but Ma does suggest that actual practice must supersede discourse and concern over esoteric technical language. Through consistent meditative praxis, the adept will gain direct experience with shifts in his or her psychosomatic condition. This involves the descent of fluids from the heart and the ascent of qi from the kidneys, which eventually leads to original qi becoming complete and the elixir of immortality forming. It also results in orb [the organs and*

their global interconnections] *harmony and a general state of well-being.*[51]

Chapter 78: How to Trust in Sincerity[52]

Within the world nothing surpasses water in tenderness and weakness.

But when it attacks what is firm and strong, nothing is able to vanquish it.

That the weak vanquishes the strong, that the pliable vanquishes the unbending.

Everybody in the Empire knows.

[But] nobody is able to act [according to it].[53]

The *Dao* is often compared to water. Water is not actually the *Dao*, but because it is fluid and infinitely flexible, having no form, no sharp edges; because it is inexhaustible and unceasing, it guides us towards the *Dao*.[54] Water acts as a model. Water is soft and gentle, yet nothing can compete with it. It is weak and pliable, yet it can vanquish the strong and hard. *The most good is like water. Water is good and beneficent towards all beings.*[55] Water provides the life force for all creatures. Nothing can live without water. It purifies and is tranquil, yet it also has irresistible force. Water *points to an inexhaustible fund of immanence.*[56] It is endlessly renewing, endlessly transforming - from water in a lake, to vapor, to clouds, to rain, and back to the lake.

Water is inactive and conforming, it accommodates itself to the container that holds it, yet at the same time it represents a potential irresistible force that without itself acting, flows toward the lowest point, following the path open to it. Water does not contend - *If dammed it stays. If let off it flows.*[57] It is non-competitive and at peace, but moves when the time is right - *For motion it chooses time.*[58] This means that it adheres to nature's terms and changes, freezing in winter and dissolving and flowing in the spring and summer.[59]

Chapter 59: How to Guard Dao[60]

In order to guard and protect the Way (*Dao*), He Shang Gong gives some very specific advice. He tells the reader to make use of heaven by harmonizing our own energies with the *Qi/Breath* of the seasons. In this way we can store up the *Jing* and *Qi/Breath,* and prevent them from escaping. When *Jing* and *Qi/Breath* accumulate and are used sparingly, then the *Dao* of Heaven can be acquired and *De* (potency; potential) can be amassed within oneself. Then there is nothing that cannot be overcome. By protecting and nurturing *Jing* and *Qi/Breath* within one's body, the breath is not heavy and the five spirits are not troubled. He Shang Gong refers to this as *the deep-going root and firm trunk.*[61] The *Qi/Breath* is the root and the *Jing* is the trunk.[62] This, combined with the inward gaze, makes life long.

Chapter 42: On the Changes of Dao[63]

Tao generates one. One generates two. Two generates three. Three generate all things.
All things turn away from yin and embrace yang.
The empty breath effects the union.[64]

Dao generates one. One generates two (yin and yang). Two generates three: the turbid-yin, the clear-yang and the harmonious. These three correlate with Earth, Heaven, and Human Beings respectively.[65] In turn these three together generate everything. All things turn toward the sun, the source of life and are a mixture of yin and yang, light and dark, fire and water. In all things there is the original breath. The ten thousand things reach their union (achieve harmony) through blending of the breaths, which in turn relies on emptiness. Within the breast are the organs, within the bones is the marrow and within plants there is emptiness. The harmonious blended *Qi/Breath* flows through and pervades them and thereby they obtain long life.[66] Here it is made clear that the free circulation of the *Qi/Breath* is ultimately the reason why emptiness or nothingness is critical to understanding the *Dao*. *The definition of the Dao as what is empty, in this regard, also means the fullness of Qi-Breath.*[67] This fullness of *Qi/Breath* in turn creates the limitless and inexhaustible changes and transformations of the natural world and the living beings within it.

Later in this same chapter of the *Dao De Jing*, Lao Zi goes on to say that: *What others teach, I also teach.*[68] I teach men to flee from strength and practice weakness, to flee from hardness and practice tenderness. The violent ones, those who do not believe in the mystery and rebel against Dao and De, do not live out their natural lifespan.[69]

Diagram of the Inner Circulation of Qi/Breath

內 經 圖

Nei　Jing　Tu

Diagram of the Inner Circulation of Qi/Breath: Nei Jing Tu

The Diagram of the Inner Circulation (*Nei Jing Tu*) depicts the inner landscape of the body. In the picture a person is seated in meditation, their body configured like a Chinese landscape painting. In the head, there are high mountain peaks; in the spine, a winding mountain path; in the neck, a many-storied pagoda; in the lower abdomen, a deep body of water. The word for landscape in Chinese is *Shan-Shui* (mountain-water). The Chinese view mountains and water as the very quintessence of nature. Hence mountains have been referred to as the "bones" of the earth, and water as it's "blood."[1]

The inner world depicted in the *Nei Jing Tu* is not just a representation. This landscape depicts the movements of the *Qi/Breath* through the human body. However, the *Qi/Breath* it depicts flows not just through the body, but through Heaven and Earth as well. What shapes and transforms the terrain "out there," equally shapes and transforms the terrain within us. When looking at a landscape, the painter sees the places where *Qi/Breath* collects and dissipates, the interplay of coming into being and fading back into the indeterminate primordial state. In Chinese landscape painting, the painting is permeated with precisely the same *Qi/Breath* that permeates the landscape itself.[2] The *Qi/Xiang* or *Qi/Breath/Image*[3] is exactly the same externally as it is "inside" the painting. In the *Nei Jing Tu* what is "outside us," perceived in terms of configurations of the *Qi/Breath* in the world around us, is depicted as simultaneously "inside us." There is no separation, because the same configurations of *Qi/Breath* bring into being and flow through everything - the world around us, the landscape, the painting of the landscape, the inner landscape of our body and even the painting of the inner landscape of our body.

This inner landscape depicts the meditator's body as a reflection of the cosmos; the human body as a microcosm of the universe itself. Inside the body are the sun and the moon, heavenly constellations, the highest mountains and the deepest seas; the farthest manifestations of Heaven and Earth. Even the breaths of the meditator are the breaths of Heaven and Earth.

Current copies of the Diagram of the Inner Circulation (*Nei Jing Tu*) are rubbings derived from an engraved stele in the White Cloud Monastery in Beijing. This monastery dates back to the Tang Dynasty and was the main temple of the Quan Zhen school of Daoism. During the Qing dynasty, the Quan Zhen school was superceded by one of its own branches, the Long Men or "Dragon Gate" school, a school that exists today and carries on the Daoist inner alchemical tradition.[4]

At the Monastery, there are two carved stone steles set into the wall near the ordination platform. One stele is carved with the Diagram of the Inner Circulation (*Nei Jing Tu*) and the other, the Chart of the Preservation of the Primary Vitalities (*Xiu Zhen Quan Lu*). These are two important images and "texts" for the practice of *Nei Dan* - Daoist inner alchemy and meditation. Reproductions of both of these charts have been produced from stone rubbings made at the Bai Yun Monastery.

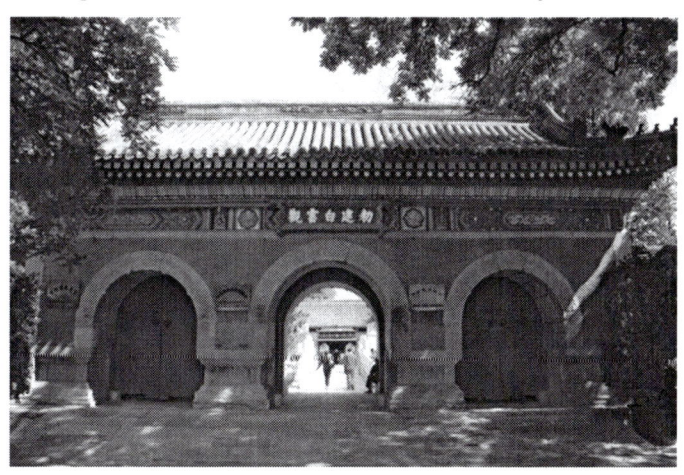

The White Clound Monastery
(photo by Valerie Ghent)

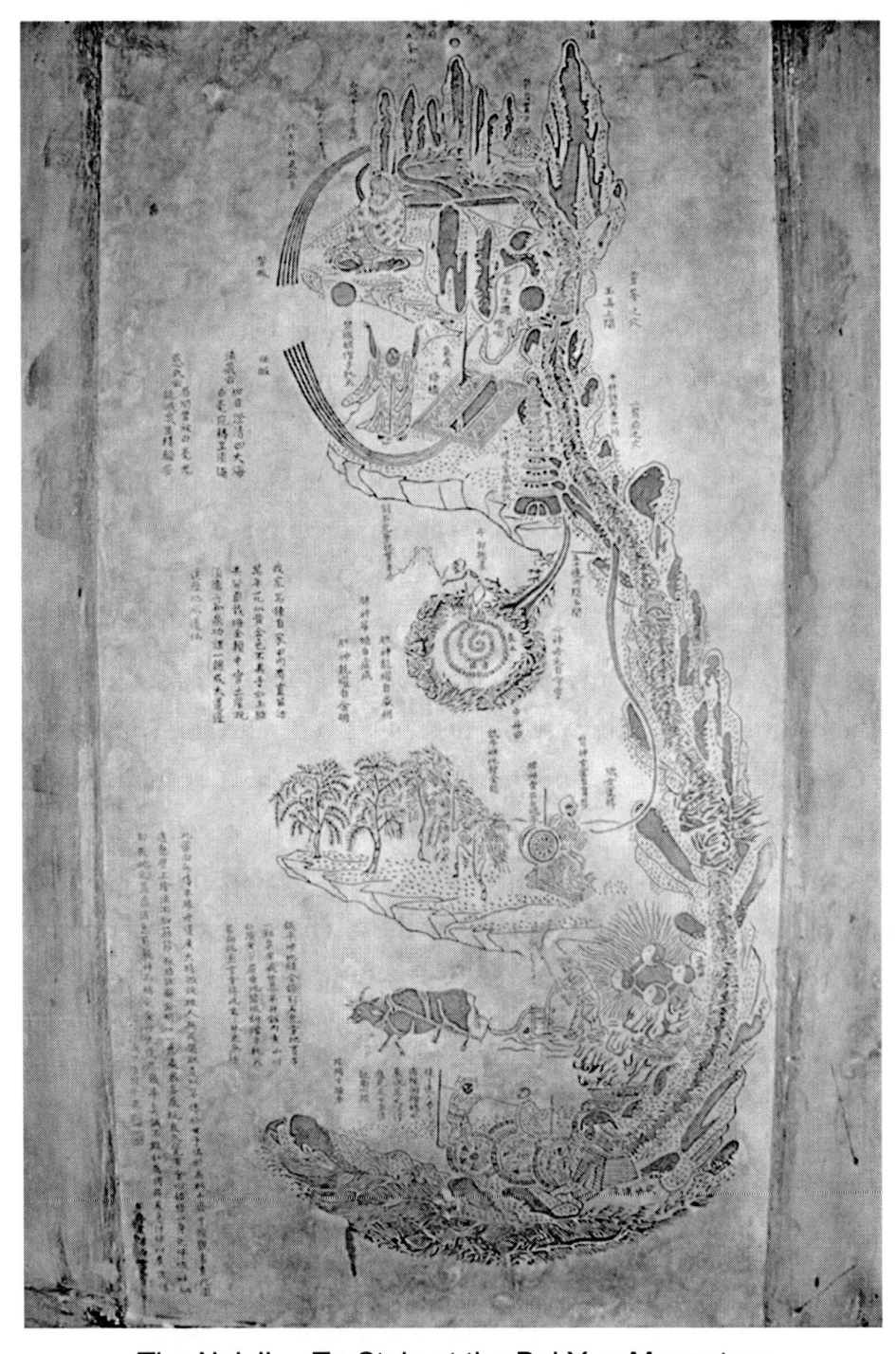

The Nei Jing Tu Stele at the Bai Yun Monastery
(photo by Valerie Ghent)

Nei Jing Tu means literally:

內	*Nei*	inner; inside
經	*Jing*	the warp in a loom
圖	*Tu*	picture; map

The Inner Circulation Diagram is meant to be an aid to those practicing Daoist meditation. It provides imagery which helps one to visualize the Micro-Cosmic Orbit and its connection with the breaths of Heaven and Earth. Understanding the meaning of the images contained in the diagram can help us in practicing the Golden Fluid Returning to Dantian Meditation.

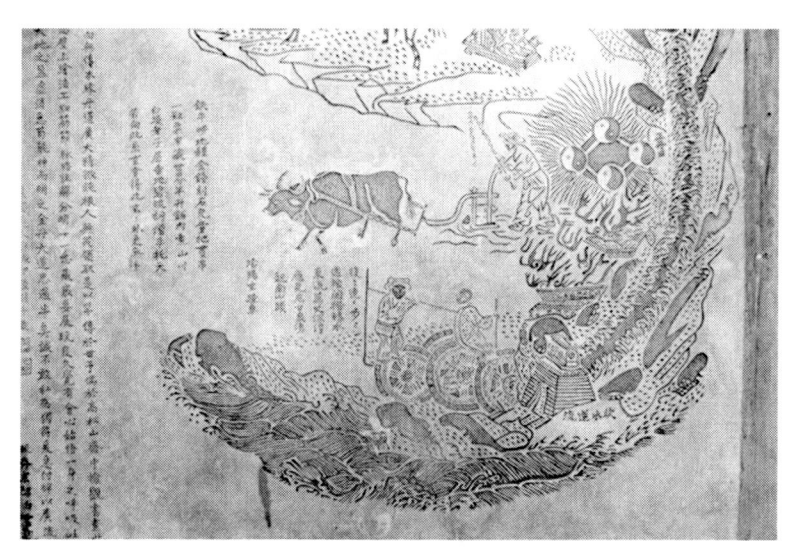

Detail from the Nei Jing Tu Stele
(photo by Valerie Ghent)

圖經內
INNER CLASSIC CHART

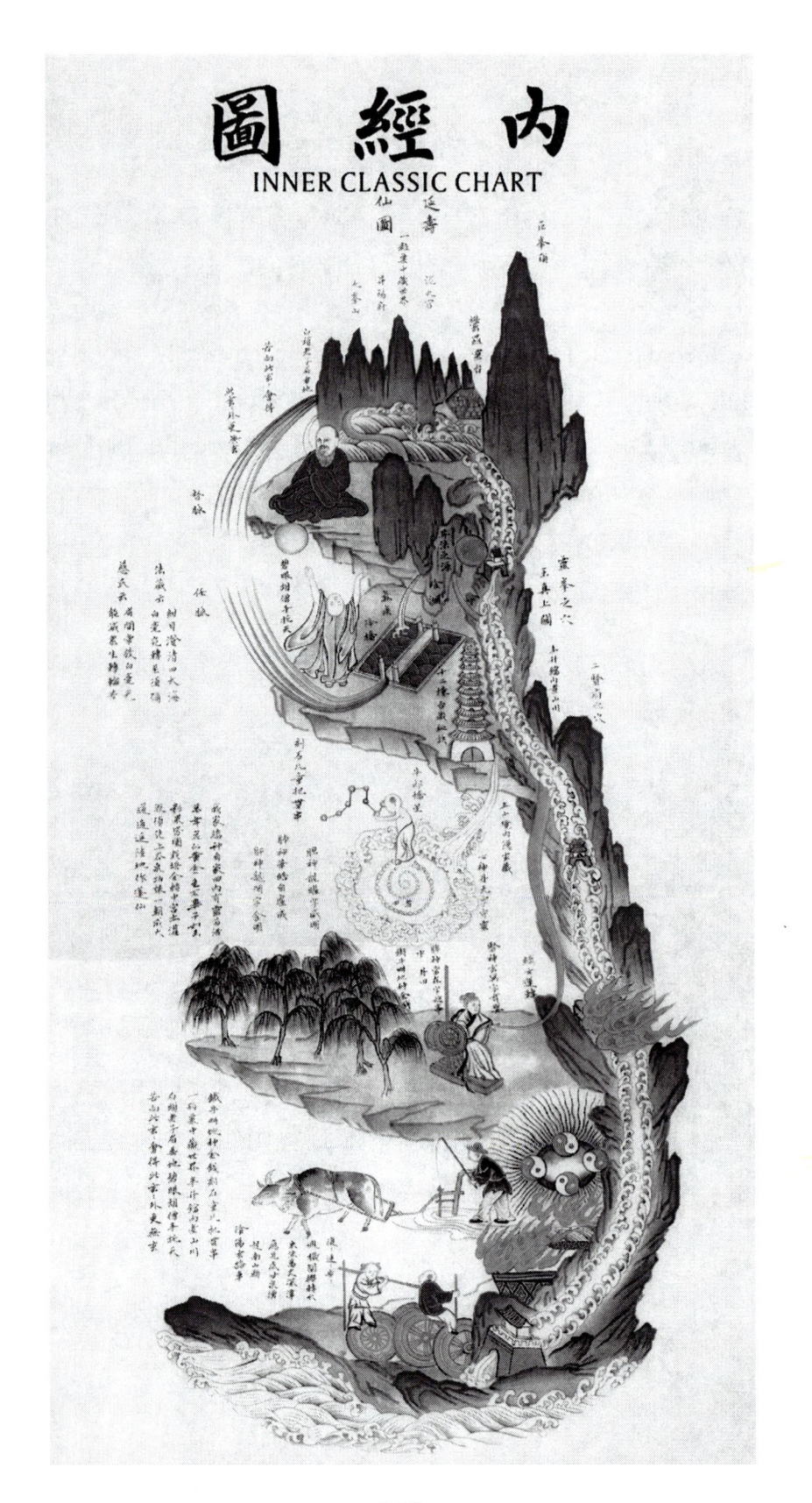

The Weaving Maiden and The Cowherd

In the center of the body, we see the weaving maiden and the cowherd. Their story was told in Lesson Seven. The cowherd holds the Big Dipper, and stands in the tranquil center of a ring of fire (the heart). Below the cowherd is the weaving maiden. Although the maiden is yin, associated with water and the kidneys, she also represents the true yang or (hidden yang) within yin, the hidden fire within Kan-Water – we see fire burning next to her along the spine. She weaves, spinning the *Qi/Breath* and the true yang qi upward behind the heart and up through the throat to connect with the Golden Fluid in the mouth, which then descends. The cowherd is yang, but also represents the true yin within yang – the hidden water within Li-Fire. Therefore, he is associated with the heart and fire. True yin moves downward to reunite with the Kan-Water, just as true yang rises upward to reunite with Li-Fire. The inscription tells us that the cowherd also represents the Gen diagram which is connected to Earth.[5] Gen can also represent the chest in Nei Gong practices.[6]

The weaving maiden also symbolizes the star Vega, the brightest star in the constellation Lyra. The constellation's name is derived from the lyre. The cowherd symbolizes Altair, the brightest star in the Aquila constellation. Altair and Vega are part of the Summer Triangle, which lies directly overhead in mid-northern latitudes during the summer months.

The stars of the dipper are also thought to be yang (male), while the dipper itself is surrounded by black (yin-female) stars. In the human body the male-yang stars of the dipper reside in the heart, while the dark-female stars reside in the brain.[7]

The Ocean in the Lower Abdomen

At the bottom of the diagram is a body of water. This represents the lower abdomen and the *Dantian* or "cinnabar field". Kristofer Schipper explains this more clearly:

> *The Cinnabar Field gives access to the deepest regions of the body, at the bottom of the ocean where a gaping hole siphons off the waters and also the vital energies of the Cinnabar Field. The most frequent names for this abyss are the Gate of Destiny, Obscure Gate, Original Pass, or Terminal Exit (wei lu). Chuang Tzu says: 'the ocean is the greatest of the world's waters, the ten thousand rivers spill into it endlessly and yet it is never too full. Its waters escape through the Terminal Exit and yet it never empties.'*[8]

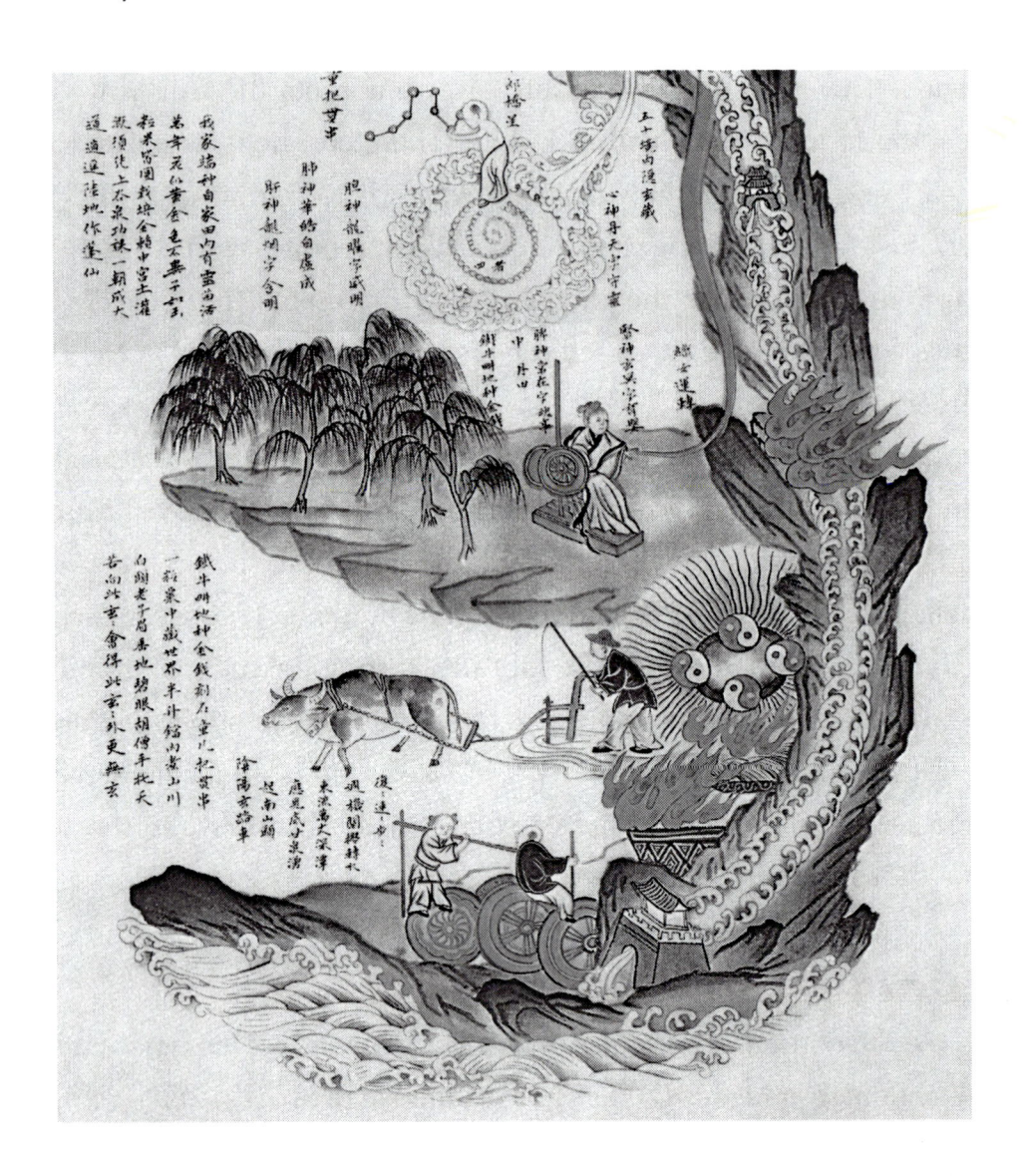

The Boy and Girl and the Treadmill

The boy and girl down at the bottom of the figure represent yin and yang and the two kidneys. They turn a treadmill (the waterwheel), whose turning represents the movement of the *Qi/Breath* and the transformation of yin and yang. The treadmill lifts Kan-Water upward, reversing its normal course. This represents the upward movement of kidney water - *Jing* - and its transformation into *Qi/Breath*.

The Cauldron and the Four Tai Ji Diagrams

The cauldron with fire burning inside it that is above and slightly to the right of the children and the treadmill, represents the fire of the *Mingmen*. Mingmen is the hidden fire within Kan-Water which converts fluids and essence to vapor. Zhang Jing Yue, a doctor from the Ming Dynasty had this to say about the *Mingmen*:

> *Mingmen has fire as a symbol; This refers to the original yang which is the fire that produces things....But how could it all come back to Mingmen? [People] do not know that the Fire in the midst of Water is none other than the First True Qi of Heaven, stored in the midst of Kan ☵. This qi rises from below, connecting to the stomach qi of later heaven to produce transformation, and thus sustains the basis of life (sheng sheng zi ben). Thus the glory of life stems from this root, the functioning of the stove pot from the firewood [beneath it]...*[9]

The four *Tai Ji* diagrams represent the five elements (water, wood, fire, earth and metal) and their associated organs and meridians. Earth is the center around which the other four revolve. It also represents the *Dantian* and its connection to the functioning of the five organs, which relies on the original yang of the *Mingmen*.

The Plow and the Ox

Next to the four *Tai Ji* symbols is a man walking behind an ox pulling a plow. This symbolizes the spleen and stomach and their interconnected processes. The spleen and stomach are associated with the earth element, which nourishes *Qi/Breath* through the intake and transformation of food and grains. The inscription says: *The iron bull tills the earth and sows gold coin.*[10] The iron ox conveys an image of strength and stolidity. The ox represents the motive power for the circulation of *Qi/Breath* and *Yi* (mind-intention) in the body. *The ox represents the physical body itself, and the physical and mental slothfulness which must be overcome to accomplish the alchemical work.*[11] Taken with the inscription, the symbolism is that internal cultivation requires the same diligence, patience and effort as cultivating crops.

The Spinal Cord (The Mountain Path) and the Three Gates

We see the spinal cord and the *Du* vessel portrayed as a twisting mountain path, barred by three gates. These gates are the San Guan or three passes (see Lesson Nine). The first pass is the *Wei Lu*, or tailbone gate. It is just beside the boy and girl on the treadmill. The second gate, the *Jia Ji* Pass, lies on the back on either side of the *Mingmen*, extending upward to the middle back. Some say it is more specifically the area *Yu Kou* located at the level of the 6th and 7th thoracic vertebrae.[12] The third gate is the *Yu Zhen Guan* (Jade Pillow Pass) at the occipital region.

The Grove of Trees

Next to the weaving maiden, on her left, is a copse of trees. The trees represent the liver and gallbladder. These organs are associated with the wood element and assist the spleen in raising the clear *Yang Qi* upward. The liver *Qi/Breath* is said to rise on the left side of the body, while the lung *Qi/Breath* descends on the right.

This hidden yang within yin of the *Mingmen* is known as the *Qing Long* "Green Dragon," or the *Long Lei Zhi Huo* "Dragon-Thunder Fire", both of which are associated with the liver. The hidden yin within yang-fire in the heart is known as the *Bai Hu*, or "White Tiger," which is associated with the lungs. The Dragon is associated with Heaven and ascends upward. The White Tiger is associated with Earth and crouches on the ground. The liver energy spreads upward like a tree, lifting *Qi/Breath* upward. Lung energy spreads downward like mist or dew covering the earth. These two create a balanced upward spreading and downward dispersing dynamic.

The energies (*Shenqi*) of the liver (the *Hun*) are born out of Kidney-Water (*Jing*). Although rooted in the blood, these energies are themselves light and airy and rise upward, just as plants and trees move upward and outward in the Spring, but are rooted in the wet earth, nourished by Spring rains.

The energies of the Lung (the *Po*) are heavier yin-fluid essences that, although rooted in the *Qi/Breath*, are drawn downward toward the earth. These fluids perfuse through the body and into the organs and tissues like autumn mists or dew spreading out over the earth and percolating into the ground.

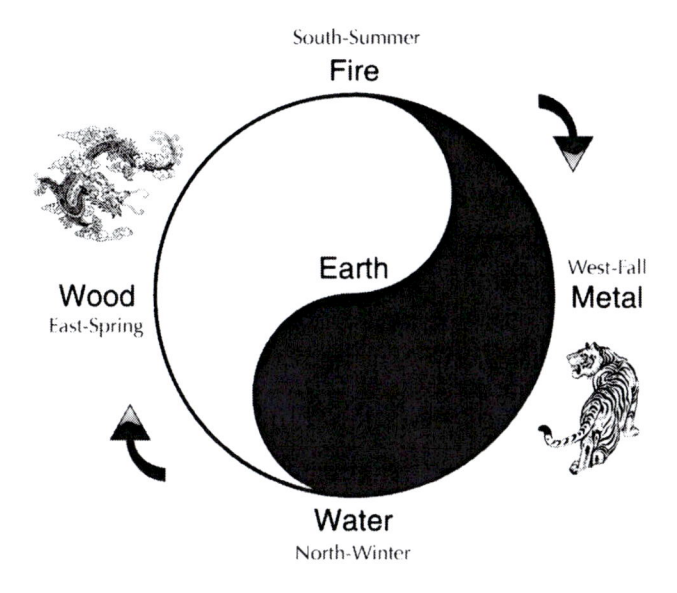

In the preceding diagram, the liver and the dragon are connected symbols, both representing movement being incited. In the spring, the Green Dragon awakens from its winter hibernation under the earth and rushes upward toward Heaven creating spring thunderstorms. In autumn, as we move toward the stillness of winter, the White Tiger crouches on the Earth. In human beings, the awakening of the dragon-thunder fire is connected to the activation and transformation of yin and yang; water and fire. This transformation is continued by the descending action of the lungs. Earth lies at the very center of this diagram, the hub around which these processes revolve. Earth is associated with the spleen and stomach, these organs themselves organs of transformation through the digestion and assimilation of food.

Normally, as in the diagram above, the energies of the liver and Green Dragon move upward on the left and the energies of the lung and White Tiger move downward on the right. However, in the Diagram of the Inner Circulation the grove of trees is on the right and on the left, fluid moves downward from the twelve-story pagoda (the throat). This represents the idea that through the practice of Daoist meditation, the normal orientation of the Five Agents, and therefore of the liver and lungs, is reversed or flipped. In this way, yin (water) and yang (fire) interact and transform, and *Jing, Qi/Breath* and *Shen* interact properly. When this reversal occurs it said that: *The liver is wood which flourishes in the west; the lungs are metal which comes forth from the east.*[13]

The Pagoda

The pagoda with its twelve tiers represents the cartilaginous rings of the trachea. The saliva or "Golden Fluid" is swallowed and passes down through the throat and trachea, following the *Ren* vessel, by straightening and extending the neck.

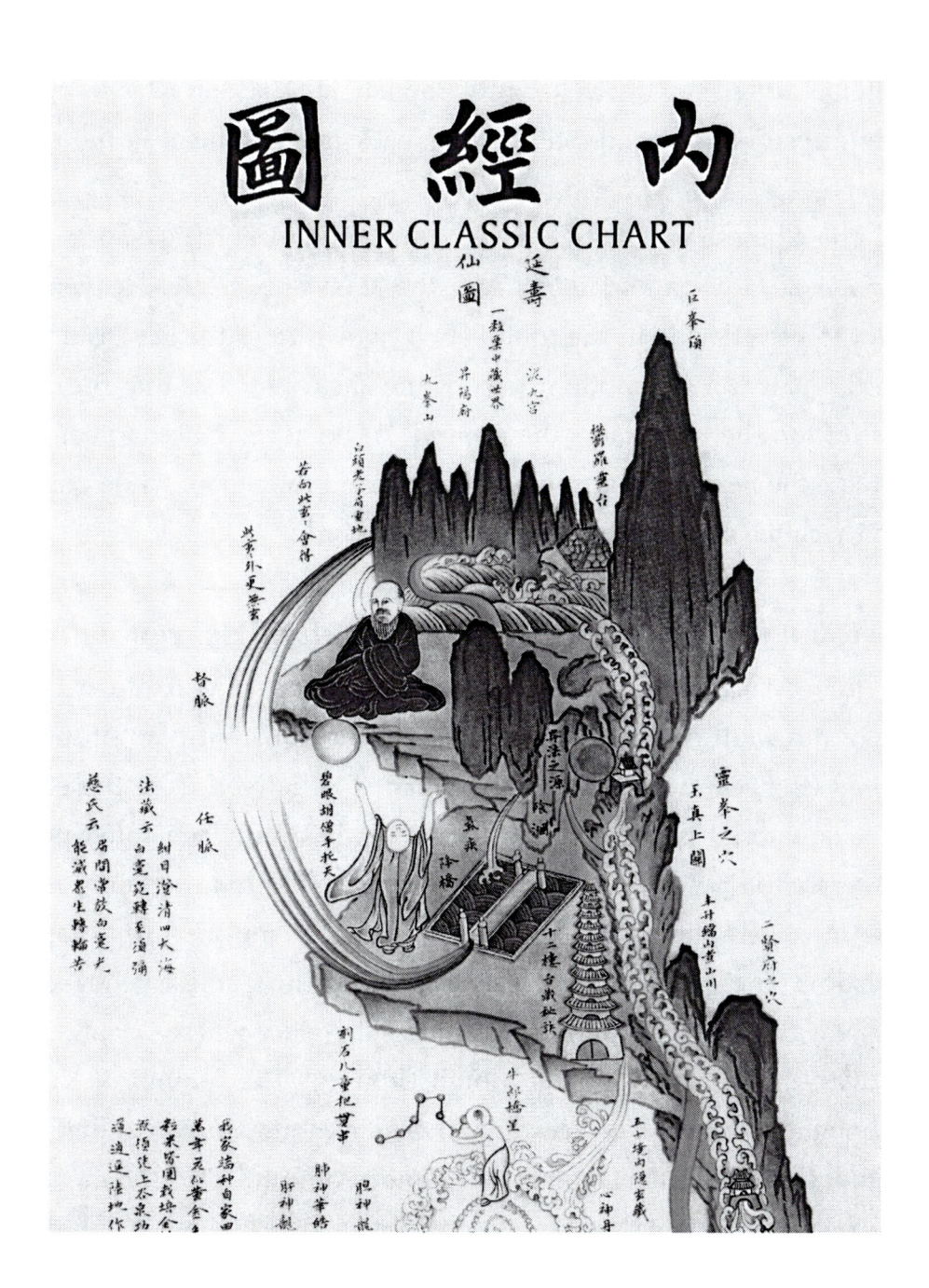

The Eyes (Sun and Moon)

The two circles in the head area of the diagram are the two eyes. The eyes also represent the sun and the moon. The left eye depicts the sun and the right eye the moon.[14] Between the eyebrows is the *Yin Tang* acupoint, which lies on the pathway of the *Du* vessel. Directly behind *Yin*

Tang is the *Ming Tang* (明堂 "Brightness Hall").[15] The character Ming (明) depicts the sun and moon. Still farther back into the head is the upper *Dantian*.

The Chinese say that "Heaven is round and Earth is square." An old image of Heaven and Earth was the shell of a turtle. Heaven was thought to be reflected in the round shell (which faces the sky) and Earth in the flat plastron (the bottom part of the shell structure that forms the "belly" of the shell and faces the ground).[16] The head of human beings is round like the heavens that contain the sun and the moon, while our feet, which touch the earth, are roughly square shaped.

The Mountains and the Head as the Vault of Heaven

John Major feels that "Heaven being round" has to do with the shape of the vault of the sky overhead and the apparent path of the sun overhead (the ecliptic). "Earth being square" is derived from the elliptic and the equatorial plane, creating four roughly evenly separated points: two intersection points which are the spring and autumn equinoxes and two points where the elliptic and the equatorial plane are farthest apart - the solstices. These four points create a square.[17] The Chinese believed that the cosmic axis, or world pillar (*axis mundi*), the place where sky and earth meet, was in Northern China at Mount Kunlun.[18] The summit of Kunlun was thought to touch the polestar.[19] The nine mountain peaks that form the top of the head can also represent Mount Kunlun.[20] Daoists often refer to the head as Mount Kunlun. In the Daoist worldview, Kunlun is a mountain of the western seas, considered to be the home of the Daoist immortals. However, it is also the name of a region in the brain, a cavern in which the *Ni Wan* (see below) resides.[21] In the Golden Fluid Returning to Dantian Meditation, we hold "Kunlun" in our two hands as we let the *Qi/Breath* circulate through the Micro-Cosmic Orbit.

At the foot of the mountains in the diagram is a river (the Yellow

River), which emanates from Mount Kunlun.[22] The water in this iverrepresents "divine water," the *yin qi* that ultimately descends to return to the *Dantian*.

The Brain and the Marrow

The brain is referred to as the *Ni Wan* ("mudball" or "sticky pellet"). In Chinese medicine, the brain is called the "sea of marrow." Some think this name refers to the Cerebrospinal Fluid (CSF) which is produced in the ventricles of the brain and circulates through the ventricles and the spinal cord. The spinal cord itself is sometimes called the "Marrow Path."[23] The marrow has a direct connection with the *Jing*, which is thought to produce both the marrow that fills the head and bone marrow.

The Daoist classic *Ling Jian Zi* says that the *Qi/Breath* of the heart is connected with the *Ni Wan* Palace. The *Ni Wan* is also called the *Huang Ting* ("Yellow Palace"). In the Daoist tradition, *Huang Ting* is the central palace of the nine palaces in the brain. This central palace is thought to be the place where the various *Shen* meet and the location of the material basis of the *Shen*.[24] The connection between the heart, the kidneys (*Mingmen* and *Dantian*) and brain is elucidated to in the following statements:

- *When marrow is full, thinking is clear.*
- *The marrow is rooted in the Jing and connects with Du Mo.*
- *When the Mingmen warms and nourishes, the marrow is full.*[25]

The Du 24 acu-point (*Shen Ting* "spirit court") is said to directly access *Ni Wan*.

The Two Monks

The old man at the top is generally thought to be Lao Zi, and the monk below him is called the "blue-eyed monk" representing Bodhidharma (Da Mo), the Buddhist Monk who traveled from India to China in the Fifth Century and is credited with transmitting Chan Buddhism to China. The old man also represents the yin alchemical agent lead, while the monk below with his arms in the air represents the yang alchemical agent mercury. The relationship of these two, in which the old man (yin) is placed over the younger monk (yang), implies that there is yin within yang and yang within yin, as well as the concept that the reversal of these energies is part of the meditation process.[26] The poem that appears nearby on the Inner Circulation Diagram says:

> *The white bearded old man's eyebrows hang down to the earth;*
>
> *The blue eyed foreign monk supports heaven with his arms.*[27]

The juxtaposition of Lao Zi and Da Mo may also be an oblique reference to the syncretic nature of Daoism and Buddhism. Legend has it that Lao Zi disappeared into the West and his teaching informed Buddhist philosophical ideas. Later, Da Mo brought Chan Buddhism to China and his teachings influenced the practice of Daoist meditation.

Another interpretation of the images of the two monks is that they are synonyms for essence (*Jing*) and spirit (*Shen*): The "white haired old man" is a code for *Jing* and the "barbarian with jade-blue eyes" refers to *Shen*.[28]

The Rainbow

The rainbow-like ribbons surrounding the two monks in the front left side of the head represent the connection of the *Ren* and *Du* vessels in the head. The lower set of ribbons represent the connection, via the tongue, of *Ren Mo* and *Du Mo* to a pool of liquid. This is the "Jade Pool". the place where the saliva collects.

The Bridge, the Spring and The Pool

Next to the monk standing with his arms upraised (Da Mo), is a pool of water spanned by a bridge. A spring pours down into the pool. This is the "Jade Pool," the place in the mouth where the saliva accumulates. The pool is spanned by the Upper Magpie Bridge (the tongue) which, in touching the upper palate, connects *Ren Mo* and *Du Mo* inside the mouth and simultaneously stimulates the flow of saliva. Once collected, the saliva is swallowed and passes through the throat to the *Dantian* where it replenishes the essence.

Keys to the Code:

Understanding Daoist Symbolism

乾　坤

Qian　Kun

Keys to the Code:

At its heart, Daoist meditation is a simple and practical method of establishing unity between our internal environment and the external world so that we can engage with life in a clear and present way. Daoist symbolism is designed to aid this process by providing images that bypass our normal thought patterns. If you understand the language of Daoism, its code, then you can read books on Daoism and Daoist meditation and understand what lies beneath the surface. What follows are a series of discussions and keys (taking a page from Joseph Needham)[1] that will help you decode and understand Daoist symbols and images. The cosmological system of the *Yi Jing* (*I-Ching*: Book of Changes), and its numerological associations, as well as Daoist alchemical metaphors, are repeatedly interwoven into the tapestry of Daoist imagery and symbolism and will be discussed in detail in this section.

The first key depicted on the following page outlines some of the associations connected with the images of Heaven (Qian) and Earth (Kun), the fundamental expressions of yin and yang. Qian is represented by three yang-solid lines. These lines, read from bottom to top, are pushing upward with vigor and strength. Kun is represented by three broken-yin lines that are open, receptive, and yielding. Qian-Heaven is the "Creative" and Kun-Earth, the "Receptive." Kun-Earth is the concrete realization of Qian-Heaven's creative impetus. Qian and Kun are like positive and negative poles, with an oscillating current vibrating back and forth between them. In human beings and in the natural world, Qian and Kun are represented by Li-Fire and Kan-Water respectively.

HEAVEN-QIAN 乾
☰

Heaven 天 (Tian)

Yang 陽

Upper, Ascending 上 (Shang)

Sun 日 (Ri)

Hard, Strong 刚 (Gang)

Movement, Action 动 (Dong)

Male 男 (Nan)

South 南 (Nan)

Head 头 (Tou)

Round 圆 (Yuan)

Light 光 (Guang)

Outer; External 外 (Wai)

Fire Trigram-Li Gua 離 卦
☲

EARTH-KUN 坤
☷

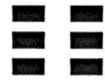

Earth 土 (Tu)

Yin 陰

Lower, Descending 下 (Xia)

Moon 月 (Yue)

Soft, Pliable 柔 (Rou)

Stillness, Quiescence 静 (Jing)

Female 女 (Nu)

North 北 (Bei)

Legs, Feet 腿 (Tui)

Square 方 (Fang)

Dark 暗 (An)

Inner; Internal 內 (Nei)

Water Trigram-Kan Gua 坎 卦
☵

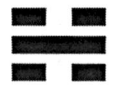

From the fundamental interaction of Heaven and Earth other oppositional forces manifest. This is represented in the "Pre-Heaven" (*Xian Tian*) arrangement of the Eight Trigrams shown below. The term "Pre-Heaven" refers to the unchanging and eternal nature of these dynamic universal forces.

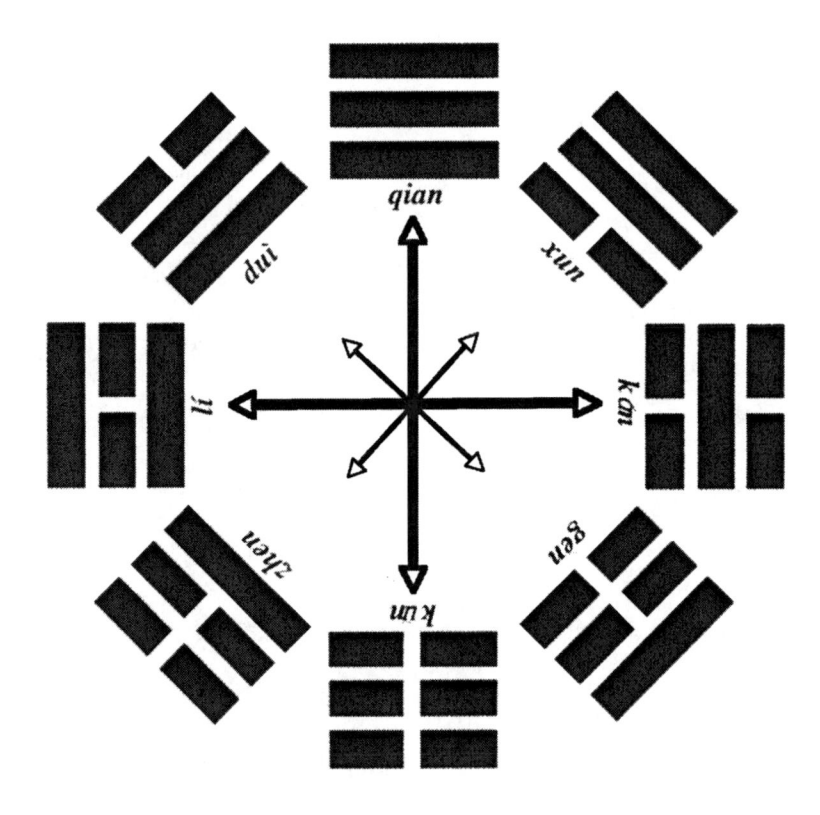

Pre-Heaven Arrangement of The Eight Trigrams

Qian Diagram: The Creative
Image: Heaven
Nature: Creativity; Strength; Vigor
Trigram: Qian is 3 links (Qian San Lian)

Kun Diagram: The Receptive
Image: Earth
Nature: Yielding; Receptivity
Trigram: Kun is Separated into Six Sections (Kun Liu Duan)

Zhen Diagram: The Arousing
Image: Thunder
Nature: Exciting; Arousing; Emerging; Renewal
Trigram: Zhen is an Upturned Jar (Zhen Yang Yu)

Gen Diagram: Keeping Still
Image: Mountain
Nature: Immovable; Stillness;
Trigram: Gen is a Toppled Bowl (Gen Fu Wan)

Li Diagram: The Clinging
Image: Fire
Nature: Attachment; Cohesion
Trigram: Li is Empty in the Middle (Li Zhong Xu)

Kan Diagram: The Abysmal
Image: Water
Nature: Enveloping; Adaptable
Trigram: Kan is Full in the Middle (Kan Zhong Man)

Dui Diagram: The Joyous
Image: Lake
Nature: Joy; Pleasure
Trigram: Dui Lacks in the Top (Dui Shang Que)

Xun Diagram: The Gentle
Image: Wind; Wood
Nature: Penetrating; Pliable
Trigram: Xun is Broken in the Bottom (Xun Xia Duan)

When these forces operate within us, in the temporal realm of change and transformation, they are arranged differently and referred to as the "Post-Heaven" (*Hou Tian*) arrangement. Rather than the trigrams acting in polar opposition, they move cyclically, representing our experience of human life that unfolds "between Heaven and Earth." In the Pre-Heaven arrangement of the eight trigrams Qian-Heaven and Kun-Earth were the fundamental operating forces. In the Post-Heaven Arrangement, Li-Fire and Kan-Water replace Qian and Kun on the vertical axis of the diagram and become the fundamental operating forces.

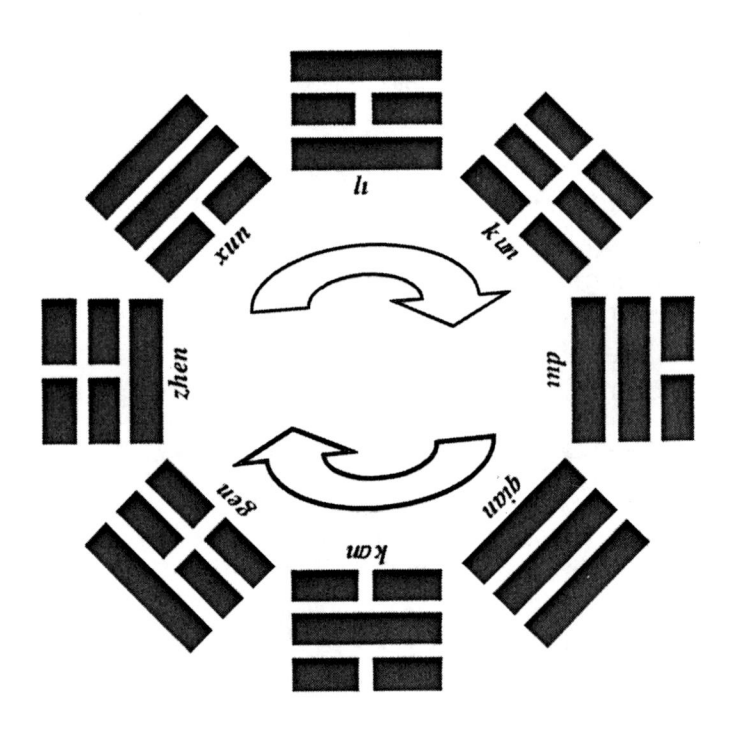

Post-Heaven Arrangement of The Eight Trigrams

When Li and Kan are used to represent Qian and Kun, they in turn take on numerous associations which can also act as alternative ways of talking about Li, Kan, Qian and Kun.

Fire-Li 離 ☲	Water-Kan 坎 ☵
Yang 陽	Yin 陰
Fire 火 (Huo)	Water 水 (Shui)
Heart 心 (Xin)	Kidney 腎 (Shen)
Upper, Ascending 上 (Shang)	Lower, Descending 下 (Xia)
Upward Transmitting 升 (Sheng)	Downward Showering 降 (Jiang)
Floating 浮 (Fu)	Sinking 沉 (Chen)
Sun 日 (Ri)	Moon 月 (Yue)
Hard, Strong 剛 (Gang)	Soft, Pliable 柔 (Rou)
Movement, Action 動 (Dong)	Stillness, Quiescence 静 (Jing)
Celestial (Ethereal) Soul 魂 (Hun)	Earthly (Animal) Spirit 魄 (Po)
Qi/Breath 氣 (Qi)	Saliva 唾 (Tuo)
Shen 神 (Spirit)	Essence 精 (Jing)
Red 紅 (Hong)	Black 黑 (Hei)
Male 男 (Nan)	Female 女 (Nu)
South 南 (Nan)	North 北 (Bei)
Mercury 汞 (Gong)	Lead 铅 (Qian)
Li Maiden 离女 (Li Nu)	Kan Boy 坎男 (Kan Nan)
Heaven Trigram- Qian Gua 乾卦	Earth Trigram-Li Gua 坤卦
Green Dragon 青龍 (Qing Long) of the Western Seas	White Tiger 白虎 (Bai Hu) of the Eastern Mountains
Vermillion Bird (Zhu Que) 朱雀 of the South	Black Tortoise (Xuan Wu) 玄武 of the North

Qian and Kun are considered to be "the door and the gate" through which change arises, and "the father and mother" of all emblems that represent change.[2] Qian entrusts its generative potential to Kun, and in so doing becomes Li. Kun receives the essence of Qian to bring it to fruition, and in so doing becomes Kan.[3] The two solid (yang) outer lines of the Li-Fire trigram embrace or act as the outer walls of Kun (true yin) represented by the broken line at the center of the Li trigram. The two broken (yin) lines of the Kan-Water trigram embrace or act as the outer walls of Qian (true yang), represented by the solid line at the center of the Kan trigram. Fabrizio Pregadio says that if the walls are curved into semi-cicles they form a wheel. The central hub of the wheel represents the emptiness from which existence and change emanate. The axle passing through the hub is the axis of Qian and Kun, and the wheels connecting to the axle with their spokes radiating outward, cyclically changing position in time and space, are Li and Kan.[4] This is represented by the Tai Ji diagram, attributed to Chen Tuan that we saw earlier in Lesson 4.

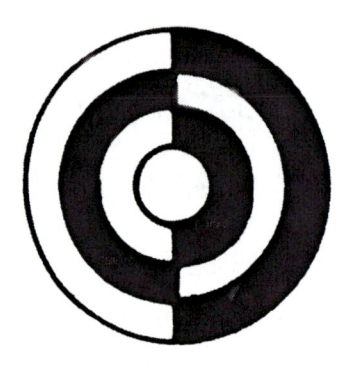

Li-Fire: Li-Fire symbolizes the clarity of consciousness and depth of feeling and warmth that is associated with the human mind and the human heart.[5] In the center of the trigram, the broken-yin line represents receptiveness and openness that is characteristic of a clear and conscious mind. However, it can also represent the mental conditioning and circular thinking that insinuates itself into the heart and mind, making us cling and attend to the external and superficial.[6]

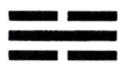

☵

Kan-Water: Water represents adaptability, fluidity, and formlessness.[7] The solid-yang line in the center of the trigram represents the original yang, the intrinsic, "real" wisdom embedded within us that often lies hidden or buried.[8]

The Five Powers

The Eight Trigrams manifest as the *Wu Xing* or *Wu De*, five dynamic interacting forces. Hence they are often called the Five Powers, Five Agents or Five Forces: Water, Wood, Fire, Earth and Metal. They are also known as the Five Elements or Five Phases, because each force both acts and is acted upon. The Eight Trigrams manifest within the Five Forces as follows:

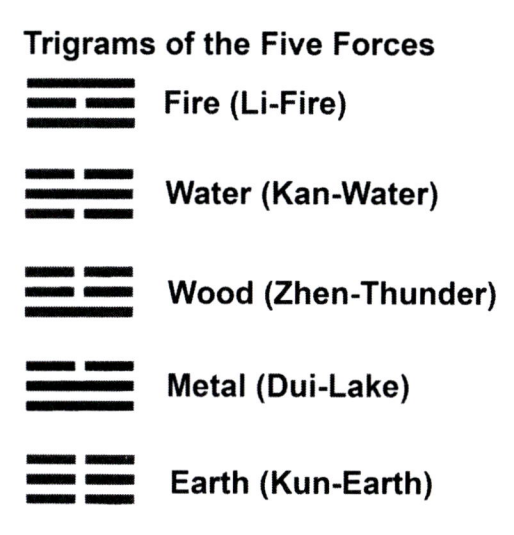

Trigrams of the Five Forces

☲ Fire (Li-Fire)

☵ Water (Kan-Water)

☳ Wood (Zhen-Thunder)

☱ Metal (Dui-Lake)

☷ Earth (Kun-Earth)

Each force has it own intrinsic movements and properties, but Earth lies at the center of their interaction and movement.

Li-Fire

Zhen-Wood

Kun- Earth

Dui-Metal

Kan-Water

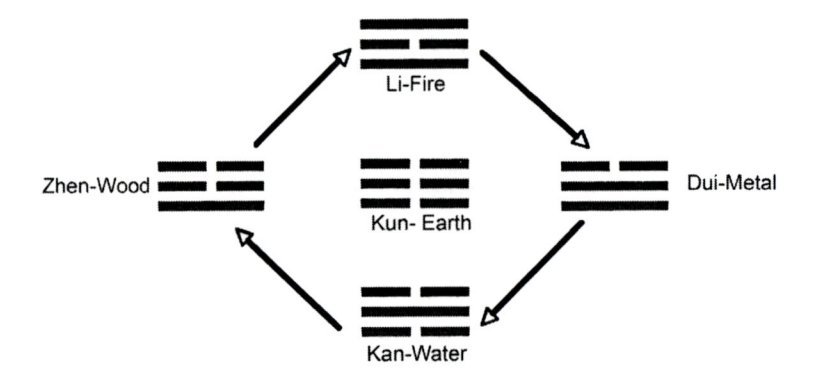

Cyclical Movement of the Five Forces

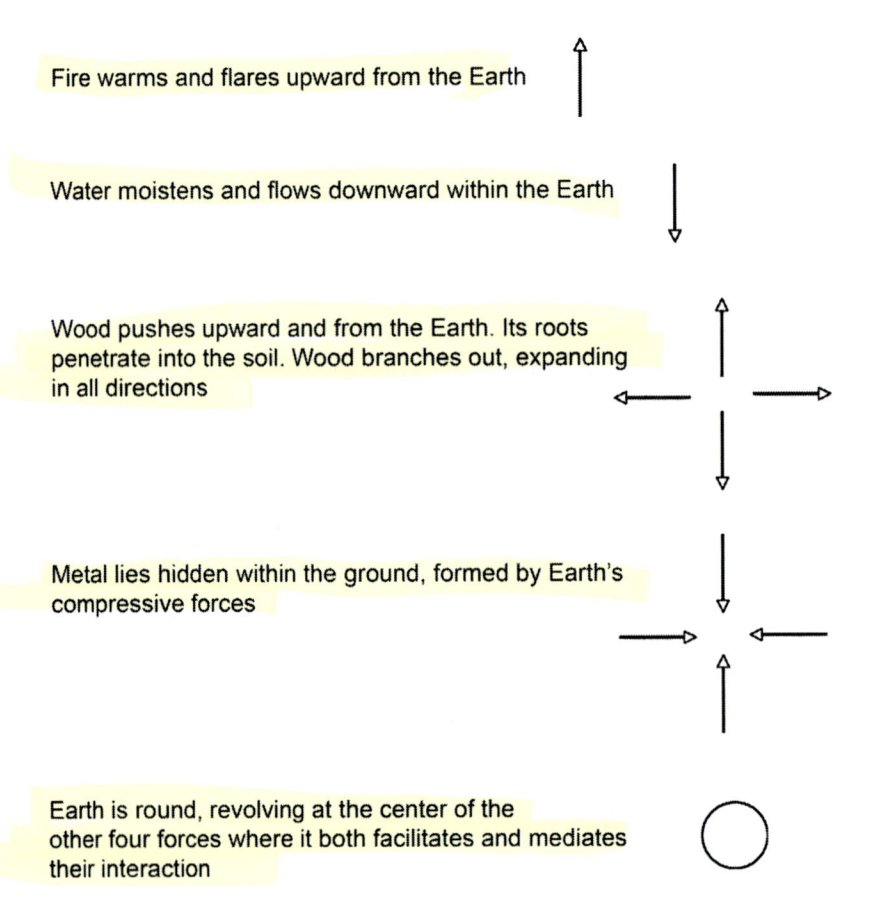

Fire warms and flares upward from the Earth

Water moistens and flows downward within the Earth

Wood pushes upward and from the Earth. Its roots penetrate into the soil. Wood branches out, expanding in all directions

Metal lies hidden within the ground, formed by Earth's compressive forces

Earth is round, revolving at the center of the other four forces where it both facilitates and mediates their interaction

Actions of the Five Forces
Adpated from *Hua Yo T'ai Chi Ch'uan: The Kung Fu of Six Combinations and Eight Methods (Liu He Ba Fa)*, by Kahn Foxx

The cyclical movements of the five forces and their association with the trigrams and the internal organs are depicted below.

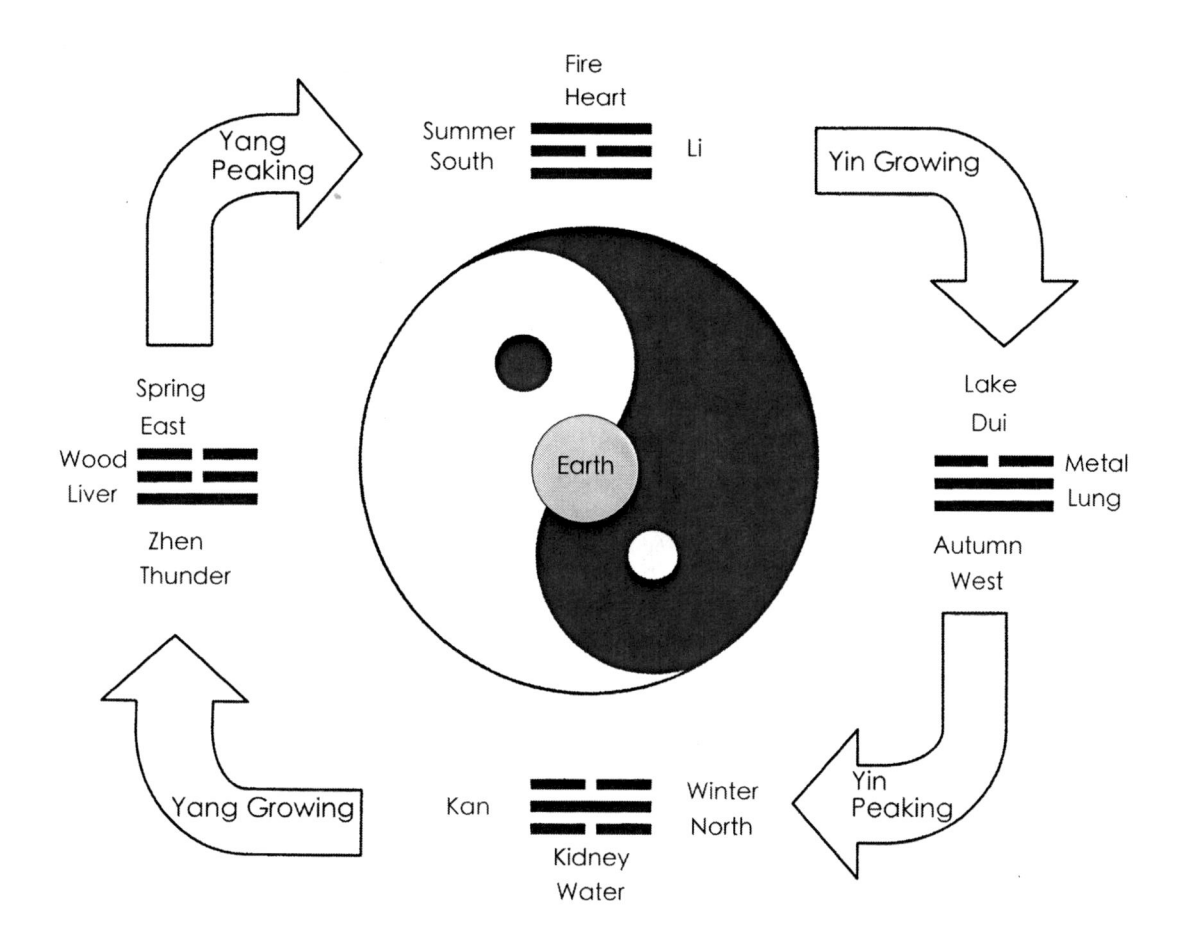

The Five Powers are sometimes obliquely referred to by using the names of the mythological or emblematic animals:

Green or Azure Dragon - Wood

Red or Vermillion Bird - Fire

White Tiger - Metal

Black Tortoise/Black Snake - Water

Yellow Dragon - Earth

The Black Tortoise/Snake is also known as *Xuan Wu*: Dark Warrior of the North. The diagram below shows the seal forms of the four emblematic animals. In the center is the ideogram for Earth.

Fire-Li (Heart)
Red Bird

Wood-Spring (Liver)
Green Dragon

Earth
Yellow Dragon

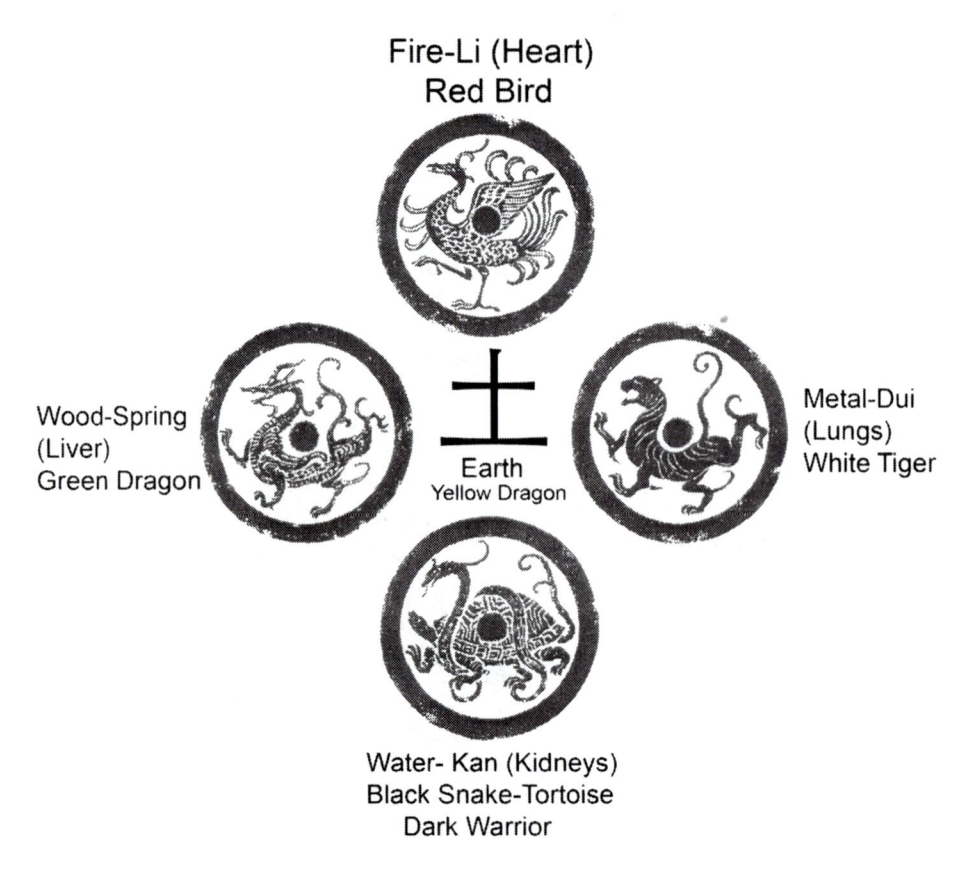

Metal-Dui (Lungs)
White Tiger

Water- Kan (Kidneys)
Black Snake-Tortoise
Dark Warrior

The Five Emblematic Animals

Dragon and Tiger

Prior to the creation of the *Tai Ji* diagram (in the Eighth Century), yin and yang were symbolized by the Tiger and the Dragon. The Dragon was associated with Heaven and the Tiger with Earth. Fire and Water are associated with the South and the North respectively. The Green Dragon is related to Wood in the East and the White Tiger to Metal in the West. Simultaneously, the Dragon and Tiger are manifestations of the two fundamental operating forces in the post-heaven arrangement of the trigrams: the Green Dragon is associated with Li-Fire and the White Tiger is associated with Kan-Water. Together they symbolize movement and change:

Wood becoming Fire - The Dragon Leaping Upward
Metal becoming Water - The Tiger Pouncing on Its Prey

The Dragon is yang. It symbolizes the movement of life growing upward and outward like a plant growing from a seed. The Green Dragon represents the spring thunder and rains that nourish living things. It represents the incitement of life and movement, hence its association with thunder. The Tiger is yin. The White Tiger represents autumn, the time when growing things begin to withdraw into the earth, when the first frost comes to kill living things. Hence the Tiger can represent death, but also the quiet and stillness of late autumn as it moves into winter. The Tiger is therefore associated with the still lake whose depths cannot be seen. In this context, the Dagon and Tiger together represent the natural cycle of life and death that moves through us and all living things.

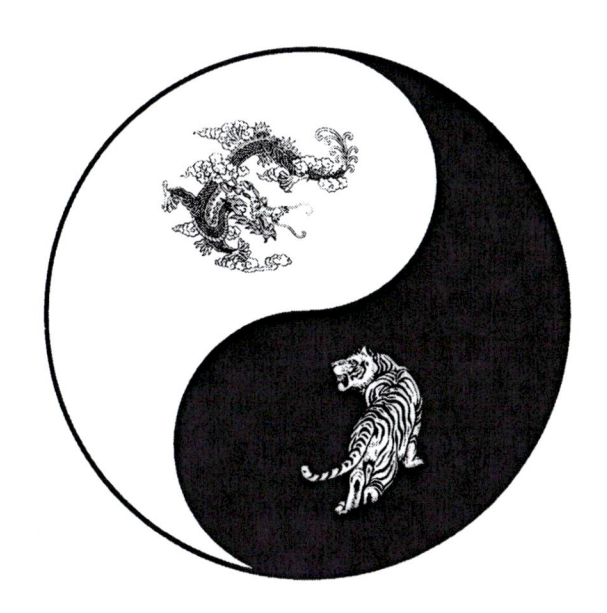

The Dragon is associated with Zhen-Thunder - excitation and movement. The Tiger is associated with Dui-Lake, which in turn represents joy, sensibility and feeling. These qualities are conveyed in the Chinese saying:

> When the tiger roars the valley wind comes.
> When the dragon arises great clouds appear.[9]

The Shen: The Five Psycho-Spiritual Faculties

Shen, in its purest form, is the spark which enters the void and creates the "One", thereby differentiating the universe into Yin and Yang. In human beings, *Shen* comes into being when the essences of the two parents meet (ie: at conception). When this spark of creative energy is formed, it activates the *Qi/Breath* and forms the *Jing*, which in turn leads to the development of the other bodily processes. *The Shen designates the very principle of life - that which transforms an assemblage of matter into a human being.*[10] *Shen* is not a single thing, but a collection of forces and manifestations rooted in the physical reality of human beings. In the *Ling Shu*, the Five *Shen* are described as follows:

> *When two seminal essences [**Jing**] strike each other, it is spoken of as spirit [**Shen**]. Following the spirit as it goes and comes is the animal spirit [**Po**]. Together with the seminal essence as it exits or enters is that which is spoken of as the human soul [**Hun**]. Those which are in accord with control of myriad things are the heart and mind. The mind has recall which is spoken of as thought [**Yi**]. Thought is that which, when kept, is spoken of as will [**Zhi**]. From will and that which is kept and changed is spoken of as consideration. From consideration of distant longings comes planning. From planning, to managing of myriad things, is that which is spoken of as wisdom.*[11]

This quote from the *Ling Shu* shows that although various aspects of the *Shen* may be differentiated, they operate collectively, and as a collective are they are referred to as "the *Shen*." However, in order to avoid confusion, hereafter the term Heart-*Shen* will refer to the psycho-spiritual faculty housed by the Heart. It can loosely be defined as consciousness.

The Five Psycho-Spiritual Faculties are difficult to define in English, but they can roughly be described as follows:

神	Shen	(Consciousness; Mind)	Housed by the Heart
魂	Hun	(Celestial Soul; Ethereal Soul)	Housed by the Liver
魄	Po	(Animal Spirit; Corporeal Soul)	Housed by the Lungs
意	Yi	(Thought; Intention)	Housed by the Spleen
志	Zhi	(Will; Original Vital Impulse)	Housed by the Kidneys

These spiritual faculties enter consciousness under the control of the Heart-*Shen*. When the heart is untroubled, then the mind and the spirit are clear. If disturbed the mind becomes jittery, cloudy, and vague, and one's memory may be faulty. The Heart-*Shen* shines out through a person's eyes. If the eyes are clear, and the gaze piercing and vibrant, then the Heart-*Shen* is calm and resides comfortably inside the heart. When the eyes are manic and staring, or cloudy, dull and lifeless, then the Spirit is disturbed.

The *Hun* and the *Po* are Yin and Yang aspects of the Shen:

Heart Shen

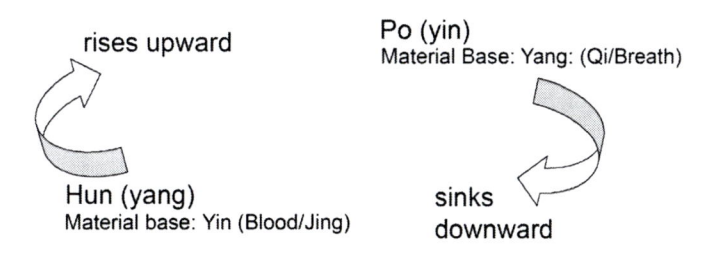

rises upward

Hun (yang)
Material base: Yin (Blood/Jing)

Po (yin)
Material Base: Yang: (Qi/Breath)

sinks downward

One view of the *Hun* and *Po* is that they exist independently of the body and unite with it at birth. They operate with the body's organic functioning and then at death separate from it, the *Po* returning to Earth with the bones, while the *Hun* returns to Heaven, merging with the cosmic yang energies. This perspective views *Hun*, *Po* and *Shen* as a micro-cosmic expression of the Three Powers: Heaven, Earth and human beings.[12] Traditional Chinese medicine generally takes the view that the Five *Shen* represent various aspects of consciousness and psycho-emotional activity that is a by-product of the physical activity of the internal organs and their organic and functional interactions. The *Hun* and *Po* are often referred to as the etheric and corporeal "souls" respectively. Although the term "souls" is often used to refer to the *Hun* and *Po*, they are better seen as two types or two groups of vital entities that are the source of life in every individual. They can be referred to as singular or plural. The *Hun* is/are yang, luminous, and volatile, while the *Po* is/are yin, somber, and heavy.[13]

The *Hun* is housed by the liver and associated with Wood. The *Hun* is tied to the spark of creativity, the ability to see with the inner eye. The *Hun* sees a course of action and sets it in motion. Like the Green Dragon, the *Hun* rise upward and *lift themselves in intelligence, knowledge, sensitivity, spirituality and imagination.*[14] The *Hun* comes and goes, moves up and down freely under the auspices of Heart-*Shen*.[15] The blood contains and holds the *Hun*.

The *Po* is stored in the lungs and is associated with Metal. It is the aspect of the lungs associated with spirit and mental functions. The *Po* is associated with the rhythm of our breath and with the unconscious life rhythms. It is yin, but is rooted in the yang of the *Qi/Breath*. The *Po* controls "*entering and exiting,*"[16] a reference not only to the endless breaths moving in and out of our body, but also to our sensations and reactions. Like the White Tiger roaring or crouching to pounce, this movement downward toward the earth is the expression of our sensations and reactions, our instinctive movements and thrusts.[17]

Some sources say that the sensory perceptions of the eyes and ears comprise the *Po*. When these become *Qi/Breath*, it is called the *Hun*.[18] The

Hun is said to have three "spirits" which are akin to the Three Treasures, and the *Po* seven "souls" which are related to the emotions and senses.

Hun
1. *Qi*/Breath
2. *Shen*
3. *Jing*

Po
1. Joy
2. Anger
3. Pleasure
4. Sorrow
5. Like
6. Dislike
7. Desire

In Daoist meditation and internal alchemy it is believed that the passions of the *Po* usually dominate the *Hun*, causing the life force to decay. In Daoist thought, by concentrating the vital forces within the body through meditative practices, one attempts to reverse this dynamic - one's emotions, passions and desires then become ruled by the *Hun*. This is another aspect of the reversal of the Five Powers, discussed later in this section.[19]   The Heart-*Shen* is consciousness, our aware and engaged mind - *the intelligence of existence.*[20] When the heart is calm, it clearly reflects the perceptions from the outside world. When the heart is overloaded or stirred up by our emotions and desires, the reflections are muddled and unclear. This is why the heart must be empty for the Heart-*Shen* to be clear and reflect properly. If the heart is overburdened or overfilled with the outside world, then the Heart-*Shen* can become disturbed.

Yi is often translated as "mind-intention." It is a manifestation of the *Qi*-Dynamic of Earth and its associated organs, the spleen and stomach. This is the transformative aspect of the *Qi/Breath* that changes and moves, processes and distributes. When the Heart-*Shen* applies itself there is intent,[21] the ability to reflect upon and put into action ideas, and express those ideas through language. The intent of the Heart-*Shen* manifests itself in speech, thought, and action.

The *Zhi*, housed by the kidneys, is the underlying driving force of the organism, the will to live. The *Zhi* is "thought which is kept." Thought and intention which endures and becomes permanent. It is the aspect of the Shen which supplies the ongoing aspirations and drives that allows us to achieve a goal. The *Zhi* supplies the underlying motive power for the *Hun* and the *Po*, which, through them, unites the will with the consciousness of the Heart-*Shen*. The *Zhi* is connected to the deeper aspects of intelligence, memory and wisdom, that are tied into the *Jing* (essence).

The interactions of the Five Psycho-Spiritual Faculties can be diagrammed in a way that resembles the Five Element cycles. The *Po, Hun* and *Yi* lie between the *Zhi* and the *Shen*:

InterAction of The Five Shen

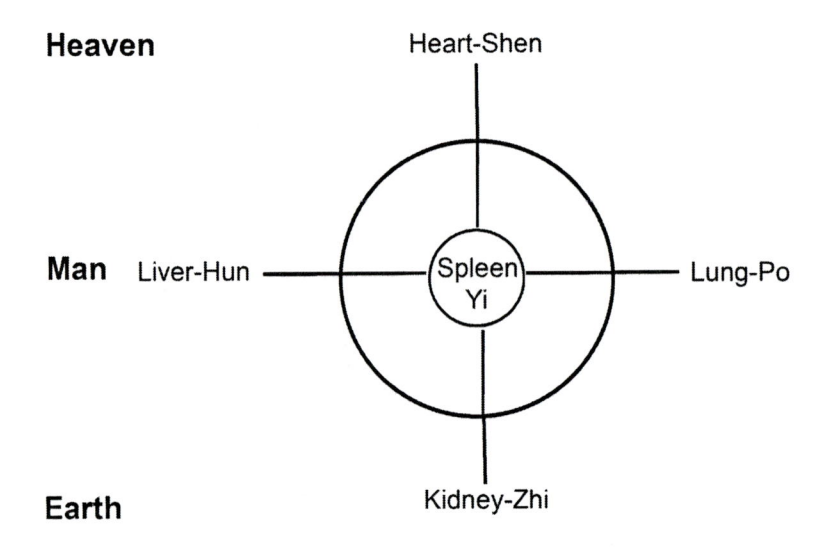

Heaven — Heart-Shen

Man — Liver-Hun — Spleen Yi — Lung-Po

Earth — Kidney-Zhi

The *Hun* and *Po* form one axis connecting with a second axis, that of the *Shen* and *Zhi*. The *Hun* and *Po* are driven by the force of the *Zhi* as it rises up to join with the Heart-Mind characterized by the *Shen*. The central hub, *Yi* (thought and reflection) ruled by the Spleen, is an extension of the Heart-Mind and acts as a liaison between the other psycho-spiritual faculties, bringing them together in thought and speech. Discussion of the Five Shen necessitates their separation into five distinct parts, but it is important to keep in mind that they represent different phases of the same continuous Heart-Mind, and therefore act as one organic whole engaging in a process of continuous transformation and change.

Alchemy: Lead and Mercury

Much like their western counterparts, Chinese alchemists also tried to transmute base metals like lead into gold. However, the focus of alchemy in Daoism was on longevity and immortality rather than wealth. It was thought that the refinement and ingestion of these transmuted metals could enhance longevity and even confer immortality. The Daoists also employed alchemical terms to describe the internal interactions of the body and mind during meditation. Hence Daoist meditation is sometimes referred to as "Internal Alchemy," a term which has led to much confusion over the centuries, in some cases leading to the ingestion of toxic metals like cinnabar in the pursuit of immortality.

Cinnabar (red mercuric sulphide), known as "red mercury," is vermillion or bright red in color. Cinnabar was mined since the Neolithic Age for use both as a pigment and for its mercury content. Through the centuries it has been the main source of mercury. To produce liquid mercury ("living metal" or "quicksilver"), cinnabar ore is crushed and heated so it is separated from sulfur, which then evaporates. Similarly, lead is usually found in ore with other metals. The ore is roasted to convert it to metallic form, and then the other metals separate out and are removed. Images of extracting pure metals from ores are metaphors for the effort, concentration and physical practice inherent in meditation or "internal alchemy." Hence the yang in the *Dantian* is often referred to as the "furnace" (*lu*) and the yin as the "reaction vessel" (*ding*).

Practitioners of internal alchemy in China felt the Fire of the heart was red like cinnabar and the Water of the kidneys was dark like lead.[22] The term *Dantian* literally means "cinnabar field" and conveys the image of fields of cinnabar in the lower abdomen, chest and head. These fields of cinnabar are thought to be alchemically acted upon by the Fire of the heart and the Water of the kidneys. Just as smelting or refining of ore produces "true mercury" (also called the Dragon) and "true lead" (also called the Tiger), this process involves the application of fire and water. True mercury is the Dragon hidden in cinnabar and true lead is the Tiger hidden within black (unprocessed) lead. Inside mercury is a radiant golden color and inside lead, a silver color. Joseph Needham says the yellow and white colors together are the "Golden Sprout" (*Huang Ya*)[23], also known as the "Golden Elixir." Therefore in "Internal Alchemy," the ingredients that produce the golden pill of "immortality" are actually not metals but the Five Forces (or Five alchemical agents) and their interactions.

The "true mercury" extracted from cinnabar is the true yin-*qi* associated with Fire and the heart and liver. It is the true yin-essence of the heart. It is also the conscious, discerning mind. The "true lead" extracted from the unprocessed lead ore is associated with Water, the lungs and the kidneys. It is the true yang-*qi* of the kidneys. It is also true, intuitive knowledge or wisdom. When mercury and lead come together, when true essence and qi unite (the conscious mind and the intuitive wisdom unite) through the refining process of meditation, then the body is regenerated, the Three Treasures unite and combine and consciousness is unified.

                    Vermillion Bird
                    Original Spirit (Yuan Shen 元神)
                    Red Cinnabar - Fire
                              2

Green Dragon   Yellow Dragon   White Tiger
Inner Nature (Xing 性)   Intention (Yi 意)   Sentiment/Quality
True Mercury - Wood   Earth   (Qing 情)
         3   5   True Lead - Metal
                                                             4

                    Black Snake/Tortoise
                    Original Essence (Yuan Jing 元精)
                    Dark Lead - Water
                              1

Associations of the Five Agents

(Derived from *Foundations of Internal Alchemy: The Taoist Practice Of Neidan* by Wang Mu - Translated by Fabrizio Pregadio). p. 126.

These concepts are brought together in the picture below, a rendering of a drawing from the *Xing Ming Gui Zhi*, an alchemical text from the Ming Dynasty. It depicts the Tiger and Dragon pouring the yin and yang energies (lead and mercury) into an alchemical vessel. The girl astride the dragon represents true yin (true lead) within yang, while the boy mounted on the tiger represents true yang (true mercury) within yin. The drawing is titled the "copulation of the dragon and tiger" or the "marriage of the dragon and tiger." The drawing simultaneously references the transmutation of metals into their pure forms, Daoist meditation and internal alchemical practices as well as Daoist sexual alchemy.[24]

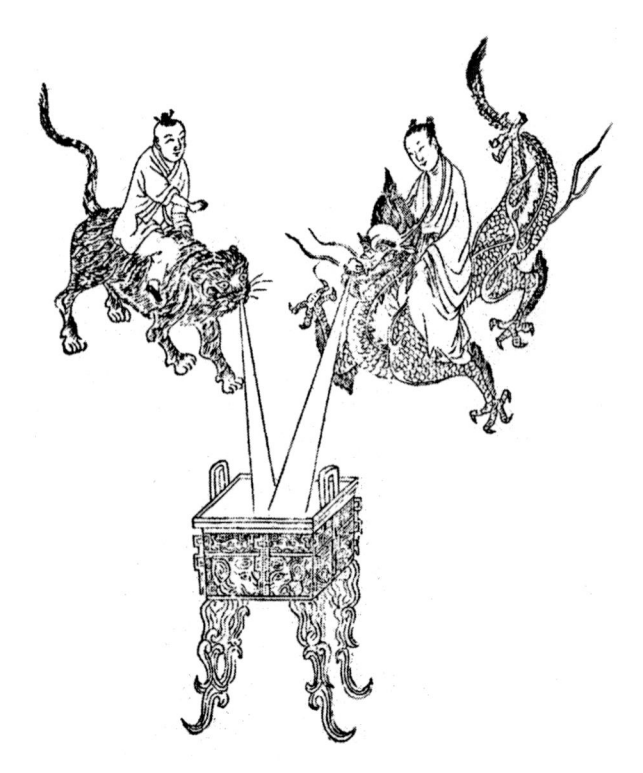

The Marriage of The Dragon and Tiger
From the Directions for Endowment & Vitality (Xing Ming Gui Zhi), a Ming dynasty text on Inner Alchemy

The reaction vessel or tripod (ding) and the stove (lu) are metaphors derived from external alchemy and the extraction of pure metals from base metals. The tripod is *Niwan* (upper *Dantian*) and the stove is the lower *Dantian*.[25] In the cyclical circulation of the *Ren* and the *Du* channels, a refining process is envisioned in which ore is removed to extract gold. This is merely another way of saying that one is refining the Three Treasures (*San Bao*): *Jing, Qi/Breath* and *Shen*.

In this context, many Daoist internal alchemical texts speak of "firing times" or *Huohuo*. This is yet another metaphor taken from external alchemy and metallurgy - adjusting the fire or heat in order to properly extract, refine and temper metal. Often these firing times were associated with the twelve sovereign hexagrams and the phases of the moon, as well as the Twelve Earthly Stems associated with two hour divisions of the day that delineate the waxing and waning of yin and yang during the 24 hour daily cycle.

The Twelve Earthly Stems

yang stems

1. 子	Zi	Rat (鼠)	11 p.m. to 1 a.m.	Fu Hexagram
2. 丑	Chou	Ox (牛)	1 to 3 a.m.	Lin Hexagram
3. 寅	Yin	Tiger (虎)	3 to 5 a.m.	Tai Hexagram
4. 卯	Mao	Rabbit (兔)	5 to 7 a.m.	Da Zhuang Hexagram
5. 辰	Chen	Dragon (龍)	7 to 9 a.m.	Guai Hexagram
6. 巳	Si	Snake (蛇)	9 to 11 a.m.	Qian Hexagram

yin stems

7. 午	Wu	Horse (馬)	11 a.m. to 1 p.m.	Gou Hexagram
8. 未	Wei	Sheep (羊)	1 to 3 p.m.	Dun Hexagram
9. 申	Shen	Monkey (猴)	3 to 5 p.m.	Pi Hexagram
10. 酉	You	Rooster (雞)	5 to 7 p.m.	Guan Hexagram
11. 戌	Xu	Dog (狗)	7 to 9 p.m.	Bo Hexagram
12. 亥	Hai	Boar (豬)	9 to 11 p.m.	Kun Hexagram

In inner alchemy and meditation, "Fire" is taken to mean the "Original Spirit" and the application of the True Intention (*Zhen Yi*) which must coalesce with the breath and the essence.[26] The hexagrams and the firing times then simply refer to the natural cyclical transformation and coalescing of yin and yang as they circulate through the Ren and Du channels, rather than specific practice times and arcane methods. This is made clear in the 11th century Daoist text *Awakening to Reality* (*Wuzhen Pi*), written by Zhang Bo Duan, in which he disparages those who misunderstand and cling to these images:

The images of the hexagrams are established on the basis of their meanings:

Understand the images and forget the words - the idea is clear of itself.

The whole world delusively clings to the images:

They practice the "breaths of the hexagrams" and hope thereby to rise in flight.[27]

Alchemical Images: Key

HEAVEN-QIAN 乾
Heaven 天 (Tian)

Fire-Li Trigram 離卦
Fire 火 (Huo)
Heart 心 (Xin)

Shen 神

Green Dragon (East) 青龍 (Qing Long)

Mercury 汞 (Gong)

Furnace (Lu) 爐

Conscious Mind

EARTH-KUN 坤
Earth 土 (Tu)

Water-Kan Trigram 坎卦
Water 水 (Shui)
Kidney 腎 (Shen)

Jing 精

Lead 鉛 (Qian)
Reaction Vessel (Ding) 鼎

White Tiger (West) 白虎 (Bai Hu)

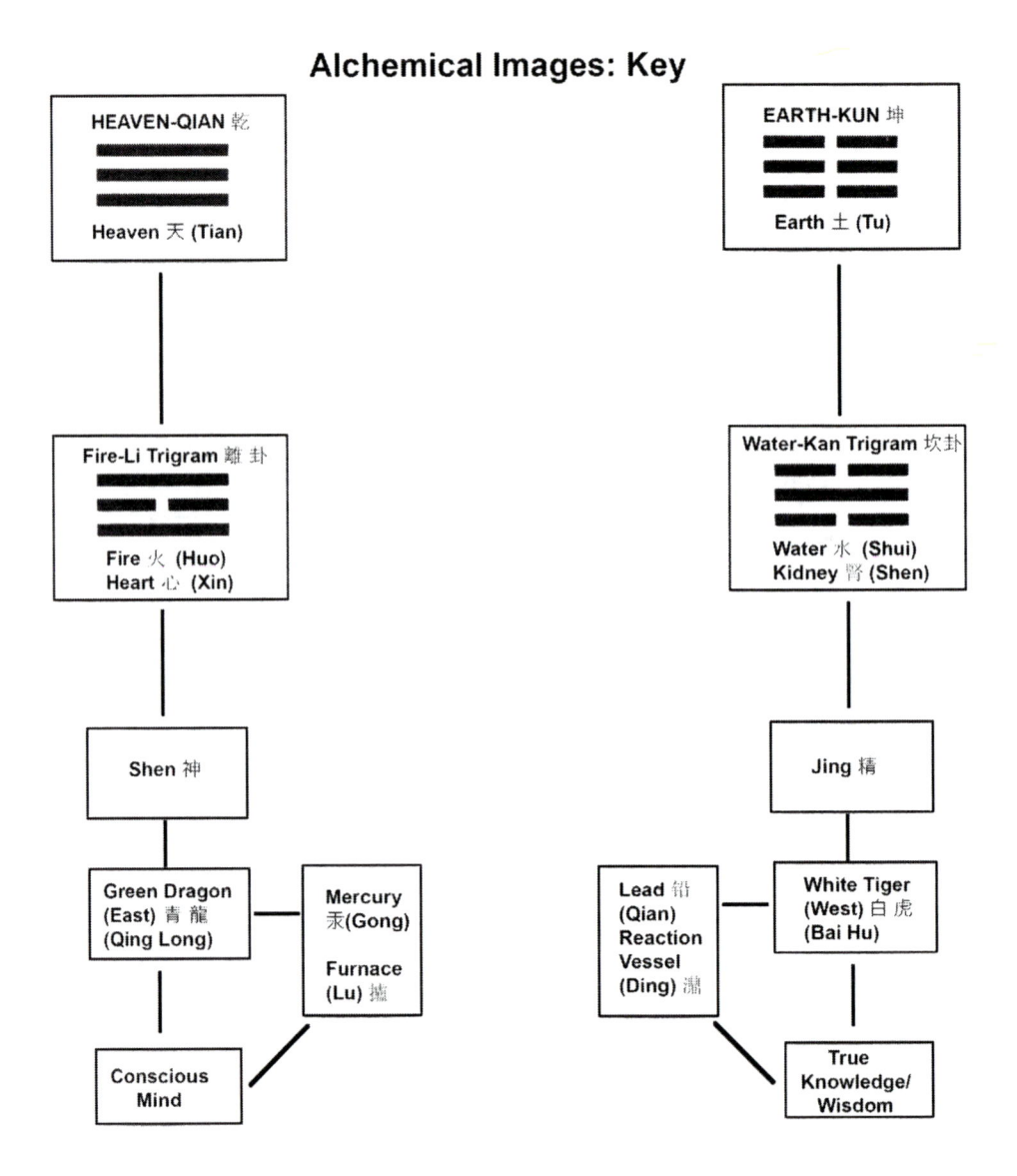

True Knowledge/ Wisdom

Reversing the Movement of the Five Powers

One of the aims of Daoist internal alchemy and Daoist meditation is a reversal of the movement of the Five Powers and the movements of the Green Dragon and the White Tiger. If yang is allowed to expand endlessly without the regressive, inward movement of yin, the cycle ultimately moves out of balance. Uncontrolled, the upward and outward movement of the liver and the downward spreading action of the lung - the action of the dragon flying upward and the tiger pouncing (i.e. undirected creativity and excitement coupled with feeling, emotion and sensation) - spirals outward, depleting the body's essence and disturbing the harmony of the spirit. In his translation of *The Secret of the Golden Flower*, Richard Wilhelm tells us that the normal movement of the Five Powers allows our passions, emotions and interactions with the external world to lead and influence the clarity of the heart-mind and spirit, thereby gradually diminishing our life energies and dimming the clarity of our Spirit. This is a kind of death.[28]

Li Dong Yuan (1180-1251), one of the great physicians of the Jin-Yuan dynasties, described this dynamic in his *Treatise on Yin and Yang, Longevity and Pre-Mature Death* from the *Pi Wei Lun* (Treatise on the Spleen and Stomach). As the title of his book implies, Li stresses the central role of the Earth Phase (spleen-stomach) in the movement of the five phases. Li tells us that with the arrival of spring, the deep-lying, hidden yin of Earth changes, stirs, begins to soar and becomes airborne above. *This is none other than the engendering and effusing qi. Upbearing to the extreme it floats. This is none other than flourishing qi.* This upward, rightward turning of the Five Phases (Five Powers) is what Li calls the *clear yang of heaven.* When yang retreats in autumn, it is downborne and falls downward to form the gathering, constraining, reducing and killing qi. At the extreme of down-bearing there is *storing and sealing.* The Five Phases therefore turn left and downward to form the *turbid yin of earth. Yin governs killing and therefore administers pre-mature death*[29].

Because yang governs life, and also long life, it must be managed so that the aspect of the Earth Phase that flourishes in the spring and summer is encouraged and does not sink to overwhelm and damage the kidneys and essence (*Jing*). If one can achieve this, then the killing energy of autumn and winter *is not imposed* and one will live out their full lifespan. Li tells us that in order to do this one must manage activity and rest (*stirring and stopping*) and eating and drinking. Most importantly, *there must be clearness [or tranquility] and there must be stillness [or quiet].*[30]

Li Dong Yuan indirectly refers to the still clarity of meditation, through which a liberation from the external takes place and with it, an upward circulation of the life energies. The body is then rejuvenated and the spirit becomes bright and clear. This is a kind of rebirth, a sloughing off of the physical body so that the spirit can ascend to become numinous. Perhaps this is the origin of Daoist images of creating a golden elixir inside the body, that acts like a fetus giving birth to a new existence. The process of gathering and storing Qi/Breath in the Dantian is sometimes referred to as: *Like a child nourished in the womb or like a hen incubating an egg.*[31]

According to Daoist Liu Yi Ming:

> Golden Elixir is another name for one's fundamental nature, formed out of primeval inchoateness. There is no other Golden Elixir outside one's fundamental nature. Every human being has this Golden Elixir complete in himself: it is entirely realized in everybody. It is neither more in a sage, nor less in an ordinary person. It is the seed of Immortals and Buddhas, and the root of worthies and sages.[32]

The diagram below is adapted from an illustration in the *Xing Ming Gui Zhi*, a Ming Dynasty text on meditation and internal alchemy. The four animals representing water, wood, fire and metal are depicted around an alchemical crucible or tripod (which represents the realized will/intention: *Zhen Yi*).[33] The tripod, the object of the gaze of the four emblematic animals, is placed in the area corresponding to earth, where the alchemical reaction, the interaction and ultimately reversal or inversion of the five phases, takes place.

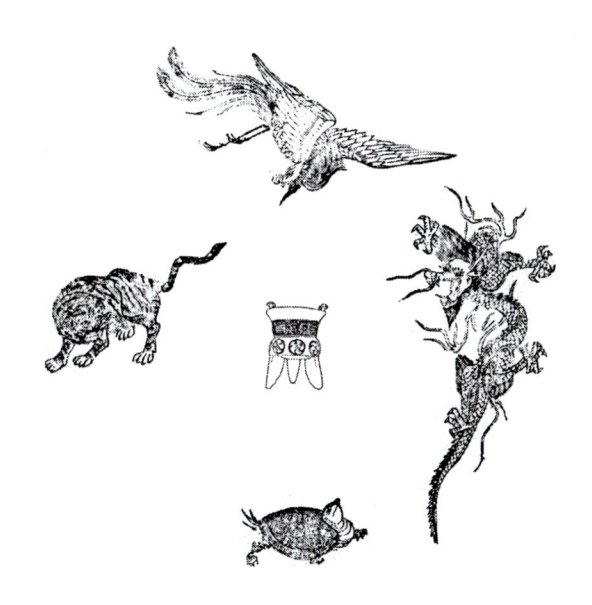

The Dragon is the yang component of the essence (*Qi/Breath*) and the Tiger is the yin component (*Jing*). Lead and the Tiger are the yang-vapor represented by the solid line within the Water trigram, while the Dragon and the mercury are the yin-fluid represented by the broken middle line of the Fire trigram. In his introduction to the *Cantong Qi*, Fabrizio Pregadio explains the alchemical model succinctly: The alchemical process is a means of retracing the stages of the generative process of the cosmos in reverse sequence in order to return to and rediscover the "One Breath":

- Black Lead is Water (Kan) and Cinnabar is Fire (Li)
- True Lead (True Yang) is Metal (Qian) and True Mercury (True Yin) is Wood (Kun)
- When the cycle of the Five Powers (Phases) reverts, Water (Black Lead) generates Metal (True Lead) and Fire (Cinnabar) generates Wood (True Mercury)
- Soil (Earth) allows the chemical process to unfold. The central position of soil is emblematic of the essential unity of True Yin and True Yang. The True Yang half of this unity is represented by the middle solid line of Kan-Water diagram. It is Qian. The True Yin

half of this unity is represented by the middle, broken line of the Li-Fire diagram. It is Kun.[34] These interactions are illustrated in the diagrams below.

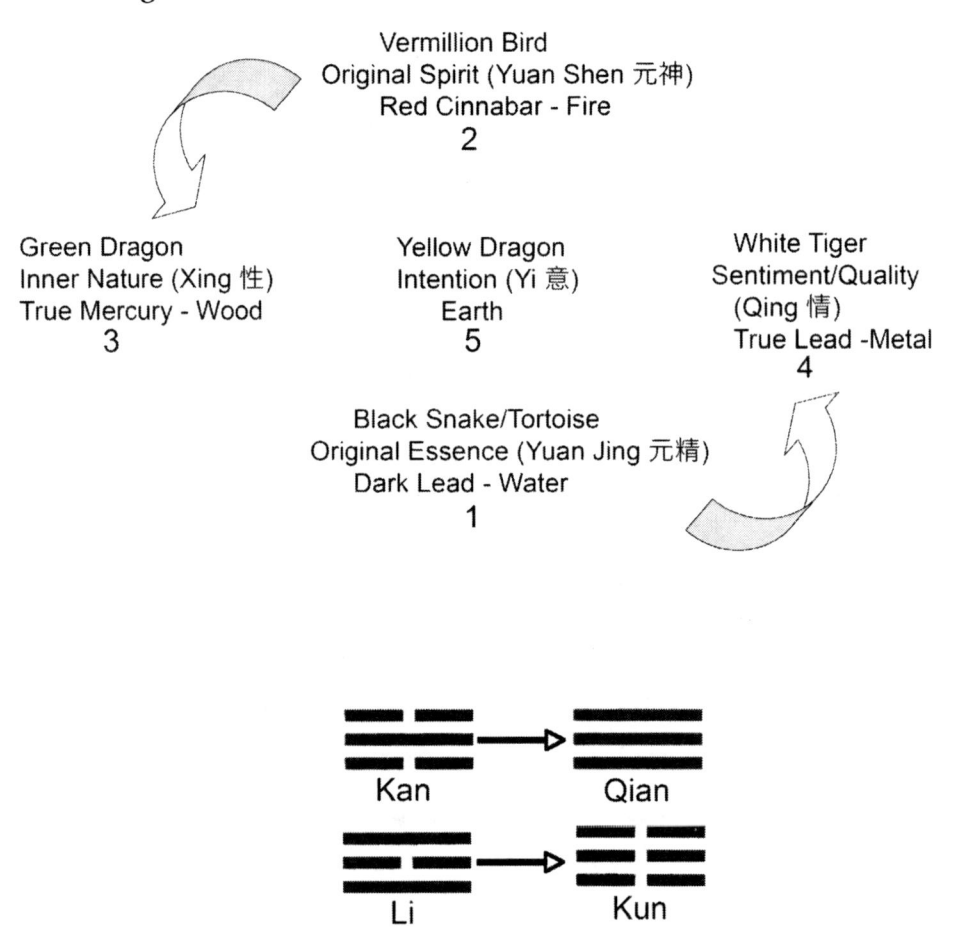

Vermillion Bird
Original Spirit (Yuan Shen 元神)
Red Cinnabar - Fire
2

Green Dragon
Inner Nature (Xing 性)
True Mercury - Wood
3

Yellow Dragon
Intention (Yi 意)
Earth
5

White Tiger
Sentiment/Quality
(Qing 情)
True Lead - Metal
4

Black Snake/Tortoise
Original Essence (Yuan Jing 元精)
Dark Lead - Water
1

Kan → Qian

Li → Kun

True Yin is the yin within yang, and True Yang is the yang within yin. They can also be represented by the black dot in the white "fish", and the white dot in the the black "fish" of the classic Tai Ji diagram:

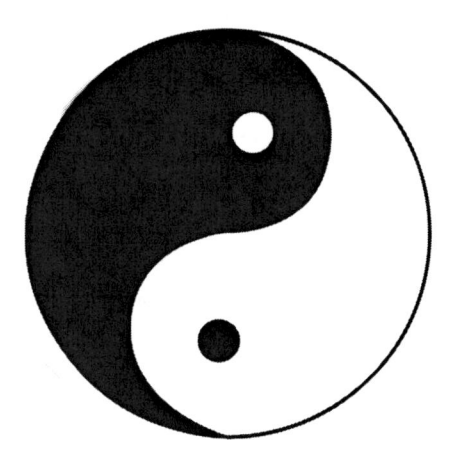

True Yang is the counterpart of True Yin, however it also represents the One Breath, the state of unity associated with the Dao. This is the state before the separation of yin and yang that is represented by the empty circle at the center of Chen Tuan's Diagram.

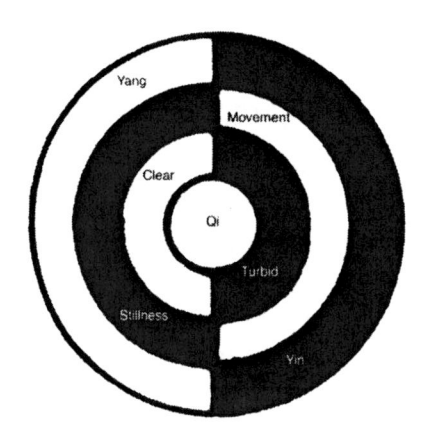

When the Five Powers, or Five Agents, are used to represent the alchemical process, Zhen-Thunder is associated with the Dragon and True Mercury and Dui-Lake is associated with the Tiger and True Lead.

☳ Zhen-Thunder (Dragon)

Although yang, the Dragon (Associated with the Zhen-Thunder Trigram) has two yin lines and therefore represents the hidden yin within the yang of Li-Fire.

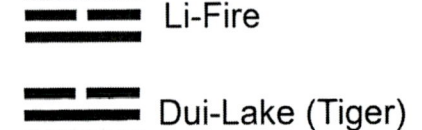

☲ Li-Fire

☱ Dui-Lake (Tiger)

Although yin, the Tiger (Associated with the Dui-Lake Trigram) has two yang lines and therefore represents the hidden yang within the yin of Kan-Water.

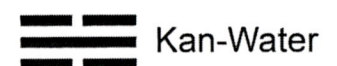

☵ Kan-Water

How does one reverse the normal cycling of the Five Powers? In his translation of the *Wondrous Scripture for Daily Internal Practice of the Great High Lord Lao,* Louis Komjathy put it quite clearly:

> *During the twelve double-hours of the day,*
> *Constantly seek clarity and stillness.*
> *The numinous tower of the heart emptied of all things:*
> *This is called clarity.*
> *Not allowing even a single thought to arise:*
>
> *This is called stillness.*
> *The body is the dwelling place of qi.*
> *The heart is the residence of spirit.*
> *When intent moves, spirit is agitated;*
> *When spirit is agitated, qi is dispersed.*
>
> *When intent is stable, spirit remains settled;*
> *When spirit remains settled, qi gathers.*
> *The perfect qi of the Five Phases*
> *Then gathers together and forms a pinch of elixir.*[35]

When the intent is stable, the spirit is settled and *Qi/Breath* gathers, the yin portion of the essence (*Jing*) and the yang portion (*Qi/Breath*) rise up the *Du* vessel, and the dragon and tiger meet and combine to nourish the spirit, forming a unified vapor that descends to the mouth and manifests in the production of a thicker, richer saliva, which is then swallowed and descends to the *Dantian*.[36] This in turn leads to a transformation or transmutation of Fire and Water and a reversal of the normal movement of the Five Powers. Now all the metaphors and images come together.

Alchemy
- Lead is extracted from its carrier, Kan-Water, to combine with the yang lines in Li-Fire.
- Mercury is extracted from its carrier, Li-Fire, to combine with the yin lines of Kan-Water.
- Lead and Mercury thus extracted produce the "Golden Pill" in the *Dantian*.

Dragon and Tiger and the Five Agents
- The Dragon and Tiger intermarry or "copulate" to exchange places.
- The yang-active impulse (the dragon) hides and coils, returning to stabilize the *Jing*. The Dragon is now in the West.
- The yin-quiescent impulse (the tiger) sits on the ground, returning to harmonize the *Shen*. The Tiger is now in the East.
- Zhen-Wood, representing True Yin, is extracted from Li-Fire. This is a reversal of the normal generation cycle of the Five Agents - Fire now produces Wood.
- Dui-Metal, representing True Yang, is extracted from Kan-Water. This is also a reversal of the normal generation cycle of the Five agents - Water now produces Metal.

- Soil (Earth) is the axis around which this transformation takes place.

Yi Jing
- Fire and Water switch places and their middle lines also switch positions creating Kun-Earth over Qian-Heaven. This is a return to the pre-heaven condition and original wisdom represented by the Hexagram Peace (*Tai*).

The Shen
- The *Hun* (our knowledge, creativity and imagination) returns to its yin root and harmonizes with the wisdom embodied in the Will (*Zhi*) - the spirit of the kidneys, which anchors not only the *Hun*, but also our feelings and emotions.
- The *Po* (our sensations and reactions) returns to its yang root embodied in the *Shen*, which is housed by the heart and whose consciousness, along with the *Hun*, then guides the *Po*.
- All of these transformations are mediated by the *Yi* (mind-intention), which gives us the capacity for clarity of thought, purpose, and sustained concentration.

The Three Treasures
- Vapor, or *Qi/Breath,* is associated with the upward movement of the yang, while the thickened saliva is associated with the downward movement of the yin.
- The process of *Jing* being expended to generate *Qi/Breath* in order to foster *Shen* is now reversed to the pre-birth state, where *Shen* guides the *Qi/Breath* to generate the *Jing*. *Jing* is then replenished and stabilized.

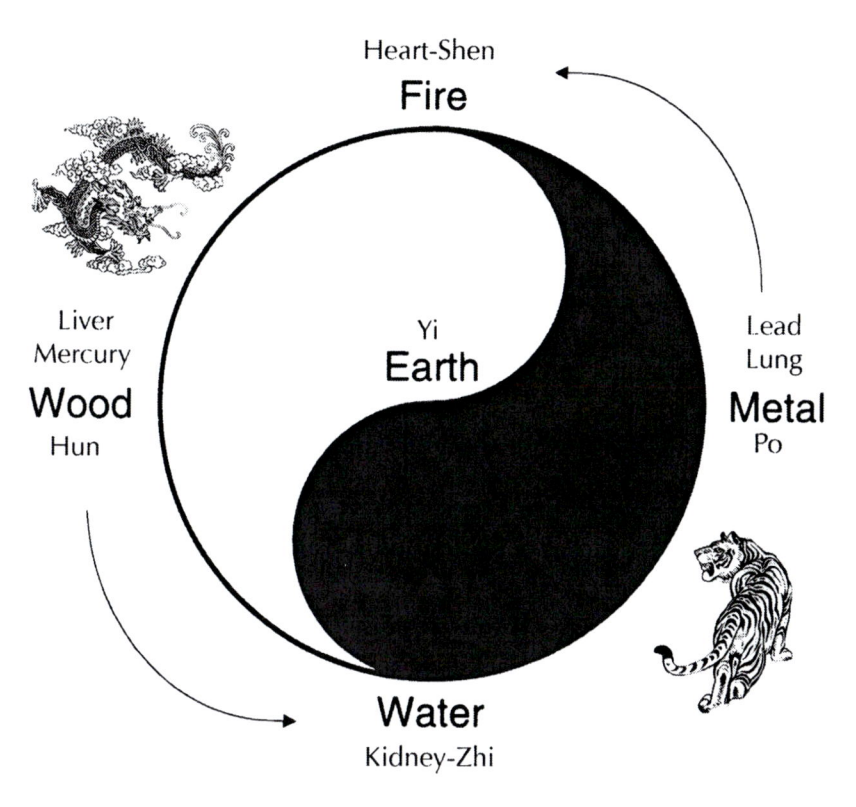

Reversal of the Five Powers:

Fire and Water are Balanced; Dragon and Tiger Meet; Lead and Mercury are Extracted; Essence is Stabilized

When the cycle of the Five Powers reverses, Water and Fire switch positions. Now Water and Fire, rather than moving away from each other (fire upward and water downward), move towards each other and interact correctly. If fire is beneath water, it creates steam and condensation which is a rarefied energy. This process can be likened to water heated on a stove, creating a vapor which rises upward only to coalesce and descend again. The two elements must act in relation to each other and be in balance. If the heat is too great, the water will evaporate. If the water boils over, the fire will be extinguished. This balance is represented by hexagram #63: Ji Ji (Completion) in which the trigram for water is above and the trigram for fire below. Here, water and fire interact and inter-transform.

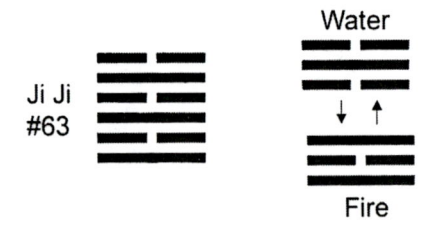

By employing proper posture, breathing and stillness of the mind, the *Dantian* acts like a stove that heats water so that it transforms into vapor which rises up to the chest and heart, where it coalesces to become water and then sinks back to the *Dantian*. Metaphorically, this plucks the yang-solid line from the center Kan-Water to fill the yin-broken line in the center of Li-Fire, thereby producing Qian-Heaven, represented by three solid-yang lines. The yin-broken line in the center of Li-Fire then moves to the center of Kan-Water, thereby producing Kun-Earth, represented by three broken-yin lines.

When the middle lines of the trigrams switch places and form the Qian-Heaven and Kun-Earth trigrams, there is a return to the original pre-heaven (before-birth) state, which in Daoist beliefs leads to a stopping of the temporal movement and therefore "immortality," or more practically speaking, a reconnection of our conscious mind with our innate wisdom resulting in a deeper connection with the world. This is represented by the hexagram that results from this transmutation of water and fire: Hexagram #11: Peace (Tai).

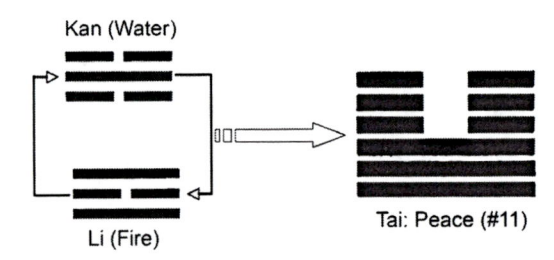

Daoist Numerology

Some of the key tools and metaphors in Daoist meditation and internal alchemy are the trigrams of the *Yi Jing* and their the numerological associations. Numbers and images are two connected codes which help us to comprehend and order the world. Isabelle Robinet gives us some insight into the importance of numbers in Daoist thought:

> *According to certain authors, the numbers preceded the images (xiang); according to others it was the opposite. In either case, images and numbers are deemed to be primordial: they appeared before ideas or concepts, and before names and forms.*[37]

In Chinese thought, numbers produce the world. The oft quoted passage from chapter 42 of the *Dao De Jing* says:

> *The Dao begets the one, the one begets the two, the two beget the three and the three beget the myriad things. The myriad things, bearing yin and embracing yang form a unified harmony through the fusing of these two vital forces.*[38]

This idea is often graphically depicted by combining the concepts of the *Wu Ji* and *Tai Ji* (Lesson Three) with imagery from the *Yi Jing*. *Wu Ji* becomes *Tai Ji*; *Tai Ji* becomes *Liang Yi* (Two Aspects: yin and yang) which in turn becomes *Si Xiang* (Four Appearences: old yang, young yang, young yin and old yin). *Si Xiang* become the *Ba Gua* (Eight Trigrams) which in turn represent myriad things.

Wu Ji

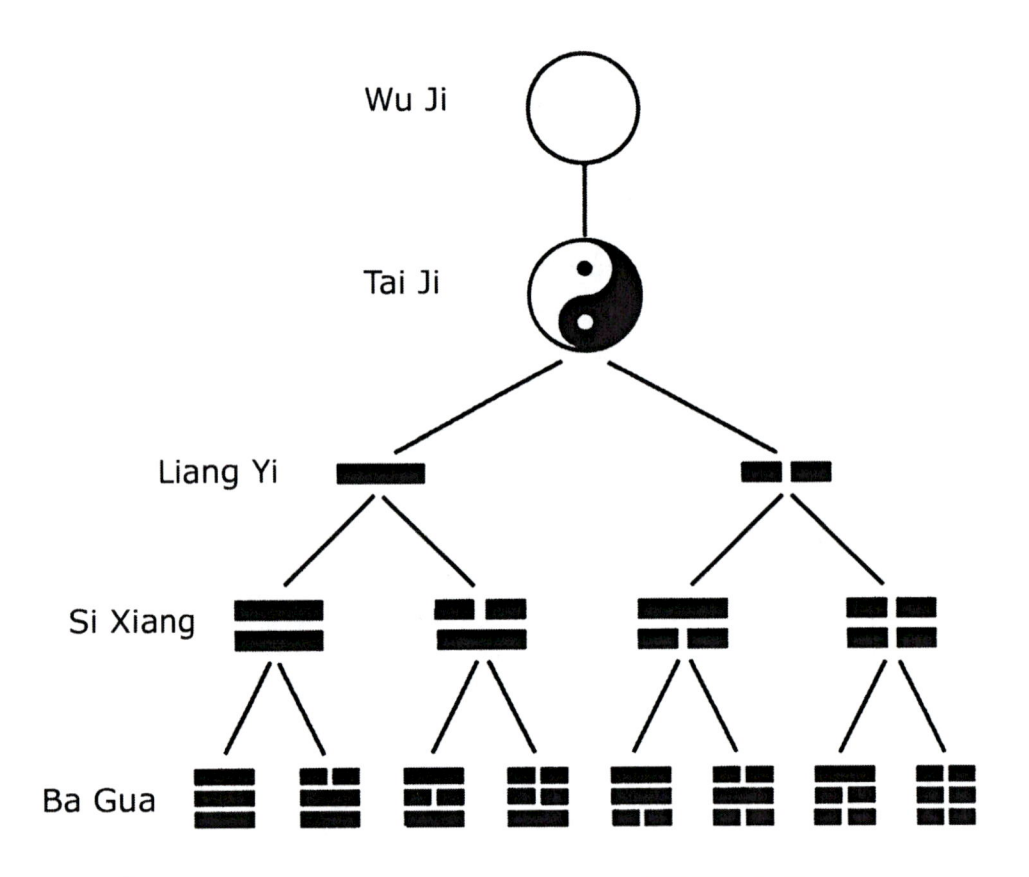

Tai Ji

Liang Yi

Si Xiang

Ba Gua

Odd numbers are considered to be yang and unstable, and therefore subject to movement and change. Even numbers are yin, stable, and capable of taking on form. One and two combined create a stable unity, a triad or trinity – movement and form combined – able to give birth to all things.

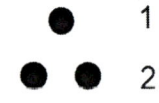

●   1
● ● 2

The Trinity
One and Two Create Three

One is often seen as the Dao, but it is also associated with Qian-Heaven, the yang principle, represented by the Qian Trigram. The origin of the world is movement which relates to yang. Two is associated with yin and Kun-Earth and pertains to phenomena and form.

(1) Qian   (2) Kun

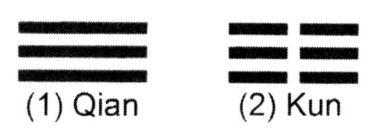

Three is the product of these two complimentary forces. It is the sign of unity restored after their separation. Three is a harmonious blending of yin and yang resulting in human beings or the human world. Thus three *is a replica of the primordial unity.*[39]

Fu Xi (the mythical sage who among other things, is said to have invented Chinese ideograms) saw a dragon-horse emerge from a river with this pattern of dots inscribed on it, and from this pattern he created the *He Tu* Diagram (map; chart).

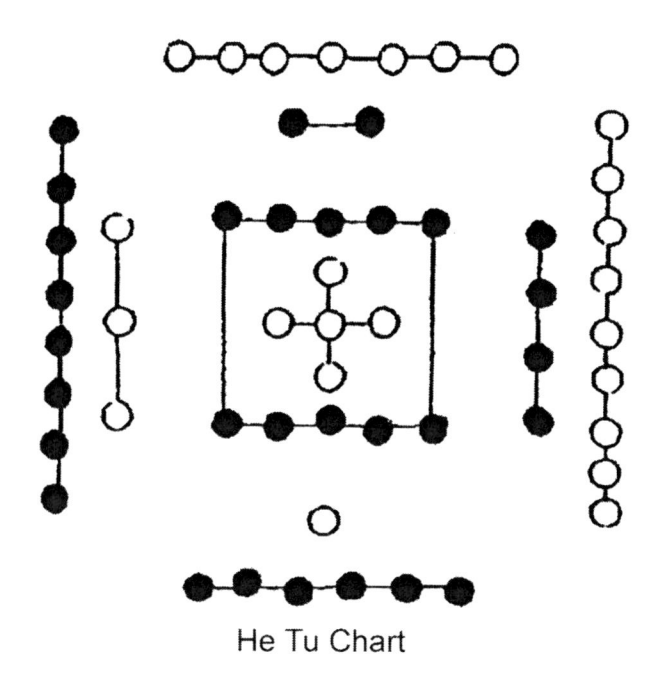

He Tu Chart

The numbers 1,2,3,4 and 5 are on the inner ring. The inner ring represents phenomena at their beginning stages when they are active and expansive. However, the latent energies of these "generative numbers" are not manifest, so they are "hidden" in the inner ring.[40] The numbers

6,7,8,9 and 10 are on the outer ring. The numbers in the outer ring are called the "accomplished numbers" or "achieved numbers." They represent phenomena that are completed or manifest. Five is the number associated with the center. It divides the emergent, generative numbers which go from one to four and add up to ten, from the accomplished numbers which go from six to nine. Five is also associated with Earth, which is at the center of the interaction of the Five Powers.

The direction of movement of the white dots – 1, 3, 5, 7 and 9 - is clockwise, expanding outward. 1 expands to 3 and 7 expands to 9. The direction of movement of the black dots – 2, 4, 6, 8 and 10 - is counterclockwise, contracting inward - 4 contracts to 2 and 8 contracts to 6. The odd numbers (white dots) are yang and associated with Heaven, while the yin, even numbers (black dots) are associated with Earth. When the ten numbers are combined, they represent the phenomena that are the result of the interaction of Heaven and Earth – the myriad things. The odd numbers have an essential role in their expression of movement: *The numbers emerge in One, are established in Three, are accomplished in Five, flourish in Seven, and culminate in Nine.*[41]

The Heavenly yang (odd) numbers and the earthly yin (even) numbers attract each other. In this way, the numbers one to five are the early stage generative numbers which create the Five Powers). The numbers six through ten represent the phenomena created after the generative numbers.

> *Heaven from 1 gives rise to Water, and Earth with 6 completes it, Earth from 2 gives rise to Fire, and Heaven with 7 completes it. Heaven from 3 gives rise to Wood, and Earth with 8 completes it. Earth with 4 gives rise to Metal, and Heaven with 9 completes it. Heaven from 5 gives rise to Soil and, Earth with 10 completes it.*[42]

The Five Powers can then be added to the *He Tu* diagram as follows:

Fire

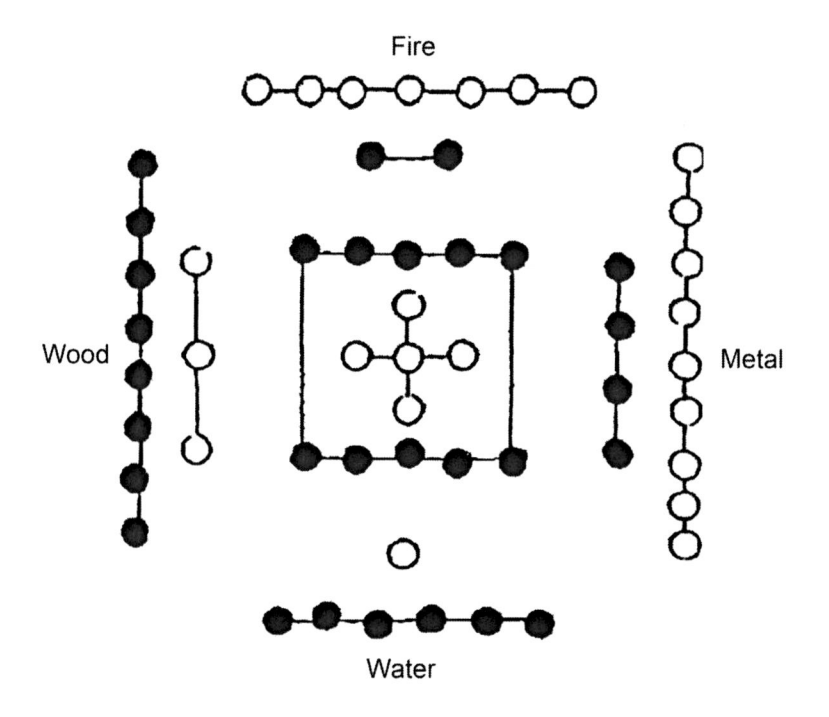

Wood · · · Metal

Water

The Five Powers and The He Tu Diagram

Earth is represented by the five white dots and ten black dots at the center of this diagram. The inner ring of black and white dots (1, 2, 3, 4 and 5) – the generative numbers - representing the generation of the five agents, is reversed in Daoist Meditation and Daoist alchemy. The four agents that revolve around earth are thereby reduced to two. Wood (3), representing the post-heaven state is reintegrated into Fire (2) and Metal (4) is reintegrated into Water. Each pair together then have a value of Five.[43]

Wood (3) (inner nature) + Fire (2) (original spirit) = 5

Metal (4) (emotions) + Water (1) (original essence) = 5[44]

Balance is achieved through the mediation of soil (earth) at the center. True yin and true yang join through the soil (intention) and the distinction between them ends.[45]

Fu Xi also arranged the eight trigrams (*Gua*) of the *Yi Jing* so that they corresponded to the *He Tu* Diagram, and the numbers became associated with the eight trigrams. These eight *Gua* illustrate the fundamental, primal forces that govern life. They reveal the polar (yin-yang) nature of the universe. The eight trigrams are said to form the outer appearance, while the *He Tu* Diagram represents the inner thought.[46] This arrangement, called the Earlier Heaven or Pre-Heaven sequence, is as follows:

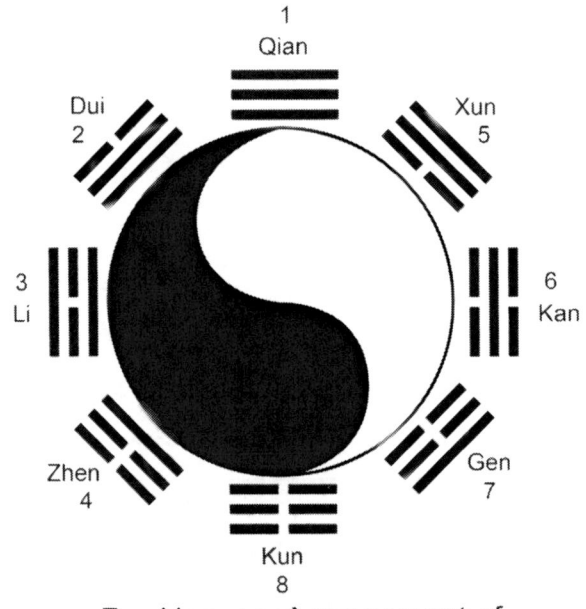

Pre-Heaven Arrangement of Trigrams and Associated Numbers

In this arrangement, the generative numbers are located on the left and the achieved numbers are on the right. Heaven (1) plus Earth (8) makes nine and similarly all of the polar opposite trigrams: lake and mountain, fire and water, thunder and wind, add up to nine. Numbers 1-4 move in a yang direction, counterclockwise, while the yin numbers (5-8) move clockwise. The yin and yang directions combined create the Tai Ji Diagram which expresses the interaction of these two fundamental forces.

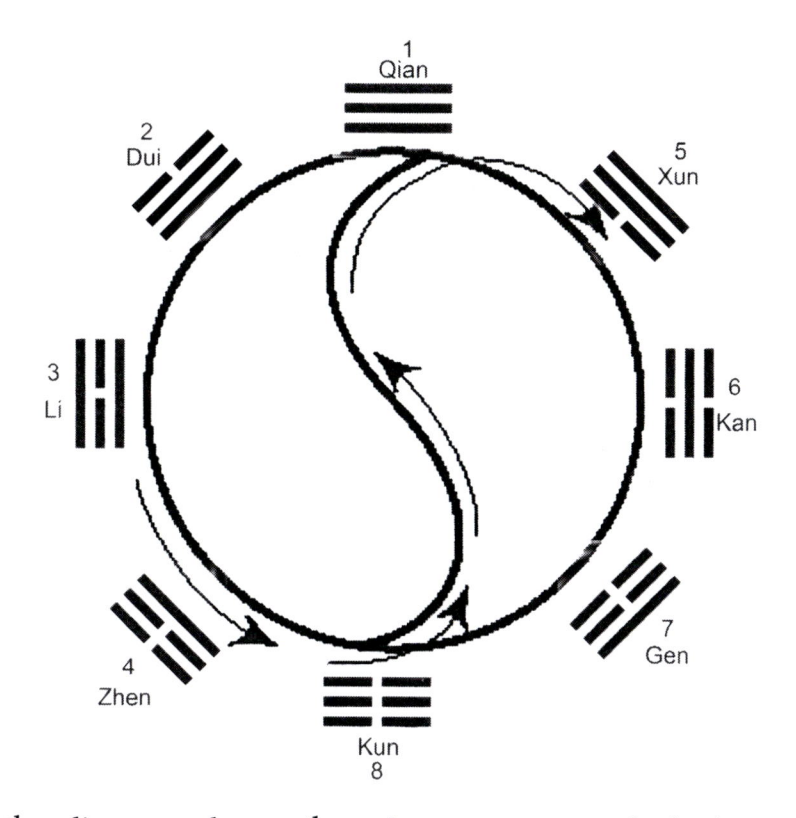

In the diagram above, there is yang counterclockwise expansive movement through the generative numbers from 1-4 and recursive clockwise contractive movement along through the achieved numbers 6, 7 and 8. The number 5 is the pivot of these two movements. This reversal takes us back to the beginning to 1, the orgin, unity, the "One" associated with Heaven. In terms of the numbers, as we have said, *The world is produced by the unfolding of the one into the multiplicity. Hence, by going back through the numbers, one goes back through time.*[47] In this way the One generates the two, which generates the three, and the 10,000 things (multiplicity). Through Daoist practices one reverses this, reversing the order of the five agents and returning back to the One.[48]

Followers of the Lung Men (*Dragon Gate*) school of Daoism practice a form of circle walking meditation called *Zhuan Tian Zun* 轉天尊 ("Rotating in Worship of Heaven"), in which the practitioner strives to find stillness in motion.[49] In this practice, they walk a circle in a manner that follows the generation and reversal of the yang and yin numbers. Modern practitioners of the martial art Ba Gua Zhang also walk in this manner as they attempt to achieve internal stillness within external motion.

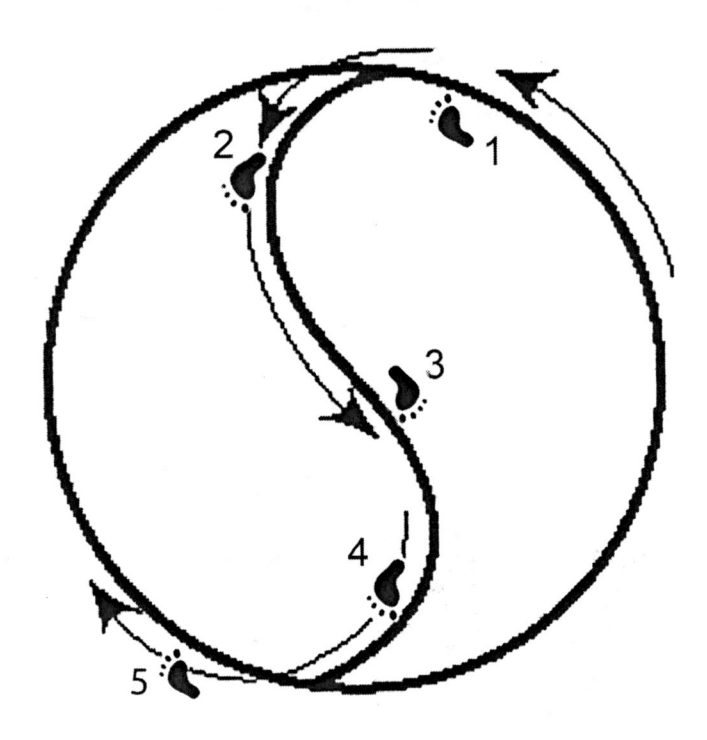

Another way to look at the movement of the Yin and Yang numbers is depicted below:[50]

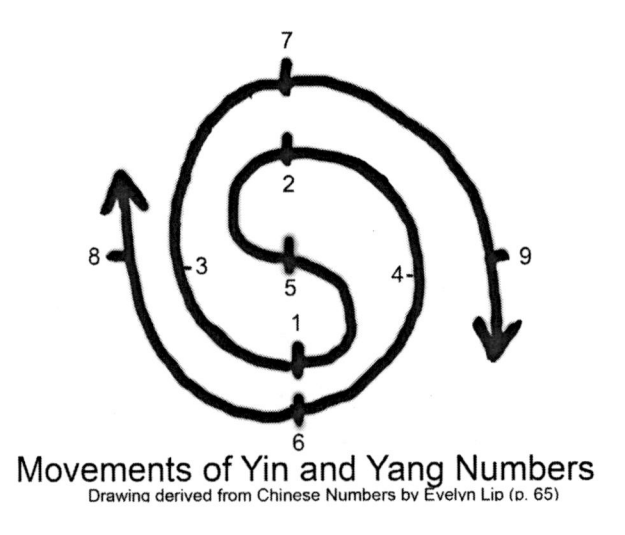

Movements of Yin and Yang Numbers
Drawing derived from Chinese Numbers by Evelyn Lip (p. 65)

316

A second arrangement of numbers is attributed to Yu the Great, the legendary sage-king who introduced flood control in ancient China. Yu purportedly observed a tortoise in a river with a design of dots on its back. This design is called the *Lo Shu* or the Lo (River) Text. The famous Neo-Confucian Scholar Zhu Xi felt that the 10 numbers of the *He Tu* symbolize a balanced immutable whole (as in the Pre-Heaven configuration of the eight trigrams), while the nine numbers of the *Lo Shu* represent change.[51]

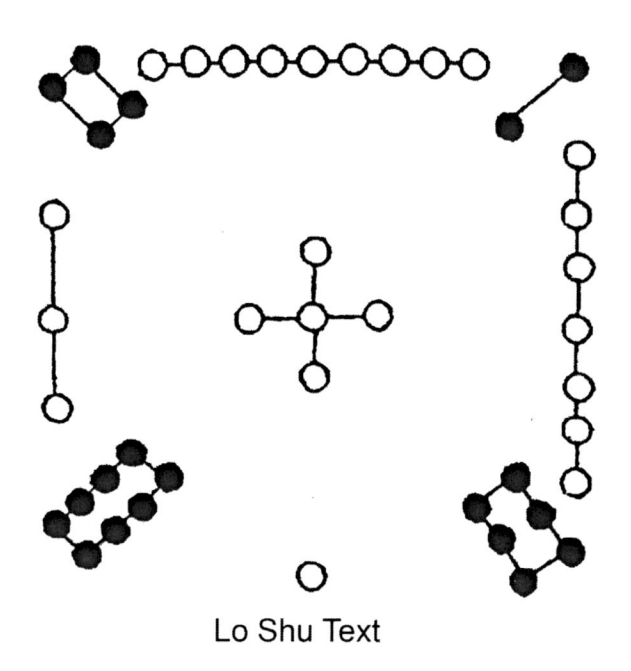

Lo Shu Text

This arrangement of dots places the yang numbers (white dots) at the four cardinal directions and the yin numbers (black dots) at the four diagonal directions. Five is at the center. When the digits are placed in rows they form a magic square in which the sum of any row or diagonal equals 15. This square is also referred to as the *Jiu Gong* (Nine Palaces).

4	9	2
3	5	7
8	1	6

King Wen used the numbers to connect this diagram with the eight trigrams, thereby creating the post-heaven arrangement pictured below. This arrangement, rather than depicting primordial unchanging forces, shows the passing of time and temporal movement of the Five Elements and four seasons. Fire (9) and Water (1) are the Post-Heaven embodiments of Heaven and Earth.

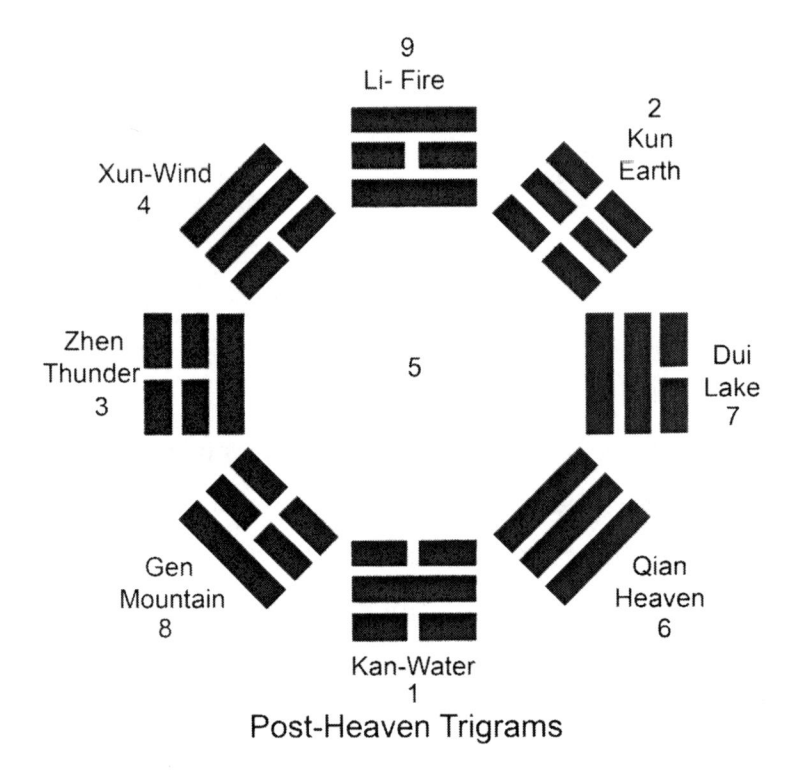

Post-Heaven Trigrams

The Nine Palaces have great significance to Daoist practitioners. 北斗(*Beidou*), the plough constellation (the Big Dipper) was the most important of the constellations because of its relationship to the pole star. The tradition of the Beidou is important in both Daoism and Buddhism and therefore forms an intricate part of the fabric of Chinese culture and spirituality.

> *Seen as a cosmic pivot, governing time and space and regulating the natural rhythms and astrological events, the Beidou stand also as the superintendent of human destiny. Cleaving to these secular Chinese astrological conceptions, Daoism held the constellation to be the abode of the One Supreme, the Dao, the site of orignation and return, as well as the arbiter of good and evil. The Great Dipper represents the north, seat of the Great Yin – Yin at its apogee – which engenders the Yang that is life. As the cosmic matrix, it presides over the nine transformations, the complete cycle of gestation.*[52]

There are said to be nine stars in the dipper of which only seven are visible. *Fuxing*, the eighth star is discernable at certain times, but the ninth star, *Bixing*, is invisible. In some traditions it is thought that only the spiritually worthy can see these two stars. Daoist priests walked the pattern of the nine stars going sequentially from 1 to 9 and then back again, returning from 9 to 1.[53] In this way the power of the plough and the Five Powers was invoked in the ritual. In Daoist ritual, this walking pattern or series of dance steps are sometimes called the Paces of Yu, named after Yu The Great.[54] This pattern is diagrammed below. This is the same pattern walked by practitioners of Ba Gua Zhang today, who ascribe strategic principles to its arrangement. Nine is also the number of birth and rebirth.[55] Hence, forward and backward movement along the nine palaces is, in Daoist Meditation, symbolic of the reversal of the Five

Powers and the stopping of time - ie: returning to the One, to primordial inner unity.

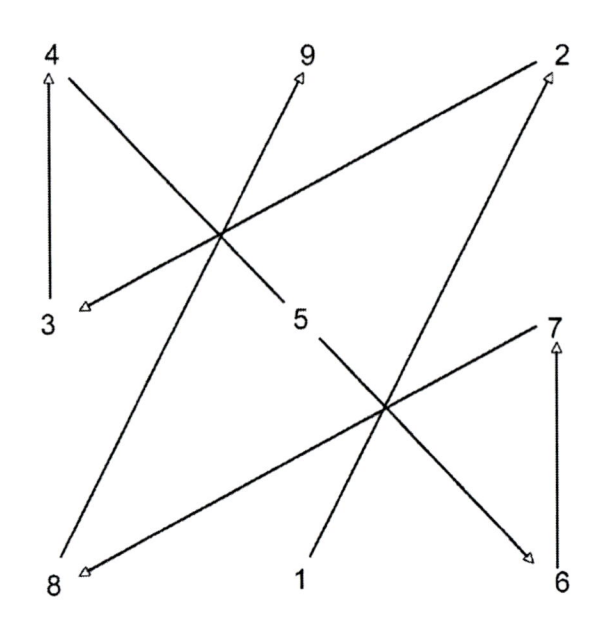

Sequence of the Nine Palaces According
to the Numbers of the Magic Square

Images of Sages and Immortals

The sage, or the immortal, represents the unified human being who exhibits the "true knowledge" of inner wisdom. In the sage, the conscious mind and the innate unconscious knowledge, what Thomas Cleary calls the "mind of the Dao,"[56] act as one. The sage can spontaneously adapt and change according to the situation. This implies a clarity of internal reflection that leads to a natural, harmonious movement through the world. Claude Larre and Elisabeth Rochat de la Valle describe this as a fundamental "knowing how."[57] Kristopher Schipper adds to this knowing how, "a refusal to be used for something." Our "being used" stems from our own imbalanced desires creating involvement with others, rather than the involvement with others being a natural extension of living within oneself. The detachment of the immortal from the cares of the world represents a calm inner detachment and acceptance within outward interactions.[58] Guo Xiang (252-312), one of most influential commentators on the Zhuang Zi, puts this another way:

> *Living in a human community, it is impossible to separate oneself completely from other people. But because of the many transformations of the human world, different behaviors are appropriate to each time. Only those who are free from any fixed intentions of their own, not insisting on their own way, can follow wherever the changes may go without bearing their entanglements as a burden.*[59]

The Ren and the Du Vessels

Ren Mo is considered to be the "Sea of all the Yin Vessels" in the body. 任 *Ren* means to "take charge of," "to accept" or "to take control." Because one of the things the *Ren* vessel takes control of is the fetus, it is often referred to as the "Conception Vessel" in English. *Ren Mo* is less a vessel than an area where yin and blood collect.[60] Both *Ren Mo* and *Du Mo* emanate from the Gate of Vitality, the *Dantian* and *Mingmen*.

Du 督 means to "superintend," "govern," "regulate" or "direct." *Du* can also mean "the capital," and is therefore the capital of the yang vessels. The *Du* vessel regulates all the yang channels in the body. *The Du may be understood in militaristic and political terms as an allusion to the imperial title of Director General (Zong Du* 總督*), a term in use since the Former Han, denoting one who is generally in charge, typically of regional clusters of two or more provinces.*[61] The *Du* also refers to being upright and centered - *Zheng Zong* (正中).[62]

The spinal cord through which *Du Mo* runs is filled with marrow and is sometimes called the "marrow path." In the internal martial arts (*Nei Jia*) and in the practice of internal exercises (*Nei Gong*), the path of *Du Mo* running from the perineum to the top of the head is also known as the *Tian Gan,* or "Heavenly Stem." The *Tian Gan* connects the yin of Earth in our body with the yang of Heaven and serves as the conduit for their energies. This axis, the *Tian Gan*, must be free of restriction in order for *Qi/Breath* to circulate freely through the *Du* and *Ren* meridians (the Micro-Cosmic Orbit). This is one reason why *Ba Gua Zhang* (Eight Diagram Palm) practitioners practice a series of "*Tian Gan* Exercises" that wring out the spine and the fascia surrounding it. When meditation and *Qi Gong* movements are performed properly, with correct form and intention, then the *Qi/Breath* can circulate through the *Ren* and *Du* meridians. In *Ba Gua Zhang* there is a poem that discusses this:

> *The chest must be kept empty, the Qi will sink,*
> *Hold up the back and drop the shoulders to extend the arm.*
> *Hold the grain duct while Qi reaches the Dantian area,*
> *Uplift the vertex to foster spirit.*[63]

This poem contains many important implications:

- In order for the *Qi/Breath* to sink to the *Dantian* area in a natural way, it is necessary to soften and empty the chest. This refers to the relative emptiness of the chest represented by the broken middle line in the Li-Fire trigram.
- In order to hollow the chest you must lift, spread and round the upper back.
- Sinking the shoulders helps to round the back and allows the two arms to extend forward by intention. (If they were extended by force the power and intention would float upward).
- Because the chest is hollow and the elbow and shoulder sink downward, one can use intention without physical force in order to guide the *Qi/Breath* downward (to *Dantian*). Then the abdomen is full relative to the chest. This is represented by the solid line in the center of the Kan-Water trigram.
- When *Qi/Breath* reaches *Dantian*, hold the grain duct (ie: gently lift the perineum upward). This makes it possible for the *Qi/Breath* to flow through *Du Mo* and *Ren Mo*.

- *Qi/Breath* ascends up *Du Mo* to the brain, where *Du Mo* connects with *Ren Mo* through the tongue. Qi-Breath enters and descends through *Ren Mo* to reach *Dantian*. In this manner *Qi/Breath* flows continuously through the whole body.
- When one meridian is opened, a hundred meridians can open and the spirit can be naturally vigorous and the whole body relaxed. This allows the formation of an internal energy directed by the intention.[64]

Clearing the extraordinary channels via the breath is one of the key parts of internal alchemy and Daoist meditation. In his *Method of Sitting in Quiescence of Master Yin Shi (Yin shi Zi Jing Zuo Fa)*, Jiang Wei qiao (1872-1995) relates his personal experience as follows:

> *When I was sitting in quiescence, I suddenly experienced a vibration. A warm energy (qi) arose from the caudal funnel [the coccyx] to the top of my head, circulated through my body along the function [ren mo] and control [du mo] vessels, passed again through the top of my head and then slowly descended through the chest, until it reached the area below the navel. After some time, this energy began to rise and descend spontaneously. By means of my intention (yi), I could move it throughout the entire body so that it permeated my four limbs.*[65]

Zhuang Zi, in discussing how to nourish life, councils:

> *Doer of good, stay clear of reputation,*
> *Doer of ill, stay clear of punishment.*
> *Trace the vein which is central and make it your standard.*
> *You can protect the body,*
> *keep life whole ,*
> *nurture your parents,*
> *last out your years.*[66]

In this context, the "vein which is central," references the *Du, Ren* and *Chong* vessels. These three vessels, although in theory separate, are considered to act as a single entity and functionally are therefore inseparable. Kristofer Schipper believes that this statement specifically refers to the *Du* vessel ("the energy channel of control").[67] The flow toward the current of the central meridian, if left to itself, is neither good nor evil and seeks neither fame nor notoriety. If not driven by doctrines and their resulting uncompromising and sustained practices which are imposed by the conscious mind, *the spontaneous fluctuations of behavior tend to normalize around the central current.*[68] The *Du* is hidden and unseen. Unlike the *Ren*, which lies in front, the *Du* is behind us and thus invisible.[69] *Hence it is opposed to the "knowing mind "and is the real controller, as opposed to the knowing mind's pretensions to control and direct life.*[70]

Francois Jullien refers to the *Du* as the *vector of vital nourishment*. He feels it defines *the line and rule of life* through its ability to renew the body via its connection with respiration.[71] Schipper adds that: only by remaining independent, by following the natural action of the spinal column can we be a free human being, standing upright within our own vital space.[72]

Daoist Meditation and the Image of the Gen Diagram

艮   卦

Gen   Gua

Daoist Meditation and the Image of the Gen Diagram

Image and Name

In the *Yi Jing* (I Ching), the "Book of Changes," the image of the Gen diagram is the Mountain. Gen refers to that which is "Stationary", and to "Restraint," "Stillness" and "Keeping Still." *In its application to man, this hexagram turns on the problem of achieving a quiet heart and mind.*[1] The Gen hexagram is simply the Gen trigram doubled - Gen above Gen. The structure of the trigram shows a solid (yang) line above two broken (yin) lines. This solid line above the two yielding lines, shows that yang has ascended to the top. With no room to ascend further, this strong moving line stops and rests. This implies restraint and stillness.

Gen-Mountain Trigram   **Gen- Mountain Hexagram**

Both the trigram and hexagram diagram movement. This movement can relate both to a situation or configuration of events and/or to movements inside the body, including the movements and interactions of the *Qi/Breath*, *Jing* and *Shen*. The structure of the diagram can best be understood by starting with the Kun-Earth Trigram. The Earth trigram is composed of three broken (yin) lines. A mountain is an extension of Earth. It is Earth raised to its highest point. The point where Earth stops, the closest it can approach Heaven, is at the top of a mountain. This is represented by the strong line at the top of the Gen Diagram.

Kun-Earth Trigram   **Gen-Mountain Trigram**

When a solid line appears at the bottom of Kun-Earth, it becomes Zhen-Thunder, representing excitation, arousal, emergence, movement and creativity. The solid line at the bottom of Zhen can advance and move upward, filling the empty space by following the unobstructed path created by the two pliable yin lines above.

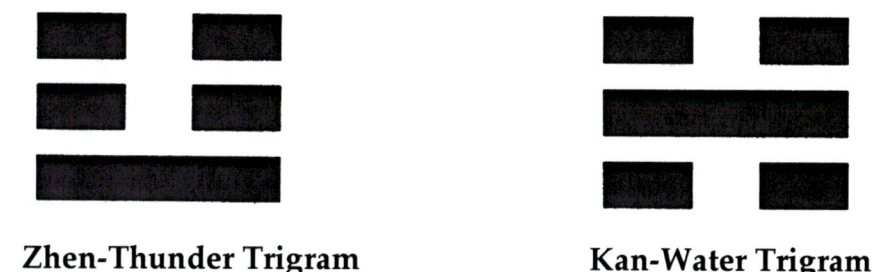

Zhen-Thunder Trigram   **Kan-Water Trigram**

As action and movement emerge, they build. The solid line advances to the central position designating Kan-Water. Its attribute is flowing, continuing - action fluidly moving and conforming to the terrain and circumstance. In the Kan diagram, the path is still open for the strong, moving central line to advance. When the solid line advances to the top movement stops. This is Gen-Mountain.[2]

≡≡ Gen-Mountain

≡≡ Kan-Water

≡≡ Zhen-Thunder

≡≡ Kun-Earth

Action must be balanced by stillness, because movement is generated by stillness, by keeping still. Stillness is in itself a type of action and all actions must be in accord with the situation. Movement and stillness must take place at the appropriate times. Too much action and things spin out of control. Too much stillness and there is stagnation and decay. In the order of the hexagrams, Gen (Hexagram 52) follows Zhen (Hexagram 51). The solid lines within each trigram of Zhen have moved upward to the top and stopped. After movement there must be stillness and restraint so that movement can start again. Jian (Hexagram 53) follows Gen. Jian signifies "gradual advance" or "gradual development." The Xun-Wood Trigram is now over the mountain trigram. Forward growth, and upward movement begin again – the third yang line moves upward slowly and gradually like a tree growing on the mountain. The movement is orderly and appropriate. Xun is also associated with Wind. Wind represents penetration and insight. Appropriate movement can only occur when overseen by the discerning penetration of wind.[3]

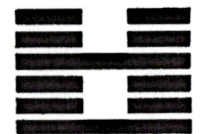

Zhen Hexagram
Hexagram #51

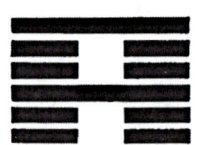

Gen Hexagram
Hexagram #52

Jian Hexagram
Hexagram #53

The upper and lower trigrams of the Gen hexagram are the same and do not interact. They stop to rest in the right time and right place.[4] In each trigram, the yang line is at the top attempting to move upward while the yin lines are below and moving downward. Yet the downward movement of the yin lines in the upper trigram is blocked by the strong yang line at the top of the lower trigram. Thus there is stillness.

In China, the mountain also conveys the idea of being solitary, like a hermit or a recluse. Traditionally Daoist recluses retreated to the mountains to practice meditation and self-cultivation. Thus there is a long association of mountains with meditation, self-cultivation and esoteric Daoist practices.

The Gen Ideogram

The Chinese character or ideogra, for Gen is 艮, meaning blunt, tough, or chewy. The upper part of the ideogram is the eye radical. Originally this character was a mirror image of 見 (见 *jian*): to see; to catch; sight of; to meet with; to be exposed to; a person with a big eye. The bottom of the character designates to turn around, as in turning around to look. Some commentators feel that this action of looking signifies "keeping still." Others say that this "turning to look" is the "inward looking" associated with meditation practices.[5]

The great commentary on the *Yi Jing* associates Gen with 止 (*zhi*):[6] stop; halt; arrive at; suppress; prohibit; stay; detain.[7] The ancient oracle bones character resembled a foot,[8] and was essentially picture of a left footprint. The toes were at the top, the heel at the bottom. *Zhi* was sometimes written so that it appeared as part of the character 走 (*zou*: go; walk; leave), 足 (*zu*: foot), and 步 (*bu*: step). *Zhi* now means "stop" (i.e.: hold the feet still).[9]

Gen: Judgment and Line Commentary

The decision or judgment related to the Gen Hexagram images the back of the body. Stillness or restraint *takes place with the back*. This leaves the eyes unimpaired so that *one does not obtain the other person*.[10] *He goes into that one's courtyard, but does not see him there*.[11] If restraint operates through the back, through not seeing the other person, then there is no face-to-face confrontation. This means that one can apply stillness and restraint without *separating the person involved from the object of their desire*.[12] Because one's eyes are not involved, one is naturally still, without effort. This also indicates the posture used in Daoist meditation. Stillness can only be supplied through the back and its connection with the *Ren* and *Du* Vessels. If the back is straight, still and aligned,[13] if the eyes look inward and do not see, then restraint and stillness can take place naturally, allowing the *Jing* and *Qi/Breath*, to move of their own accord.

The following line commentaries primarily quote the Richard John Lynn translation (*The Classic of the Changes: A New Translation of the I Ching as interpreted by Wang Bi*, pp. 468-70):

Line 1 - First Yin: *Keeping Still (restraint) takes place with the toes, so there is no blame and it is fitting that such a one practices perpetual constancy.* Stopping the toes and feet is the way to keep the whole body still. This is a yin line in a yang place; keeping still is the way to prevail. The feet are the location of the most yin acu-point *Yong Quan*, the "bubbling well" point, from which yin Earth energy enters and wells up in the body. Stopping, standing still and being quiescent allows yin to grow and flourish in the body.

Line 2 - Second Yin: *Keeping Still takes place with the calves, which means that this one does not raise up his followers. His heart feels discontent.* The calves and the heel tendon are the root of the *Yin Qiao* and *Yang Qiao* Extraordinary vessels. The calves allow us to spring into movement. However the calves cannot raise up and move because below the toes are still and above the strong yang line holds the dominant position. Although this is a yin line in a yin place it is subordinate to the third strong line. Therefore it can neither move nor be still. This can stagnate movement within the *Qiao* vessels leading to disturbance of the inner spirits. *Not only is he unable to raise up his followers, he cannot withdraw and obey the call to quietude.*[14]

Line 3 - Third Yang: *Keeping Still with the midsection, which may split the back flesh, a danger enough to smoke and suffocate the heart.* Keeping still and restraint here imply a disconnect between the upper and lower trigrams, symbolizing a split between those lines above and below this place. In terms of meditation it implies a disconnect between mind and body, heart and kidneys, *Jing* and *Shen*. If there is blockage and restraint in the middle of the body, the *Qi/Breath* cannot move and transform. This damages the center and the back, causing the heart-fire to burn too hot, thereby suffocating the spirit. It can also represent someone who stays still in the extreme, preventing harmony with the four other yin elements that surround this line.[15] In the Wilhelm-Baynes translation of the *Yi Jing*, the commentary reads

> *Keeping his hips still.*
> *Making his sacrum stiff.*
> *Dangerous. The heart suffocates.*[16]

The hips are the boundary of yin and yang, and in Daoist meditation the sacrum is the first gate through which the *Qi/Breath* must pass in order to rise up the spine and the *Du* channel. If there is tension or rigidity here the heart will ultimately feel suffocated and blocked.

Line 4 - Fourth Yin: *Keeping Still takes place with the torso. There is no blame.* The torso here refers to the area in the chest where the heart lies. The yin line is in a yin position and the yin element has an open and empty space in the center. This helps the heart to be calm and still. Upper and lower, fire and water and *Jing* and *Shen* are connected and the *Qi/Breath* can move freely. A quiet and open heart is one of the conditions for meditation.

Line 5 - Fifth Yin: *Keeping Still takes place with the jowls, so this one's words have order and regret vanishes.* The mouth does not say arbitrary things, but knows where and when to talk and to stop talking, so that one's speech is appropriate. When one chooses one's word carefully, the inner spirits are calm and the circulation of the breath is not disturbed. This facilitates the inter-transformation of *Jing*, *Qi/Breath* and *Shen*.

Line 6 - Sixth Yang: *This one exercises Restraint (Keeping Still) with simple honesty which results in good fortune.* The top yang line is at the peak of stillness and restraint. This weight at the top needs honesty and modesty to reinforce it so that it does not topple or fall into errant practice. One should not consider matters that are beyond one's position, things that are the concerns of others. Instead, focus on the business at hand, your own inner stillness. Then you can find the serenity of the still mountain[17] and your interactions with others become appropriate and honest. This top line of the hexagram can also represent the sage. Chapter 66 of the *Dao De Jing* is titled, "How to Put the Self Behind."[18] The text reads:

If therefore the Saint wants to be above the people,
He by his words submits to them.
If he wants to precede the people,
With his personality he puts himself behind them.
When therefore the saint dwells above, the people are not weighted down
When he stands forth, the people are not hurt.
Therefore the empire is glad to push him on and gets not tired of him.
Because he does not contend,
Therefore nobody in the empire is able to contend with him.[19]

The Gen Diagram and Daoist Meditation

The Gen hexagram, mountain over mountain, designates stillness or stopping doubled, like a mountain range impeding forward movement. Gen has often been associated with the stillness of meditation and contemplation. While sitting in meditation, one is shaped like a mountain.[20] In meditation, one sits quietly without movement, attending to the breath, and letting the movements of the mind become still, letting the heart become tranquil. The mind turns inward, oblivious to one's surroundings, resembling the pristine purity and stillness of the mountain. Movement, represented by the strong yang line at the top of the trigram, stops. There is still movement but it is the movement of the body within the body; internal, inwardly directed movement.

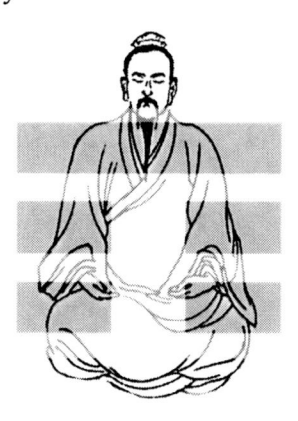

In the Ming Dynasty, Lin Zhaoen established the syncretic "Three Teachings School", which was characterized by an interweaving of Daoist, Buddhist and Confucian thought. Lin used imagery from the *Yi Jing*, particularly the Gen hexagram, to help image and explain a nine-stage process of Daoist meditation.[21] The back is related to water, to the kidneys and the north. Water is pushed up the back (through the *Du* and *Ren* Channels) to reach the heart. In this way fire and water and *Jing*, *Qi/Breath* and *Shen* can connect and inter-transform. Lin advocated imitating the Gen hexagram in order to seek stillness and calmness so that Kan and Li (Water and Fire - the kidneys and heart) and Qian and Kun (Heaven and Earth - the brain and *Dantian*), could connect. Thereby the *Qi/Breath* could freely flow.[22]

The Gen hexagram is shown below superimposed on the body of the meditator. The first two lines in the lower trigram represent the stillness of the legs (knees and ankles) in the meditaion posture. The third (yang) full line symbolizes the concentration of *Qi/Breath* and intention in the lower abdomen and the opening and holding power of the *kua*. This also represents the full middle line of the trigram Kan-Water, which is the lower "inner trigram" (see discussion below). The middle line of Kan-Water also represents the True Yang hidden within yin. The empty torso and chest, symbolized by the two yin lines in the upper trigram, are the empty and quiet heart and spirit. The fifth broken (yin) line represents the True Yin hidden within yang - the middle line of the Li-Fire trigram. This relative emptiness in the chest gives the *Shen* a place to reside. When the heart is calm and there is stillness and emptiness inside, the strong third and sixth lines can move freely - the *Qi/Breath* can circulate from *Dantian* upward into the brain and back to *Dantian* following the Micro-Cosmic Orbit.

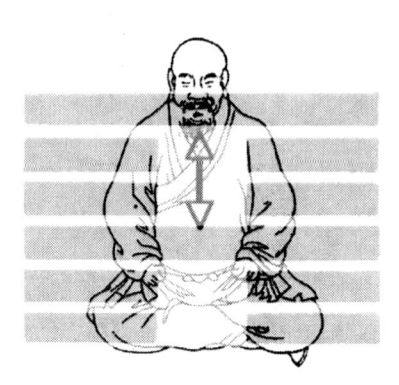

Gen: The Inner Hexagram

Each trigram is said to have an inner or nuclear hexagram that expresses the original hexagram's essential, internal nature and qualities. This central, inner quality can be expressed or remain latent, depending on the circumstances.[23] The inner hexagram is formed by creating a "lower inner trigram" from lines 2, 3 and 4 and an "upper inner trigram" from lines 3, 4 and 5. The inner trigrams for the Gen hexagram as diagrammed below are Zhen-Thunder over Kan-Water. This forms Gen's Inner Hexagram: Jie. Jie can mean: release[24]; relief; disentanglement; setting free; unfastening.[25]

Gen: Inner Trigrams

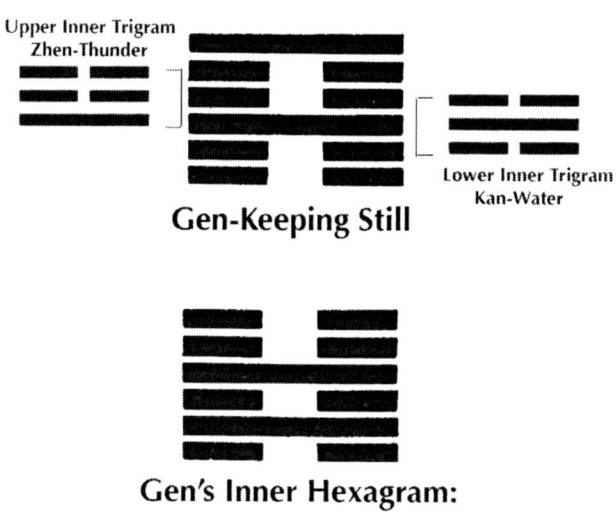

Gen-Keeping Still
Upper Inner Trigram Zhen-Thunder
Lower Inner Trigram Kan-Water

**Gen's Inner Hexagram:
Jie-Release**

Thunder above Water indicates thunder and rain. When Heaven and Earth allow release, the result is thunder and rain which breaks a deadlock or obstacle. The dark and wild storm indicates a release of pressure that has built up, creating danger and obstruction. Now the skies clear, the clouds are gone and the pressure is relieved. All living things (i.e. plants and trees) have been nourished and rejuvenated by the rain.

Thunder represents movement and Water can indicate danger. Through movement, one avoids danger and finds a safe place. This is indicated by the strong fourth line which now can freely move upward away from danger and impasse. Once one is out of danger it is useful to pause, to consider the situation in stillness so that one can appropriately move in a new direction.

Jie also means to untie or unfasten. In relationship to meditation this implies untangling the knots and entanglements in one's life which create impediment and restrict forward movement. These impediments are akin to the clouds that gather and obstruct the clear sky.[26] They cannot be forcefully cleared, but must be released and let go. This release is initiated through inner observation, stillness and letting go. *Thunder and Rain perform their roles: this is the image of Release. In the same way, the noble man forgives misdeeds and pardons wrongdoing.*[27]

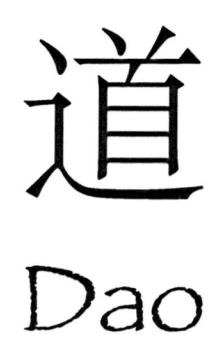

The Message in the Code

道
Dao

Conclusion: The Message in the Code

The Daoist images and symbols we have decoded here and throughout the lessons in the book reveal the keys to practicing meditation as a way of deeply engaging with our life. For Daoists, the physical, mental and spiritual planes (body-mind-spirit) are one. The psychic manifestations of *Qi/Breath*, *Jing* and *Shen* cannot be separated from their physical manifestations. Engagement can only come about through practice - practice that engages body, mind and spirit as one unified whole. Louis Komjathy explains this as follows:

> *Internal alchemy practice frequently involves two related processes. The first is the dual cultivation of innate nature (xing) and life-destiny (ming). In terms of "Daoist etymology," the character for innate nature symbolizes the heart-mind with which one was born, while the character for life destiny depicts the two kidneys viewed from the back. In one interpretation, innate nature refers to mind or consciousness, and thus to related meditation practices; life-destiny refers to physical vitality and longevity, and thus to related "nourishing life" (Yang Sheng) practices. One is advised to maintain a balanced cultivation regimen through the use of both movement (Dong), physical discipline, and stillness (Jing), mental discipline. Closely associated with this is the process of alchemical transformation, which centers on the Three Treasures (San Bao), namely jing, qi and shen. The first, preliminary stage in internal alchemy practice involves establishing the foundations (zhuji). Adepts seek to replenish vital essence and qi through specific stretching and qi circulation practices. Internal alchemy practice proper is a threefold process: (1) refining vital essence and transmuting it into qi (lianjing huaqi); (2) refining qi and transmuting it into spirit (lianqi huashen); and (3) refining spirit and returning to emptiness (lianshen huanxu).[1]*

Through breathing, aligning the *Du* vessel and emptying the mind we can unite our innate knowledge with our consciousness and life-destiny, resulting in a penetrating inner clarity. Simultaneously the physical body is rejuvenated. One cannot happen without the other and each reinforces the other. The "secret" hidden within the panoply of Daoist imagery is actually quite simple to understand:

1. Align the body and the *Du* vessel.

Through relaxed sitting and standing in correct posture and body alignment, the central *Du* (Governing) Vessel is open and unobstructed thereby allowing the *Qi/Breath* to move smoothly through it. This in turn will open the *Ren* and *Chong* vessels so that these vessels operate together as one central channel. Once the *Qi/Breath* can move freely in the central channel, it will move freely in all the meridians.

2. Focus the attention on the Qi/Breath.

Focusing the attention on the *Qi/Breath* as it moves in and out of *Dantian* helps to quiet the mind and aids the movement of the *Qi/Breath* through the central channel of the body. By focusing on *Dantian* without force and without effort, the breath will spontaneously harmonize and become refined. This allows *Jing* to transform into *Qi/Breath*.

3. Empty the mind and observe the internal landscape of the body.

As we saw earlier, every movement of the mind is a movement of the *Qi/Breath*. When the mind is quiet, extraneous movements of the *Qi/Breath* and the blood are curtailed. Thoughts and emotions that lead the *Qi/Breath* away from circulating in the central channel do not predominate. Focusing on Breath and *Dantian* allow the mind and body to settle themselves. When they settle themselves, *Qi/Breath* becomes refined and transforms into *Shen* (spirit).

This, in a nutshell, is the "secret" of the practice of Daoist meditation. The lessons in this book are a guide to take you there.

The method is simple and easy, but people will just not put forth the effort. If you can practice it consistently for a long time, you will surely 'penetrate metal and stone,' 'walk on water and fire,' and 'comprehend heaven and earth.'[2]

APPENDIX I
Reactions to Daosit Meditation & Nei Gong

氣 偏 差
Qi Pian Cha

Reactions to Meditation and Nei Gong

Students often worry about experiencing negative reactions (*Qi Pian Cha* or "Qi Deviations") to meditation and *Qi Gong* or *Nei Gong* exercises. In a sense, such reactions are inevitable because the process of activating and regulating the innate energy of the body involves adjusting your practice as you experience different sensations. This is much like the normal functioning of the various homeostatic mechanisms of the human body. For example, a "negative" reaction such as feeling short of breath tells you that either you are forcing the breath, or that there is tension in the diaphragm chest and upper back. Only by knowing that there is tension, can it be dispelled. Knowledge about the theory and practice of meditation and *Qi Gong* will help you to understand and rectify "negative" reactions.

In lesson two we covered the three harms and it is useful to review them now:

1. <u>Forced Breathing</u>: Forced breathing can cause the lungs and the muscles of respiration to be tense, creating shortness of breath.
2. <u>Labored Use of Strength</u>: Tension in the body, especially if focused on one part of the body, creates blockages in the *Qi/Breath*.
3. <u>Throwing out the Chest and Sucking in the Abdomen</u>: This posture prevents the *Qi/Breath* from sinking to the lower abdomen and the *Dantian*.

When you catch yourself forcing the breath, you will often notice that the diaphragm or the muscles of the ribcage, upper back and chest are tight or tense. By focusing your attention on the *Dantian*, without any other intention, the *Qi/Breath* will naturally sink down without effort. Tension in the body can be difficult to release because we are often unaware that we are tense. Throughout the nine lessons you have been working to detect and release tension, particularly during the standing meditation practices in Lessons Four to Six. Detecting and realsing tension is an ongoing process. As the *Qi/Breath* begins to move smoothly through the body, you will discover deeper, more subtle areas where the *Qi/Breath* does not move easily and smoothly. The very process of discovering these areas is how they release. This process happens in its own time, It cannot be forced and is different for each individual.

Sensations You Might Experience When Practicing Qi Gong and Daoist Meditation

Dizziness/Headache

Dizziness and headaches are usually the result of an over-focusing of the mind, or leading *Qi/Breath* upward and not letting it descend to *Dantian*. Let the mind relax and observe without forcing the application of the mind-intention. Focus on the *Dantian* and let the *Qi/Breath* move naturally.

An Upward Surge Of Qi From the Lower Abdomen

This physical sensation can occur if one focuses the mind-intention too much on movement of *Qi/Breath*. Relax mentally and let the breath be natural.

Tension and Heaviness in the Upper Back and Shoulders

Usually this is due to noticing that upper back and shulders are tense, and then trying too hard to relax them. The simplest way to correct this is to work with the other alignments: the head lifting as though suspended, the tail sinking, drawing up the back while dropping the chest and letting *Qi/Breath* sink to *Dantian*. Correcting these other alignments will help you to relax the shoulders and upper back.

Accelerated Heartbeat or Palpitations

An accelerated heartbeat and palpitations is a result of tension in the chest and unnatural or forced breathing. It can also be the result of focusing the mind intention too strongly in the chest area. Focusing on the **whole** pattern of the body alignments and letting the breath be easy and natural will usually resolve this problem

Abdominal Distension

A sensation of abdominal distension is the result of forced deep respiration or holding the breath, both of which can compresses the *Qi/Breath* downward. Returning to natural unforced, breathing and remembering that the diaphragm does not push the air down, but drops and lets the air flow into the lower abdomen, can help.

Insomnia

Insomnia usually occurs when one practices *Qi Gong* or meditation at night before going to bed. For some meditating before bed is relaxing, for others it is too activating. Although Daoist meditation can be practiced in the morning or the evening, if you experience insomnia, try moving your practice to the morning right after you get out of bed. Another possible reason for the insomnia is that the *Qi/Breath* is rising up the *Du* channel to the head, awakening the mind and over-exciting the nervous system. Focusing on the *Dantian* and letting the breath be relaxed and quiescent will help.

Feeling Light or Heavy in the Body, Sensations of Cold or Heat, Itching or Numbness

These are signs the *Qi/Breath* is being activated. They are normal and will come and go, change and eventually disappear.

Slight Swaying/Shaking

There may be slight swaying or vibration or other small spontaneous movements of the body during the performance of meditation and *Qi Gong*. These are indications that the *Qi/Breath* is being activated. This is a good sign and is beneficial. The sensations should not intensify and should disappear with practice as the *Qi/Breath* moves more smoothly.

Swaying/Shaking/Staring Eyes/Twitches

Stronger swaying and shaking, twitches and staring eyes are symptoms of *Qi Gong* illness from the *Qi/Breath* ascending and not descending. If these sensations are experienced, the *Shen* (spirit) can be disturbed. The spirit is "housed" by the heart and can only be clear in its perception, by having space in the heart. If you experience these symptoms it may be that the heart is too full. This is usually a result of the *Qi/Breath* being forced up the *Du* vessel. It is not uncommon to develop these symptoms in the incorrect practice of Kundalini Yoga, or when martial artists practice internal exercises with too much *Li* (force) and shock-power. Meditation and *Qi Gong* must develop in their own time and cannot be forced. These sensations should not occur if practice proceeds naturally and is unforced. If they do occur, stop practicing and they should dissipate. If they do not dissipate, then see a trained practitioner of traditional Chinese medicine.

Other Considerations

Fatigue:

If you feel tired and unfocused stop for the day or simply do less. When one is tired, just attending to Kidney Breathing (Lesson Two) or standing in the *Wu Ji* posture (Lesson Four) can re-energize and relax the body.

Clothing

Wear loose clothes that does not constrict retard the movement of the *Qi/Breath*.

Cultivate a Calm Attention

Unless you are practicing on a mountaintop, it may not be possible to insulate yourself from sudden noises or outside disturbances. Try to find a quiet place where you will not be startled. Cultivating a calm mind-intention that is directed internally, yet also externally aware. This will prevent sudden disturbances from affecting you. If you are startled during meditation, keep the eyes half-closed and continue practicing.

After Meditating

Immediately after meditating, do not engage in sudden physical activity. Leave space for the body and mind to adjust, or practice slow moving exercises like stretching, Yoga, *Tai Ji Quan* or *Qi Gong*.

Keep the Feet on the Floor

In sitting meditation, the feet are either on the floor as when sitting on a chair, or folded on the floor, as in sitting cross-legged.

Rubbing the Meridians

Massaging the meridian pathways after meditating can smooth out the flow of *Qi/Breath* to the four limbs and can prevent *Qi/Breath* from getting blocked. Massage from the shoulders to the tips of the fingers on the back of the arm, and then from the fingertips to the chest on the inside of the arm. Repeat nine times on each side. Then massage from the buttocks and hips down the back and side of the legs to the tops of the feet with both hands and then up the inside of the legs from the inside of the ankle to the groin. Repeat nine times. This was mentioned and illustrated at the end of Lesson Nine.

APPENDIX II
Body Configurations for Daoist Meditation and Nei Gong

體　式
Ti　Shi

Body Configurations for Daoist Meditation & Nei Gong

The body alignments are a very important aspect of practicing Daoist meditation and *Nei Gong*. By having the body aligned and open, the muscles are relaxed, the joints line up and the meridians are open and unblocked. This allows *Qi/Breath* to be nourished and gather in the lower abdomen. This gathering, in turn, engenders internal movement and transformation of *Jing*, *Qi/Breath* and *Shen*. The life gate (*Mingmen*) and the *Dantian* connect with the kidneys and the reproductive organs, which in turn hold and produce *Jing* (essence). This area of the body includes the lower portion of the sacrum, the first gate through which the *Qi/Breath* must flow in micro-cosmic orbit circulation. This is where Kan-Water resides. Kan contains the true yang hidden within yin.

As *Qi/Breath* gathers in this area it can easily leak out through the lower orifices - the anus and urethra. Hence it is important to "gather the anus" or "lift" the perineum (the Lower Magpie Bridge) in order to prevent this leakage. This was discussed in Lesson Two. However, restraining *Qi/Breath* from leaking is not just a matter of lifting the perineum. Preventing leakage comes from engaging with all of the body alignments simultaneously: lifting the head and upper back, retracting the chin slightly and sinking the tail aid the lifting of the perineum, while simultaneously opening *Du* Channel. The lifting actions also create a counter movement that allows the *Qi/Breath* to sink downward. For this sinking to occur naturally, without using force or encountering obstruction, the chest must be relaxed and soft or relatively empty, the shoulders and elbows relaxed and sinking, the mind quiescent and empty, but aware. The breath is slow, steady, even and deep.

Yi Jing Body Images: The Dui Trigram and the Jie Hexagram

The open hips and rounded position of the crotch, kua, hip and sacrum in sitting, combined with the gathering of the anus and perineum, create a bowl-like configuration that "holds" and stores Kan-Water, Qi/Breath and Kidney Essence. This is often understood by using *Yi Jing* Imagery. The Hexagram Jie: Restraint is composed of Kan-Water over Dui-Lake. Dui is like an upturned bowl, its two solid lines forming the bottom of the bowl, and the empty yin line at the top representing the empty space within the bowl that can contain and hold. Dui also represents the bowl-like shape of a lake filled with water. Kan-Water is solid in the middle surrounded by two yin lines. The outer yin lines represent the malleability of water, its ability to conform to the shape of its container, while the inner yang line represents the hidden yang strength of water. Water can penetrate into the smallest crack, wear away a mountain and can gather to create a wave of unstoppable power.

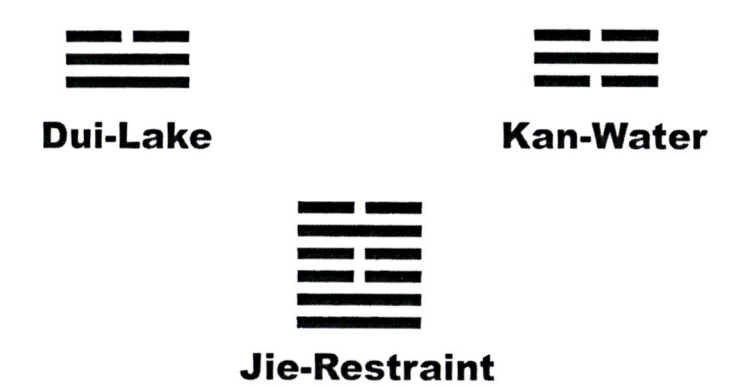

Dui-Lake   **Kan-Water**

Jie-Restraint

In the Jie Hexagram, the lower trigram, Dui, represents the crotch, kua, hips, sacrum and perineum and their rounded bowl-like shape that holds and restrains the overflow or leakage of Kan-Water.[1] This image also helps us to understand other methods of restraining the leakage of *Qi/Breath* in order to strengthen the kidneys and essence.

349

Supplemental Method for Strengthening the Kidneys and Restraining Leakage to Nourish the Qi-Breath

When *Qi/Breath* gathers in *Dantian*, one can have a sensation of needing to urinate or defecate. At the moment *Qi/Breath* is gathering, passing waste will also drain out the *Qi/Breath* that is coalescing and gathering in the lower abdomen, resulting in depletion of the kidneys and defeating part of the purpose of meditation and *Qi Gong*. Try and urinate or pass stools apart from the time of practice.

In general, when you pass pass urine or have a bowel movement, the following techniques can help you minimize the leakage of *Qi/Breath*:

1) **When Urinating:** Lift the heels, close the mouth and lightly clench the teeth. Try and inhale as you urinate. After passing urine, gather and lift the anus for 30 seconds to one minute.

2) **When Moving the Bowels:** close the mouth, clench the teeth, put the tongue on the upper palate, and do not speak.

Yi Jing Body Images: The Zhen and Gen Trigrams

The *Nei Gong Zhen Chuan* uses the images of Zhen and Gen to represent the ribs and chest respectively.

The chest is exemplified by Gen. Gen is mountain. One yang stops above two yin, the resulting image is the mountain. In the human body, this is the chest. For example in terms of Heaven, that which ascends is called qi; in terms of Earth, that which descends is called form. Qi has a tendency to float, therefore it must be restrained. This is what happens in the chest. Form has a tendency to sink; therefore it must be lifted. This is what happens outside of the chest. Chest qi flows upward to the head and neck. This is the Qian diagram, Heaven.[2]

The ribs are exemplified by the Zhen trigram, which expresses movement and thunder, one yang moving below two yin. When thunder issues out it does so in an upward direction as do the ribs. What is above the ribs is related to Heaven, while what is below the ribs is related to Earth. When the upper and lower body are unified, qi and blood flow and the power emits outward. Qi from the ribs moves upward to intersect with the head, like thunder meeting with Heaven and increasing in power. Here the Zhen Qi rises up to the head and neck, strengthened by motion and becomes even more powerful. Qi from the ribs also moves downward to intersect with the feet, like thunder meeting the earth and becoming content. Here the Zhen Qi moves downward and intersects with the feet and knees, flowing smoothly thereby the spirit and qi are content.[3]

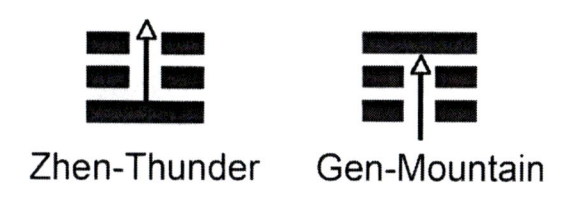

Zhen-Thunder   Gen-Mountain

Qi/Breath has a tendency to float relative to the body form. The action of lifting the *Qi/Breath* and other bodily substances upward is aided by the ribs and spine, represented by Zhen-Thunder. In the Zhen diagram, the strong yang first line is free to move upward, unobstructed through the open path created by the two yin lines. However, this movement must not float too high. It must be restrained, so that *Qi/Breath* can sink to *Dantian* and to the *Yong Quan* (KID 1) on the bottom of the foot in order to rise upward again. This can only happen if movement and restraint operate properly, if the moving yang line in the Gen and Zhen diagrams operates appropriately.[4]

The ribs are said to open and close like a "fish gill", allowing *Qi/Breath* to ascend and descend. In closing *Qi/Breath* descends; in opening *Qi/Breath* ascends.[5] When the ribs open, *Qi/Breath* goes upward to reach the heart and brain like thunder flying into the sky, reaching Heaven.

When the ribs close, *Qi/Breath* moves downward to reach Earth and *Qi/Breath* flows into the kidneys and *Dantian* and can reach the feet. The ribs, represented by Zhen-Thunder, are the intermediaries between the heart and kidneys, fire and water - the Post-Heaven manifestations of Heaven and Earth.

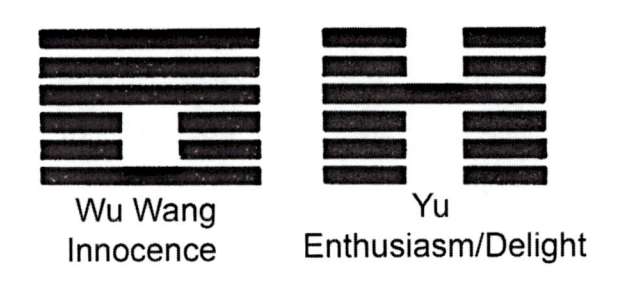

Wu Wang
Innocence

Yu
Enthusiasm/Delight

Thunder under Heaven is Hexagram #25: *Wu Wang* (Innocence). The bottom moving line of the Zhen trigram moves upward to combine with the Heaven's three strong moving lines. This represents blending one's *Qi/Breath* with the natural force of Heaven, allowing one to increase and further one's intention and vital force, just as the energies of living things move under Heaven in the spring. This same interaction is reflected in nature's creative activity - plants and animals sprouting and growing.

Thunder over Earth is Hexagram #16: *Yu* (Enthusiasm or Delight). Here Zhen's moving yang line is completely unobstructed. It can go upward toward Heaven or downward to reach the Earth. Yang energy influences and moves the yin elements and substrates of the body through the inciting power of Zhen-Thunder and the ribs. This brings delight, just as thunder and rain over the earth brings nourishment and happiness to living things.

Da Xu
Great Accumulation

Qian
Modesty/Humility

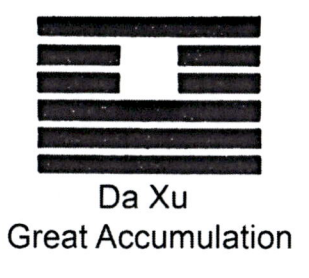

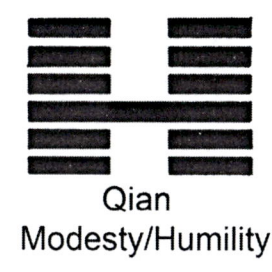

Gen's restraining influence can be represented by Hexagram #26: *Da Xu* (Great Accumulation); Mountain over Heaven. The Mountain (the chest) checks the upward movement of Heaven's three strong moving lines so that strength is not dissipated, but accumulates and is stored. The image is one of rain clouds around mountain peaks - energy accumulating and waiting to be released.

Gen's restraint in relation to Earth is represented by Earth over Mountain. This is Hexagram #15: *Qian* (Modesty or Humility). Mountain's strong yang line is hidden within yin, so that action, movement and creativity are contained within stillness and receptivity. The chest expands with the breath, but this expansion cannot be too extreme, it must be hidden and imperceptible within the stillness and receptivity represented by Earth.

The ribs are underneath the chest. When Zhen is beneath Gen, Hexagram #27: *Yi* (Nourishment) is formed. The Chinese word *Yi* means self-cultivation and nourishment.[6] The *Yi* ideogram 頤 means chin; cheek; jaw; to nourish. Thunder is movement and Gen mountain is stillness. The lower jaw (Zhen) moves against the still upper palate (Gen) to chew or talk (nourishing others through instruction and teaching). Zhen and Gen can also represent physical and spiritual nourishment. The upper trigram (Gen) represents spiritual nourishment that you give to others, and the lower trigram (Zhen), the physical nourishment you provide for yourself.[7]

Gen-Mountain

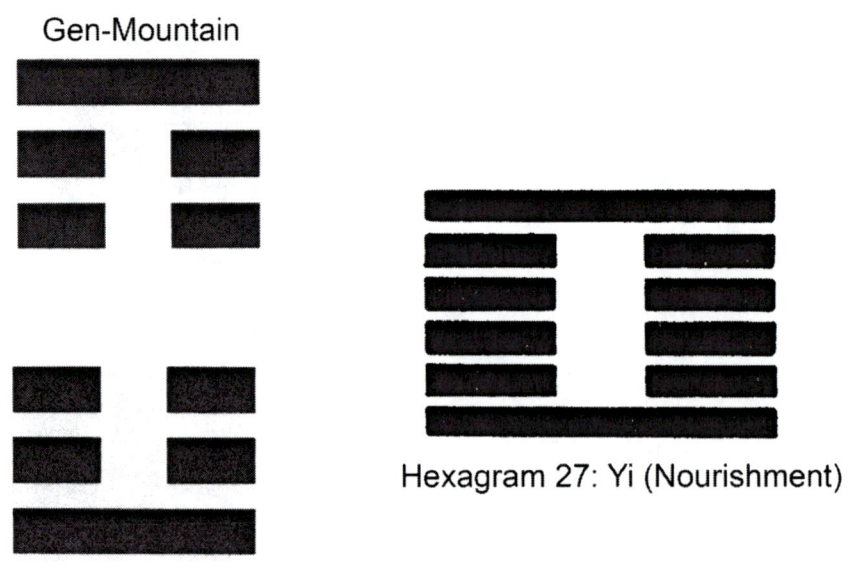

Zhen Thunder

Hexagram 27: Yi (Nourishment)

When engaged in meditation, there is emptiness inside just as the center of the *Yi* Hexagram is empty. Outside one is as stable and calm as a mountain, while inside there is movement and change. The empty center allows the moving lines to communicate and interact. Heaven's creativity interacts with Earth's receptivity; Fire and Water circulate and inter-transform, and the heart and kidneys communicate.

Traditional Mnemonic for the Body Alignments in Nei Gong and Daoist Meditation

These trigram and hexagram images can be used in conjunction with the alignments listed below. They are often memorized as a mnemonic that can be recited to set the correct position for practicing meditation or *Nei Gong*. These are not just a set of postural alignments, but a set of body patterns or configurations which are at the same time internal and external as well as energetic and structural in nature. When properly maintained, the pattern creates a web of interconnections.

全 身 放 松
Quan Shen Fang Song
Whole body released slackened (loose-relaxed)

接 头 松 开
Guan Jie Song Kai
Joints slacken (relax) open

中 正
Zhong Zheng
Centered and erect (upright, correct)

顶 头 悬
Ding Tou Xuan
Supported from the crown, the head hangs suspended

顺 项 提 顶
Shun Xiang Ti Ding
Straighten neck, uplift vertex

虚 灵 顶 劲
Xu Ling Ding Jing
Empty awareness and alert intelligence ascend to the crown of the head with vitality

舌 顶 上 腭
She Ding Shang E
Tongue goes to upper palate

溜 臀 收 肛
Liu Tun Shou Gang
Smooth the buttocks, gather the anus

松肩沉肘
Song Jian Chen Zhou
Slacken shoulder, sink elbow

氣沉丹田
Qi Chen Dantian
Qi sinks to *Dantian*

实腹畅胸
Shi Fu Chang Xiong
Solid (substantial; full) abdomen, unimpeded chest

含胸拔背
Han Xiong Ba Bei
Contain (like something held in one's mouth) the chest and draw up the back

松腰松胯
Song Yao Song Kua
Slacken the small of the back and the Kua (front of the hip)

尾閭提
Wei Lu Ti
Lift the coccyx (tail gate)

用意不用力
Yong Yi Bu Yong Li
Use intent, do not use force (do not exert oneself physically)

Appendix III: Extract on Daoist Meditation From Sun Xi Kun's *Ba Gua Quan Zhen Chuan*

八卦拳真传

About Sun Xi Kun

Sun Xi Kun 孫錫堃 (1883-1952) was one of the few disciples of the famous Ba Gua Zhang practitioner Cheng You Long. Sun's book *Ba Gua Quan Zhen Chuan* 八卦拳真传 (Genuine Transmission of Ba Gua Zhang) is one of the few records of Chen You Long's method. In addition to teaching Ba Gua Zhang and other martial arts, Sun Xi Kun also studied Daoism. He established the Morality and Martial Arts Society in Tianjin. He moved south during WWII, eventually traveling to Hong Kong and later to Taiwan where he lived and taught until his death. The treatise on Daoism below, extracted from Sun's book *Ba Gua Quan Zhen Chuan*, is a transmission of Daoist Nei Dan meditation practice. In Parts Five and Six, Sun discusses Daoist practices specific to women in detail. The translation from the Chinese and the accompanying commentary was done by Huang Guo Qi and Tom Bisio.

Part 1: Authentic Cultivation of Taoism

The essence of cultivation is to understand the methods for realizing (enlightening) the heart-mind and one's essential nature. Empty prattle about cultivating the Way (Dao) will not lead to real awakening to truth. Buddhism's empty, obstinate sitting cultivates *Xing*, but does not cultivate *Ming*. In Daoism, both *Xing* and *Ming* are cultivated.[1] But, few people can get authentic instruction. I have heard that the path to immortality has no fixed methods and no fixed phases (time period). Careless sitting can easily cause illness. If attachment to the bonds of the world is unfinished, one cannot research deeply. Those who study the

---

[1] This comparison of *Xing* 性: inner nature; character; disposition; property; quality and *Ming* 命: vital force or life, refers to two methods or "schools" of Daoist cultivation: *Xing Gong* and *Ming Gong*. *Xing Gong* refers to self-cultivation which employs quiet seated meditation to cultivate the mind, while *Ming Gong* trains the body through *Qi* cultivation exercises. These two methods or schools are complimentary. *Xing* and *Ming* are the *Qi*/Breath and the *Shen* (spirit). *Xing* relates to Earth and *Ming* to Heaven. *Xing* and *Ming* must circulate and unite.

Dao are as numerous as hairs on an ox, but those who reach attainment are as rare as a *Qilin*.[2] Those who believe and practice sincerely and painstakingly are few, and those who boast and seek fame are numerous. Coming in through the side door, one can go astray.

Of course in cultivating the Dao, there are those who cultivate movement (*Dong*) and those who cultivate stillness (*Jing*). For those who cultivate Daoism from motion, it is first necessary to strengthen *Wai Dan* (external elixir)[3], by first refining grain into essence (*Jing*) and cultivating a Pine Resin (*Song Jiao*) body[4], and then training *Nei Dan* (internal elixir).[5] For those who cultivate tranquility, one must first realize one's inner nature and then cultivate Nei Dan. The training methods are different, but the achievements are same. The real principle is to first nourish Post-Heaven (*Hou Tian*) and then return to Pre-Heaven (*Xian Tian*). Without the strong body of an *Arhat*[6] how can there possibly be an immortal baby Buddha that is vigorous and perceptive?

People today fail to understand and cultivate the Dao. Three Key Points must be understood: longevity (*Shou*), achievement (*Gong*) and Dao (the Way). These three are interrelated. The first stage of cultivation is to prevent disease and prolong life. The second stage in cultivating the *Tai*

---

[2] The *Qilin* is often equated to a unicorn. However, the *Qilin* (*Kirin*, in Japanese) is a mythical animal with the head of a dragon, the horns and body of a deer, the hooves of a horse and the tail of an ox. Other descriptions depict the *Qilin* with the scales of a carp, the hooves of an ox, the tail of a lion, and the head of a dragon. In some depictions the *Qilin* has two horns and in others, only one.

[3] *Wai Dan* (Outer Elixir): External exercises in which *Qi* is built up externally, usually through movement, and then led internally.

[4] This may be an oblique reference to *Bigu* (辟谷), which literally means avoiding grains. *Bigu* is a Daoist fasting technique associated with achieving transcendence or immortality. It is sometimes understood as not eating certain foods or in other cases as not eating any foods and subsisting on the breath and various herbs, one of which is pine resin.

[5] *Nei Dan* (Inner Elixir): Internal exercises, often involving stillness or tranquility, in which qi is accumulated internally and then led externally. Part of *Nei Dan* involves cultivating the Three Treasures (*Jing, Qi/Breath* and *Shen*) and refining and transforming them into the "internal elixir" (*Nei Dan*).

[6] In Buddhism, an *Arhat* is a practitioner whose spiritual practice is advanced and has attained liberation.

Gong (great achievement) is to lay a foundation by collecting the medicines[7] that forge *Dan* (elixir) so as to consolidate the *San Bao* (Three Treasures).[8] Then one can begin to talk about the Dao. In human life the bones and sinews change after sixty years. At that point the functioning of the internal organs has decayed. Even if one is able to prolong life, one is already half-dead. The ancients say that once a sixty-year cycle has passed, one has passed over the gate of hell. Therefore, people should accelerate their cultivation before becoming old and weak and maintain the health of their bodies.

Although there are three thousand and six hundred side doors and seventy-two heterodox paths[9], they are nothing more than just refining grain to transform into *Jing* (essence), cultivating and transforming essence into *Qi*, cultivating and transforming *Qi* into *Shen* (spirit) and then refining spirit so it can return to emptiness. One who cultivates only their nature does not cultivate life. Even if they see through the vanity of human affairs and discipline their temperament, sitting still, worshipping Buddha and chanting scriptures - they are cultivating *Xing*, but not *Ming*.[10] Obstinate empty sitting only dries up the cooking pot in an attempt to eliminate illness and prolong life. All of these methods deviate from the true instruction that is passed down. If the true doctrine of the Great Dao is sought, one must return to true awakening. *Xing* and *Ming* must be cultivated simultaneously. Because the root of the heart is the spirit, and the spirit resides in the heart and life. (*Ming*) [resides] in the kidney, essence (*Jing*) is *Yuan Qi*. Refined essence is transformed into *Qi* and refined. *Qi* is transformed into spirit and refined spirit returns to

---

[7] The "medicines" or "herbs" refer to *Qi* and *Jing* (essence) which must be gathered like herbs in order to be refined ("cooked") internally by a process of extraction and transformation. This "cooking" of the "medicinal substances" is a metaphor for cultivation of the internal elixir - Nei Dan practice.

[8] The *San Bao* 三宝 are *Jing* (essence), *Qi* (Qi-Breath) and *Shen* (spirit). In *Nei Dan* self-cultivation practices, *Jing*, *Qi*/Breath and *Shen* transmute and inter-transform in order to return to the Pre-Heaven state of emptiness.

[9] In effect: many methods and unorthodox doctrines.

[10] See footnote #1.

emptiness. Nourishing Pre-Heaven is based upon this. Therefore *Xing* is cultivated in death and *Ming* cultivates life. After *Xing Gong* is realized there are no distracted thoughts in the heart. Then one can begin to cultivate *Ming Gong*.[11] Nevertheless, *Xing Gong* and *Ming Gong* progress together simultaneously. This is exactly what simultaneous cultivation of Nature and Life means.

The heart belongs to the fire and resides in the south, a manifestation of the trigram Li. The kidney belongs to the water and resides in the north, a manifestation of the trigram of Kan. In Daoist cultivation, the principle is to use fire to boil water so that water transforms into *Qi*. *Qi* transforms spirit and spirit transforms into emptiness. The *Dan* (elixir) Classic says to "subdue the dragon and vanquish the tiger".[12] The dragon is *Xing* and the tiger is *Ming*. A calm heart is the dragon returning to the sea. Letting go of emotion is the tiger hiding in the mountain. This is the cultivation of both *Xing* and *Ming*. There are three steps in Daoist cultivation: (1) prevent disease and prolong life; (2) seek immortality; (3) cultivate the Great Dao. Therefore, those who cultivate the Dao, regardless of what situations they encounter, should avoid the pull of material desires. Upon encountering things they desire, they should withdraw the heart-mind - their conscious perception (awareness). From conscious perception to no perception to true (realized) perception. This is cultivation of the Li [trigram] palace. For one who attains the true Way, *yin-shen* (invisible spirit) appears. *Yang-shen* (visible spirit) does not appear, especially a ghost being.[13]

Both in ancient times and today, for those who cultivated the Dao, it is difficult to cut off the Licentious Root. Longevity is impossible, unless

---

[11] See footnote #1.
[12] 降龙伏虎 *Xiang Long Pu Hu*. Literally: lower; descend or subdue the dragon and hide; lie down or tame the tiger. Can also mean to overcome powerful adversaries, or in Daoism - "to conquer one's passions."
[13] This seems to refer to *Yang Shen* (yang spirit) and *Yin Shen* (yin spirit). These are projections of the spirit out of the body. Some Daoists say that the *Yang Shen* is a sign of achievement in meditation, while others posit that *Yin Shen* is the sign of achievement.

Ma Yin Zang Xiang (Penis Hidden in the Abdomen) is trained.[14] Female Daoist practitioners should first cut off the Red Dragon.[15] Male Daoist Practitioners should first subdue the White Tiger.[16] Women can cultivate the Dao faster than men, because the woman's body is the offspring of pure yang. Only the lower private parts belong to yin. A man's body is the offspring of pure yin. Only the lower private parts belong to yang. The so-called Red Dragon is between the two breasts. When the breasts are trained to emptiness, the Red Dragon is cut off. Therefore, women train form and men train *Qi*. *Ren Mai* arises from *Hui Yang* which is located slightly in front of *Huiyin* (CV 1), inside the root of the kidney (external genitalia), and ends at *Chengjiang* (CV 24) below the lower lip. *Du Mai* arises from *Huiyin* (CV 1) and ends at *Renzhong* (GV 26), in the groove above the upper lip. *Shenqi*[17] starts here and flows between the two *mai* without stopping. This is the Heavenly Circle achievement (*Zhou Tian Gong*).[18]

In cultivating the Dao and training *Dan* (the elixir),[19] it is necessary to collect the medicine to put on the stove, in order to nourish Dan to pass through the barrier, and to conceive the fetus to give birth to the spirit.[20]

---

[14] This seems to refer to a Daoist practice in which a man's "outside yang" (penis) shrinks so that *jing* (essence) is not lost and therefore *qi* can be refined internally.

[15] The "red dragon" refers to menstruation. Sun Xi Kun references Daoist practices that aim to stop menstruation so that female practitioners stop the monthly loss of blood which impacts on their essence (*Jing*).

[16] Subduing the White Tiger refers to techniques of sexual *neigong* or inner alchemy in which semen (*Jing*) is transmuted into *Qi*.

[17] *Shenqi* 神气: qi and spirit ; the aspect of *qi* that transforms into spirit.

[18] 小周天 *Xiao Zhou Tian*: "Small Heavenly Circulation" or the "Micro-cosmic Orbit." Internal transformation of the Three Treasures practiced by Daoists and martial arts practitioners, in which qi is circulated through the Ren and Du Meridians. Part of Nei Gong practices and Daoist inner alchemy.

[19] *Lian Dan* 炼丹: "Refining the elixir"; "concocting pills of immortality". In *Neidan* practices this means creating a "pill" inside the body by refining *Jing, Qi/Breath* and *Shen*.

[20] This again refers to refining *Jing* to *Qi/Breath* so that the *Qi/Breath* can move through the three barriers (*San Guan*) in the *Du Mai* and transmute into spirit. Then in passing through *Ren Mai*, spirit replenishes *Jing* forming a "fetus" inside the body which in turn gives birth to spirit.

After that one is free and unfettered and can become a contented immortal.

Cultivating the Dao occurs in the human body; the outside body is not the Dao. It is divided into three passes (*San Guan*), respectively in the front and in the back. Namely: upper Dantian, also termed *Shang Huang Ting* (Upper Yellow Court), i.e. the brain; the middle Dantian, also termed *Zhong Huang Ting* (Middle Yellow Court), i.e. the spleen, located 1.2 cun below the umbilicus, and the Lower Dantian, *Xia Huang Ting* (Lower Yellow Court), i.e. the lower abdomen. The posterior three passes are the *Yu Zhen* (Jade Pillow), i.e. the occipital bone, *Jia Ji* Pass, i.e. the spine, and *Wei Lu* Pass, i.e. the coccyx. Those are the barriers that must be passed through in refining and transforming *Qi*.

It is said in the *Dan* Classics that after going through the three mountains (three passes), one can attain immortal spirit. If those who cultivate the Dao want to understand the true way, they must seek out the wise.

Part 2: The True Formula of the Dao Elixir Secret Treasure

In the nose there are two acu-points linking with the mouth, and from the mouth to the throat, the lung and the heart. Under the heart, there is an aperture named *Jiang Gong* (Crimson Palace). Another 3.6 *cun* further below *Jiang Gong*, is a site named *Tu Fu Zhong* (Earth Cauldron Center), in which there there are two apertures, one linking with the left liver and another one linking with the right liver.[21] About 1.2 *cun* inside this area, there is the place to store *Qi* and refine Earth's elixir. Another 3.6 *cun* further down toward the umbilicus, directly opposite to *Sheng Men* (Gate of Life), there are seven apertures linking with the external genitalia, where the *Jingshen* (essence-spirit) can leak and empty. 1.3 *cun* below *Ming Lu* (Famous Stove), is called *Dantian*, a place for storing *Jing* (essence) and

---

[21] The left and right lobes of the liver.

collecting the medicine.²² The three passes in the front are *Ni Wan* (Mud Ball) (i.e. brain, the house of the mind), *Xu Guan* (Empty Pass) acu-point and *Tu Fu* (Earth Cauldron) (i.e. the spleen). *Ni Wan* (Mud Ball) is named *Shang Dantian* (Upper Dantian), with an area of 1.2 cun, a place to store the *Shen* (spirit). Its acupoint is 1 cun entering inside the space between the eyebrows. The true middle is *Tian Men* (Gate of Heaven). One *cun* further inward is *Dong Fang Gong* (Chamber Palace). One *cun* further inward is *Ni Wan Gong* (Mud Ball Palace).

To learn the fundamentals of cultivating the Dao, there are three important elements: 1) Heart and body are empty, bright and incorruptible; 2) Strictly guard the *Jing* and avoid blame and offense; 3) accumulate achievement and virtue through good deeds. Once the *Yuan Shen* (Original Spirit) is flourishing, the *Yuan Qi* (Original Qi) can grow, and the *Yuan Jing* (Original Essence) will consolidate and be solid. There is only one method to refine *Dan* (the elixir), namely to refine the temperament,²³ i.e. to train temperament (the liver, lung, metal, wood, dragon, tiger, Hun and Po), the heart and kidney (lead, mercury), nature and body (stove and tripod), and *Jing* and *Qi* (medicines, herbs).²⁴ When the five elements (*Wu Xing*) assemble in the *Zhong Gong* (Middle Palace), three origins unite as one, *Dan* (elixir) coalesces into the embryo, one becomes immortal and flies away. This is the *Jin Dan* (Golden Pill) that

---

²² *Yao* 药: can mean medicine, drug or herb. In this context, is not literally a Chinese herb, or medicine, but something that acts like a tonic herb. In Daoist inner alchemy the *yao* are *Jing* and *Qi*/Breath.

²³ *Xing Qing* 性情: literally *xing*: "character" or "nature"; *qing*: "emotion" or "feeling".

²⁴ Here Sun Xi Kun references the five elements and the internal organs with Daoist code words and imagery. The liver is associated with wood and the dragon as well as the Hun, an aspect of the spirit sometimes known as the "ethereal soul", which is associated with the *San Bao* (*Jing Qi* and *Shen*). In turn, the lung is associated with metal, the tiger and the Po, an aspect of the spirit known as the "corporeal soul", which is associated with the seven emotions. Mercury and lead are metaphors for the liver and lung and their connection to the heart and kidney in Daoist thought, and the stove and tripod (a cooking vessel) reference the lower and upper *Dantian* and the refining process (Daoist practices) that involve the mind and body. Herbs and medicines are a reference to the cultivation *Jing* and *Qi*, which then act like herbs to create transmutation and change.

gives birth to the Great Dao (*Da Dao*). The authentic transmission of the correct formula for *Nei Dan* has four steps:

1. *Xuan Pin* (Mysterious Female)[25]
2. *Yao Cai* (Medicinals)
3. *Huo He* (Firing Times)
4. Four Season conservation and adjustment of the *Xuan Pin* (mysterious female).

Namely, there is an aperture in the middle of the human body that is the source of creation and transformation, the origin of *Hun Dun*[26], the returning root of the Great Void, an aperture for revival of the life and the gate of the life and death, a dark and mysterious pass (*Xuan Gong*)[27] for

---

[25] *Xuan Pin* 玄牝: The "mysterious female" or "black female" - "black" in this context means something dark, profound, and incredible. The dark female is mentioned in chapter 6 of the *Dao De Jing*: *If one nourishes the spirits one dies not. This is called the dark and the female. The gates of the dark one and of the female, they are called the root of heaven and earth.* The commentary on this passage by He Shang Gong states that the Dao of immortality is contained within the dark one and the female. The dark is Heaven, and in humans, forms the nose. The female is Earth and forms the mouth. Through the nose, the breath, and the five atmospheres associated with Heaven enter and form the *Hun* ("spiritual Soul; ethereal Soul). Through the mouth the five tastes enter and nourish the stomach and form the *Po* (the corporeal soul). The gates of the dark one and of the female are therefore the gates through which the original breath flows. *Ho-Shang-Kung's Commentary on Lao-Tse,* translated and annotated by Edward Erkes, Switzerland: Artibus Asiae, Ascona, 1950, pp. 21-22.
Xuanpin is also a gate or passage way situated at the junction of being and non-being, the place where yang opens and yin closes. It also stands for Qian and Kun, the trigrams associated with Heaven and Earth. The Inner mysterious female is also associated with *Zhen Qi* (True Qi) and the outer mysterious female is associated with *Zhen Shen* (True Spirit), which are also called the inner and outer medicines, *Nei Yao* and *Wai Yao*. Xuan can also be the upper *Dantian* and *Pin* the lower *Dantian*. *The Routledge Encyclopedia of Taoism Volume II: M-Z*, edited by Fabrizio Pregadio, London and New York: Routledge, 2008, pp.1138-9.

[26] 混沌 *Hun Dun* has many meanings although usually it refers to a cosmogonic stage of development in the fundamental division of previously undifferentiated matter (chaos) into yin and yang. In Daoist *Nei Dan* (inner alchemy) texts, this chaotic state (*Hun Dun*) is the origin of the reshaping of the inner and outer universe - both the elixir and the Original (*Yuan*) Qi of human beings and the universe. (*The Routledge Encyclopedia of Taoism Volume I: A-L* edited by Fabrizio Pregadio, London and New York: Routledge, 2008, p 525).

[27] 玄關 *Xuan Guan,* the "mysterious pass" represents the moment *Xing* (the inner nature) and *Ming* (the vital force) come together, or return to a state of oneness. *Xing* and *Ming* are also known as Dragon and Tiger; Lead and Mercury etc. The mysterious pass is the "door of life and death", the place between being and non-being. It is also a synonym for the *Xuan Pin* (Mysterious Female) and the *Hun Dun*. This is the place where

the *Zhong Huang Gong* (Middle Yellow Palace)[28], the aperture of the gate of the *Xuan Pin* (Mysterious Female), nature's inexplicable mystery. Its form is like a chicken egg, black and white in appearance and one cun in length. After ten months, the fetus[29] comes out of its bag, white like cotton, moving like a 1.2 cun ring, the guiding mechanism of the human body, within which the pure essentials fuse and release, but which cannot be used unless the heart-mind is fully concentrated. This requires the emergence of fetal breathing (ie: "heel breathing" or "whole body breathing").

When *Shenqi* joins with feeling, when the mind and *Qi* communicate, it is possible to observe its mystery. In the *Dao De Jing* it says: "When there is no desire, it is possible to see the mystery." If one observes inside, then the upper, middle and lower are also observed and can link together. The classic says: if you attain one thing, all things will be accomplished. Once *Yuan Jing*, *Yuan Qi* and *Yuan Shen* meet, *Dan Gong* (Elixir Achievement) is achieved. Then in the dark mysterious pass, the aperture of *Xuan Pin*, and the origin of yin and yang, the *Shenqi* resides. *Shenqi* is the medicine of *Xing* and *Ming*. Fetal breathing is the root and consolidates the base. The fetus is the storehouse of the *Shen*. Breath is the origin of the fetus. Breath gives life to the fetus. Breath grows because of the fetus. Without the breath, the fetus will not have spirit and can not form the pill of immortality. Like a fetus in the mother's womb, innocent[30] and without knowledge or form. Therefore, in going back to the root and

---

transcendence and unity can occur in Daoist practices. *The Routledge Encyclopedia of Taoism Volume II: M-Z*, edited by Fabrizio Pregadio, London and New York: Routledge, 2008, pp. 1131-2.

[28] 黄宮 *Huang Gong* or *Huang Ting*: is the "yellow palace" associated with Earth and therefore lies at the center. In the body, this can be the center of the head ("Upper Yellow Palace") or the center of the *Dantian* ("Lower Yellow Palace").

[29] This "fetus" is not a real fetus, but a metaphor for the fusion of spirit and breath.

[30] This is again 混沌 *Hun Dun* (see footnote #25), but in this context can also mean the innocence of a child.

returning[31] to the beginning, one gives birth to the five viscera (*zang*), reestablishes the skeletal structure. When no substance gives birth to substance, then the Sage fetus can form. The ancient classics say: "pass on the medicine, but not the fire".

The secret that must be passed down, but cannot be passed down, are the firing times (*Huo Huo*)[32] for collecting and refining the medicine. The central fire possesses its own medicine. Know where to gather the medicine. Fire binds and wraps it to become *Dan* (elixir). This cannot be passed on through tradition but must be sensed. The medicines are yang within yin and the firing time is yin within yang. Once the theory of yin, yang and fire is clearly understood and the medicine is gathered in the place of origin, why does it need to be passed on orally?[33]

---

[31] 復 *Fu*: Returning; return to normal or to the original state. This references the Fu Hexagram in the *Yi Jing*, in which the return is symbolized by the single yang line which appears at the bottom - yang returning again after the ascendance of yin.

[32] Many Daoist internal alchemical texts speak of "firing times" or *Huo Huo*. This is yet another metaphor taken from external alchemy and metallurgy - adjusting the fire or heat in order to properly extract, refine and temper metal. Often these firing times were associated with the twelve sovereign hexagrams and the phases of the moon, as well as the Twelve Earthly Stems associated with two hour divisions of the day that delineate the waxing and waning of yin and yang during the 24 hour daily cycle. In inner alchemy and meditation, "Fire" is taken to mean the "Original Spirit" and the application of the True Intention (*Zhen Yi*) which must coalesce with the breath and the essence.[32] The hexagrams and the firing times then simply refer to the natural cyclical transformation and coalescing of yin and yang as they circulate through the Ren and Du channels, rather than specific practice times and arcane methods.

[33] This whole discussion involves a number of concepts. 炼 *Lian*: "refining", refers to heating with fire in order to transmute the body's substances. This means refining essence and breath by harmonizing the heart and sitting in emptiness. This replenishes essence and transforms it into spirit. This replenishes the supply of the *San Bao*, (Three Treasures) and is achieved by combining *Xing* (nature) and refining spirit with *Ming* (life; vital force) and refining qi and essence. The medicine is the essence, and *Qi*/Breath, which are replenished through this process. Fire is Metaphor for the Original spirit (*Yuan Shen*). When this spirit merges with the breath (*Qi*) and essence then they circulate along the Ren and Du Mo (the Micro-Cosmic Orbit or Small Heavenly Circulation). "The true fire is one's own spirit; the true times are one's own breathing. Refining the Medicine by means of fire in order to form the elixir means the Spirit driving the breath in order to return to the Dao." Thoughts arising cause fire to scorch and intention dispersing causes "cold." So the 'fire" (the original spirit) and the intention must be regulated - this what is meant by the "fire times."

The method of refining the elixir is no different than walking, sitting and lying or like a chicken laying an egg - the time spent is the amount achieved. The foundation of the heavenly circuit can be established in one hundred days. In ten months, the fetus can be conceived; fire and water can support each other; metal and wood can combine. [All] the changes in the heaven and earth relate to this breathing. If meticulously refined during the twelve time periods of a day, in a short time there will be *Gong Fu*. In one year of *Gong Fu* you can seize Heaven and Earth and 3,600 years' destiny, because the Supreme Origin (*Da Yuan*) comes from one's own nature. Practitioners of the *Dan* (elixir) must conserve and guard the Ancestral Aperture (*Zhu Qiao*).[34] This means to stop distracting thoughts, namely to refine one's nature.

When a fetus is in the mother's abdomen, first the nose grows and after that, the eyes. The tongue links with the Du Vessel and inside the mouth is a blood cake that is inner nature and life force (*Xing* and *Ming*) connected by qi to the navel. The lung is small and the liver is large. When the navel is cut off life ends. The inner nature (*Xing*) carries *Qi* to enter the heart while the life force carries *Qi* to enter the kidney. They are 8.4 cun apart.[35] When the blood cake (*Xue Bing*) is swallowed to go downward, the blue pupils disperse.[36] This is a post heaven event. On the palate there

---

Foundations of Internal Alchemy: The Daoist Practice of Neidan by Wang Mu. Translated and Edited by Fabrizio Pregadio, Mountian View CA: Golden Elixir Press, 2011, pp 75-77.

[34] The Middle Cinnabar Field (*Zhong Dan Tian*). The Yellow Court (*Huang Ting*) and the Ancestral Aperture (*Zhu Qiao*) or the Cavity of the Ancestral Breath (*Zhu Qi Xue*) are all the same - located above the navel and between the navel and the heart. *Foundations of Internal Alchemy: The Daoist Practice of Neidan* by Wang Mu, pp. 21-24. Other sources locate the *Huang Ting* below the navel, indicating that it is synonymous with lower *Dantian*, and that *Jiang Gong* (Crimson Palace) is the "Middle Cinnabar Field" or Middle *Dantian*. (*The Method of Holding the Three Ones: A Taoist Manual of Meditation of the Fourth Century A.D.*, translated by Poul Anderson. London: Curzon Press, 1980. pp. 50-51.

[35] The distance between the heart and navel is 8.4 *cun*. The Ancestral Aperture is in the middle of this distance 4.2 cun from the heart and 4.2 cun from the navel. See previous footnote.

[36] The newborn infant or the infant still in the womb is a prominent metaphor for many Daoist practices. The infant is a metaphor for returning to the One, to the Dao because the infant has not yet begun the depleting process of living in the adult world of desires and cares. The fetus does not breathe through the mouth, but once the umbilical cord is

is an acu-point and under the tongue there are two acu-points that produce body fluids (*Jin Ye*), a treasure of the human body. Saliva goes down 1.2 *cun* under the heart to the *Jiang Gong* (Crimson Palace) at the root of the liver and becomes blood. When blood descends 1.3 cun below the navel it changes into *Qi*. The Great Dao is nameless and without form, it is the integrated pre-heaven One-*Qi*. What is refined is precisely the true nature. Unless *San Hua Wu Qi*[37] are refined to the utmost, the truth cannot be the complete truth. When *Zhen Qi* (True *Qi*) is sufficient, *Yang Shen* emerges. If there is no leakage [of *Zhen Qi*)], one can be called an immortal. This is the small refining, and it is achieved after one year. After nine years of refining, then one can return to emptiness. Only when there are true *Jing-Qi-Shen* can there be True Earth. When there is True Earth there can be real intention (*Yi*). Only when there is true intention can one guide and gather together (fuse) yin and yang, and harmonize and integrate *Si Xiang* (the Four Appearances or Four Phenomena).[38] The heart refers to the Pre-Heaven One-*Qi*.

In short, without stillness/tranquility (*Jing*) and emptiness (*Kong*) the Dao cannot be reached. Therefore tranquility is the lifeblood of the three religions.[39]

---

cut, the fetus changes from Pre-Natal to Post-Natal breathing which occurs through the mouth and nose. The "blood cake" represents the residual fluids from the umbilicus that, when cleared from the mouth immediately after birth, signal the start of Post-Natal, (Post-Heaven) life, which is characterized by respiration. The *Du* and *Ren* channels now can only be connected by the tongue touching the upper palate. This passage also mentions that in the transition from Pre-Heaven (before birth) to Post-Heaven, a baby's eyes change color from blue to brown (or another color).

[37] The *San Hua* are the Three Magnificent Things, another name for the Three Treasures (*San Bao*: *Jing Q/Breath* and *Shen*). The *Wu Qi* in this context are the so-called five spirits: *Hun*, stored in the liver, *Po*, stored in the Lungs, *Shen*-Consciousness, Stored in the Heart, *Zhi*-Will, stored in the Kidneys and the *Yi*-Intention, stored in the Spleen. All of these are really one spirit (*Shen*).

[38] In Daoist cosmogeny, the *Wuji*, (no limit; void) produces the "Great Limit" or "Ultimate Limit" - the *Taiji*. The *Taiji* produces 2 Forms (*Liang Yi*) - Yin and Yang. Yin and Yang in turn produce Four Phenomena (*Si Xiang*) - these are called *Shao Yang* (Lesser Yang; Young Yang), *Tai Yang* (Greater Yang; Old Yang), *Shao Yin* (Lesser Yin; Young Yin) and *Tai Yin* (Greater Yin; Old Yin).

[39] Daoism, Buddhism and Confucianism

Part 3: The Method of Quiet Sitting - Oral Instruction

Sit silently and burn incense to stop distracting thoughts. Letting go of emotions and intention, the spirit becomes lively. Sit on a thick cushion and loosen the belt and clothing. At the time of *Zhi Shi* (first Earthly Branch: 11pm to 1 am), sit cross-legged facing east. Hold the body straight and the back upright with the lips and teeth closed and the tongue touching the palate. Stop up the mouth and ears so as to invert listening.[40] Open the eyes slightly, with eyelids drooping down in order to brighten the *Shen*. That is, so that the light reflects back [and inward] from the *Yuan Gong* (Original Palace) to below the navel.

Sitting in a quiet room without disturbance or noise and burning incense, with honesty and sincerity, it is possible to connect to the mysterious *Qi*. Stop distracting thoughts. Extinguish all rash thinking. If even a few scattered thoughts exist, the spirit is not pure yang. One who forgets emotion becomes unconscious of the boundary between oneself and the external world. Forgetting emotion one's forgotten nature is recovered, the mind becomes bright and sharp. Close the heart (heart-mind) and use the breath to forget the heart (heart-mind) and to enliven the *Shen,* so that the heart (heart-mind) is sharp and clear. Sitting on a thick cushion keeps the body from tiring. Loosening clothing and belts, allows the *Qi* to flow freely. The time of the first earthly branch is the moment yang energy emerges and grows.

A person should start each day like this, facing east, sitting cross-legged, gathering and enlivening the *Qi* and gathering and consolidating the spirit. Hold the fist so that the thumbs pinch the crease of the third finger [in the palm] and with the four fingers holding the thumb. Hold the body level and the back straight, so that *Qi* can flow smoothly without obstruction. Closing together the lips and teeth. Lifting (propping up) the

---

[40] Listen to the inside of the body rather than to outside sounds.

tongue to touch the palate enables the throat to be without disease.[41] The mouth is an aperture of *Qi*.[42] If the mouth opens, *Qi* is dispersed. Therefore it must be closed. The ears are also blocked so as to reverse the hearing. The ear is an aperture for the *Jing* (essence). Listening to sounds consumes *Jing*. Therefore, make the ear deaf to sounds. Opening the eyes slightly means not to sit under the dark earth. Moreover, the eyes are the aperture of the spirit. If the eyes are look around at colors, the spirit will disperse. If the eyes open widely, the spirit is expressed (revealed) and if closed completely, the spirit is hidden (can also mean "dim"). Therefore, the eyes should be open halfway. This also prevents dizziness. The vision from *Yuan Gong* (Original Palace), reflects back to below the navel. The second lunar month belongs to yang, just as the light of the sun and moon give birth to all living things.

By regulating the breath continuously day and night, *gong* (achievement-skill) will be pure, and [one] will collect a little bit of true yang from the kidney. From this the heart and kidney will connect and interchange, joining so that *Shenqi* promotes fire. Through reflecting light back, a little bit of True Yang from the kidney will go up and join together with the heart-*Shen*. Self-cultivation of the breath is one exhalation and one inhalation. This breath is *Qi*. When intention and breathing are interdependent, true water and fire are reinforced and supported, creating a continuous return to the root; *Ming* returning[43] so as to nourish *Shenqi*,

---

[41] The throat is referred to here as a building. In the Daoist conception of the internal landscape as in the *Nei Jing Tu* (chart of the Internal Circulation) the trachea and throat are sometimes depicted as a many storied pagoda. If the mouth is closed, pathogens cannot enter the throat.

[42] *Qiao* 窍: This word is frequently used in Chinese medicine. In English, it means a hole, aperture. In fact, it implies a close relationship between the internal organ and external physiological or pathological signs. In Chinese medicine there is saying: 心开窍于舌(*Xin Kai Qiao Yu She*). Literally, this sentence can be translated into "The heart opens an aperture into the tongue". Actually, it means the tongue is a window to see the condition of the heart. In common Chinese, it also implies an enlightenment of the wisdom.

[43] This is 復 *Fu*: Returning; return to normal or to the original state. This again references the Fu Hexagram in the *Yi Jing*, in which the return is symbolized by the single yang line which appears at the bottom. Yang returning again after the ascendance of yin.

causing warm *Qi* to extend and link. If this is interrupted, nurturing and transformation will be difficult to achieve. In practicing this skill, a warm sensation rises, gradually gushing upward from the abdomen. If this happens, it is the motion of the true Yang *Qi*. Ordinary *Qi* in the middle of the body is Yin *Qi*. When Yin *Qi* is refined to the utmost, *Zhen Qi* (True *Qi*) is created. Control its mechanism of excited upward movement. Then it is transported through the *Wei Lu* (Tail Gate)[44], the twin *Jia Ji Guan*[45] and upward to the *Ni Wan* (Mud Ball)[46], to join and communicate with the spirit (*Shen*). After this joining, [True *Qi* and *Shen*] are transformed into sweet dew (*Gan Lu*)[47] from the Magpie Bridge (*Que Qiao*)[48] which goes downward to the throat and then to the heart and to the *Zong Gong* (Central Palace).[49] One rises, one falls, mingling at the Mysterious Pass (*Xuang Guan*) for transformation.

Except to bathe at Earthly Branches four and ten, it is vitally important that the refining be continuous and uninterrupted. Otherwise, the medicines are consumed and squandered and the firing time (ie: the critical moment) is missed, so the elixir cannot be formed. *Du Mo* in the center of the back comes upward and belongs to *Zi* (First Earthly Branch). *Ren Mo* in the front goes down and belongs to *Wu* (7th Earthly Branch).

☷

In Daoist meditation, this can also represent yang beginning to grow, as breath is regulated and *Jing* is transformed by *Qi* to move upward through the body to connect and transform into *Shen*.

[44] The *Wei Lu* 尾闾: is the first of the three gates or barriers (*San Guan* 三 關) that the *True Qi* must pass through as it ascends up the *Du* channel. Sometimes it is simply translated as tailbone.

[45] *Jia Ji Guan* 夹脊: Backbone gate, the area behind the heart and the second of the *San Guan*.

[46] *Ni Wan* 泥丸: "Mud Ball"; "Clay Pellet" – ie: the brain.

[47] *Gan Lu* 甘露: Literally "Sweet Dew" (i.e. Saliva).

[48] *Que Qiao* 鹊桥: "Magpie Bridge" This "bridge" is the connection of the tongue to the upper palate which connects *Ren Mo* and *Du Mo* so that they make a circuit. The "Lower Magpie Bridge" is created by lifting and gathering the perineum so that True *Qi* does not leak out through the anus ("Grain Duct").

[49] It is unclear if the reference to *Zong Gong* 中宮 (Middle Palace) here means the area in the middle under the heart, or if the term is being used an alternative way of referring to the lower *Dantian*. In this context, it seems to refer to lower *Dantian*.

The withdrawal and addition (ie: the regulation) of *Zi* and *Wu* (of the *Ren* and *Du*) represents the Heavenly Circulation (*Zhou Tian*) fire times. Fire times implies fire and water in the body, one ascending and one descending. Ascending means promoting fire to withdraw (extract) lead (*Qian*). Descending means to give back the tally and add mercury (*Gong*). Lead is the True Yang *Qi* of the kidneys. Mercury is the True Yin Essence of the heart. The marvel lies in [their] natural withdrawal and addition, advance and retreat. So, essence, *Qi* and spirit can gradually concentrate and can migrate and reside.[50] Sitting and lying down in concentration is like a baby hiding in its mother's belly following inhalation and exhalation. By swallowing the tranquil empty *Qi* of great harmony, there is *Gong* (achievement/skill) in ten months.

When yin and yang connect and interchange and fetal breathing is sufficient, *Xuan Zhu* (the Mysterious Pearl)[51] is formed, becomes the sage fetus, and transforms into true spirit. Through careful and sufficient regulation of the spirit for three years, form and spirit become wonderful and subtle and can change and transform at will. One becomes a sage and returns to the origin, transcending the worldly and attaining the Dao. By refining again to return to the void, one rises another level.

---

[50] Daoists often employ alchemical terms to describe the internal interactions of the body and mind during meditation. Hence, Daoist meditation is sometimes referred to as "Inner Alchemy". Using alchemical metaphors, yang in the *Dantian* is often referred to as the "furnace" (*Lu*) and the yin as the "reaction vessel" (*Ting*). The "True Mercury" extracted from cinnabar is the True Yin associated with Fire and the heart and liver. It is the True Yin Essence of the heart. It is also the conscious, discerning mind. The "True Lead" extracted from the unprocessed lead ore is associated with Water, the lungs and kidneys. It is the True Yang *Qi* of the kidneys. It is also true, intuitive knowledge or wisdom. When mercury and lead come together, when True Essence unite (the conscious mind) and *Qi* (intuitive wisdom) unite through the refining process of meditation, then body is regenerated, the Three Treasures combine and unify and consciousness is also unified.

[51] The Mysterious Pearl 玄珠: Can refer to the Dao itself and to the idea of transformation and change contained in Daoist thought. The phrase may also refer to the Records of the Mysterious Pearl (*Xuan Zhu Lu*) or the Mysterious Pearl Mirror of the Mind (*Xan Zhu Xin Jing*), two teachings in the Daoist Cannon. (*The Routledge Encyclopedia of Taoism Volume II: M-Z*, edited by Fabrizio Pregadio, London and New York: Routledge, 2008, pp. 1142-3).

These are all the methods of training the *Gong*.[52] In a hundred days the foundation is built. It is called the *Xiao Zhou Tian* (Small Heavenly Circulation; Micro-Cosmic Orbit). The yang time period rules advancing. Only by inhaling and exhaling for 36 yin time periods, ruling return, withdrawal and storing for the 24 periods of the year in which *Shenqi* is consumed[53], can the Pre-Heaven *Qi* be sufficient and the *Shen* vigorous enough for the *Da Zhou Tian* (Large Heavenly Circulation; Macro-Cosmic Orbit). After the Small Heavenly Circulation is fully actualized, opening and closing are performed day and night for seven days, following close behind the fire time (i.e.: the critical moment) of the Large Heavenly Circulation.

Part 4: Discussion of the Medicine Collecting Method

Medicine means Pre-Heaven One *Qi*. What is Pre-Heaven One *Qi*? Before Heaven and Earth, there was no Heaven and Earth. This *Qi* appeared naturally in the *Hun Dun* (primordial undifferentiated state). The root of yin is the root of *Wu Ji* (no-limit) and *Tai Ji* (great limit). Then *Tai Ji* gave birth to yin and yang. This *Qi* spreads and moves and prevails, giving birth to human beings and all living things. The fetus in the mother's belly is Pre-Heaven. After the mother gives birth [to the fetus] it [the fetus] gradually suffers loss, becoming Post-Heaven *Jing, Qi* and *Shen*. Because they wither, only one who does not die can see this.

By using the method of refining and cultivating like a child ascetic, the True Yang does not leak and is consolidated. As for middle-aged and old people, using the pure Qian (Heaven - the Creative) diagram - yang going through to the pure Kun (Earth - the Receptive) diagram - Qian

---

[52] Ability or achievement.
[53] In this passage, Sun seems to be referring to reversion of the cycle of nature and the progression of the seasons. Rather than *Shenqi* being consumed through the natural cycle of life (the 24 periods of a year and their natural fluctuations of yin and yang) it is stored and withdrawn (returned) so that the vital substances and energies of the body are not consumed, but are transformed stored and increased, leading to long life, wisdom and the immortality of the sage.

transforms into Li (Fire; Clinging) and Kun transforms into Kan (Water; The Abyss). When the foundation is refined (trained), [one] takes from Kan to fill in Li, especially as one waits for the medicine to form.[54]

When does the medicine form? Through inner reflection, drooping the eyelids and clenching the fists like a great mountain[55] the heart is still like water. Internally observe the heart. There is heart without heart.[56] In the outside appearance and form, there is form without form. In looking at things from afar, there is no thing within things (no objective within the objective). If these three things are realized, only emptiness is seen; emptiness without emptiness. Then the heart (heart-mind) is bright and clear, existing in the center of great emptiness, dark and undifferentiated, like a baby inside its mother's belly, not knowing, not recognizing, without others and without self. The center of emptiness gives birth to

---

[54] In the post heaven configuration of the Yi Jing Diagrams, Qian-Heaven is replaced by Li-Fire and Kun-Earth is replaced by Kan-Water. Li and Kan, then become emblematic of yang and yin in cyclical temporal movement of living things through the seasons and in the post-heaven progression from conception and birth to aging and death. In Daoist meditation the trigram Kan represents the Kidneys and Dantian. Kan is full in the middle (it has a solid yang line in the middle). The yang line in the center indicates that there is a true yang-fire within yin-water. Li represents the heart and chest. Li is empty in the middle. This symbolizes the hidden true yin-water within yang-fire. Normally, fire is light and rises to the chest and water is heavy and sinks to Dantian. This is the post-heaven state whose trigram configuration moves temporally from birth to death. However if fire is brought beneath water, they mutually restrain each other and interact. This creates steam and condensation which is a rarefied energy. Then the middle lines of the trigrams switch places and the Qian trigram and Kun trigrams (Hexagram 11: Tai) are formed creating the original pre-heaven state, which in Daoist beliefs leads to stopping of the temporal movement and therefore "immortality".

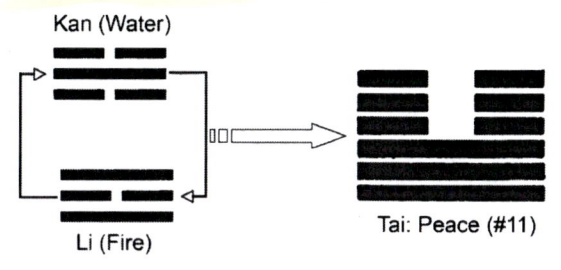

Kan (Water)

Li (Fire)

Tai: Peace (#11)

[55] Great Mountain, (*Tai Shan* 太山): can also refer to Mount *Tai Shan*.
[56] Although this phrase 心无其心 (*Xin Wu Qi Wu*) may literally mean "heart without its heart" or "no heart within the heart". In context it means that there is emptiness inside the heart or "no mind within the mind" and "no intention within intention."

tranquility and to its polar opposite - movement.[57] This [movement] is True Yang. The *Zi* time period (First Earthly Branch: 11pm to 1 am) is the firing time (the critical moment). Collect the medicine immediately and be sure not to let the intention wander.

Da Mo said: "Rein in the yang pass and regulate the external medicine through *Er Hou Cai Mo* (two steps to perceive the essence)[58] and the treasure sword joins the three roads."[59] Master Huang taught him the method of reversing the flow of water. The normal flow gives birth to sons, while reversing the flow gives birth to the elixir. For longevity, one must return (turn back) essence to nourish the brain. In this way *Qi* is returned to the stove and refined. Through the firing times it is cooked and refined to become the elixir, the priceless treasure of the body.

Part 5: Woman's Seated Meditation Method for Cultivating the Dao

In *Kun Gong*[60] seated meditation, shut the mouth and hide the tongue, with the tongue touching (propping up) the palate. On the palate, there are two holes. They are called *Tian Chi* (Mountain Lake) acu-points, which go up to link directly with the brain. Above the brain is the *Bai Hui* acu-point (DU 20), which is exactly at the top of the head (vertex). This is the "upper leakage." If the *Qi* leaks upward, it is not possible to extend life. Touching the tongue to the palate prevents leakage of brain *Qi*. Under

---

[57] In this sentence *Zhong* 中 "center" or "middle", can also mean "between the two extremes", between the two poles of the *Tai Ji*, the ultimate division or supreme polarity. From emptiness comes tranquility and automatically its opposite - movement.

[58] *Er Hou Cai Mo Ni* 二候采摩尼: one step to contain the essence through intention after the medicines (*Jing* and *Qi*) are produced, and another step to return the medicines to the stove for consolidation.

[59] The Chinese Sword (*jian*) was viewed by Daoists a sacred implement that could embody the primordial energy and act as a microcosm of the human body. Here the treasure sword and the three roads probably refers to the three treasures co-mingling and inter-transforming.

[60] *Kun* - the Receptive: referencing Earth and the Kun trigram, whose respond and receives the qi of Heaven (Qian trigram). Kun is also the female. *Kun Gong* is a metaphor for woman's achievement or women's practice.

the tongue, there are two acu-points. The left one is called *Jian Jing* (*Jin Jin*). The right one is called *Shi Quan* (*Yu Ye*).[61] By touching the tongue to the palate, fluid (*Jin Ye*) is copiously produced. The water throughout the body is salty. Only the water in the Magnificent Pool (*Hua Chi*), under the tongue, is sweet. Saliva is a treasure of the human body. When the mouth is full [of saliva], the tongue should still touch the upper palate and gulp the saliva down through the throat to the area 1.2 cun under the heart (The root of the liver: *Jiang Gong* - Crimson Palace), to transform it into blood. For women, *Jiang Gong* is the Pre-Heaven *Ming*, which connects down via *Ren Mai* to a site 1.3 cun below the navel known as *Jin Lu* (Golden Stove), also called the *Zhen Qi* (True Qi) acu-point. Here blood changes into *Qi*, and *Qi* is a woman's Post-Natal *Ming*.

When in the mother's belly, the two eyes are opposite and the tongue connects to the outer line of Du Mo. Inside the mouth is a blood cake. *Xing* and *Ming* combine in the same place and link with the mother's breathing through the umbilical cord. After the baby is born the umbilical cord is cut off. (In the Pre-Heaven state the lung is small and the liver is large). Pre-Heaven *Qi* is cut off. The infant is forced to breathe Post Heaven *Qi* through the mouth and nose. The lung expands and enlarges, and *Xing* and *Ming* separate from other. *Xing* takes *Qi* into the heart. *Ming* returns *Qi* to the kidneys.[62] In the middle of the 8.4 cun distance between them is *Qian Zi Li* ("child cavity field"). When the blood cake in the mouth is swallowed down, the black pupils of the eyes are dispersed.[63] Thereafter in this Post-Natal state, the respiration does not link with the original ancestral *Qi*. Through training and cultivation one can accumulate essence and abundant *Qi*. Food and drink can also generate *Qi*, but it [this *Qi*] can

---

[61] *Jin Jing* 肩井: "Golden Well"; *Jin Jin* 金津: Golden Fluid"; *Shi Quan*: 石泉: "Rock Spring"; or *Yu Ye* 玉液: Jade Liquid"
[62] *Xing* 性: Inner Nature; *Ming* 命: Life-Destiny which is associated with *Qi*/Breath. *Xing* is related to *Shen* (spirit) and *Ming* is related to the life force, the *Qi*/Breath. Therefore *Xing* is related to the heart-mind and *Ming* to the kidney and the *Jingqi*.
[63] See footnote #35 above.

only sustain the physical body. If accumulated it cannot prolong life. If let go of, life is not shortened.

The great and wonderful methods of augmentation teach one to cultivate and refine the quest for long life. It is known that the two nostrils under the nose are for respiration. This is because they can correctly grasp Heaven and Earth. In exhalation, one's own internal *Yuan Qi* exits. In inhalation Heaven and Earth's correct (positive) *Qi*, from outside, enters. When the body is strong and healthy it is possible to take in this correct *Qi* of Heaven and Earth so that one's lifespan can be lengthened. If the *Jing Qi* is weak and feeble, the correct *Qi* of Heaven and Earth will disperse and escape with exhalation, and the body's *Yuan Qi* (Original *Qi*) will not return and will be taken by Heaven and Earth. Everyone fails to understand that *Qi* is the true medicine for prolonging life and cannot find the gate to enter. If one wants to return to the Pre-Heaven state, one must recognize the original appearance (true form). Metal-Male and Wood-Female must merge.[64] Before the parents give birth, with the sun in the west and the moon in the east [there is] Pre-Heaven concentration and intention drops to gather in the ancestral aperture.[65] In the *Wu Ji* state, the nose develops first, and then the two eyes. The spiritual *Qi* of the eyes comes from the brain. The manifestation of intelligence in the brain is generated by the heart. Therefore, the ancestral aperture (this aperture exists before the body) must be refined skillfully in order for the eyes to perceive the moment the light of wisdom appears. Namely to observe the

---

[64] Metal-Male and Wood-Female is a reference to alchemical terminology in which Metal-Male is the true yang within yin and Wood-Female is the true yin within yang. To return to the Pre-Heaven state, these elements must be extracted and combined though internal cultivation practices.

[65] The Ancestral Aperture (*Zhu Qiao*) is the cavity of the Ancestral Breath and is located either between the navel and the heart or in the *Dantian*. Some Sources mention and upper and lower ancestral aperture one in the chest, associated with the heart and one in the *Dantian*, associated with the kidneys. Here the sun in the west and moon in the east reference reversal: the return to the Pre-Heaven state.

truth in the emptiness of the Mysterious Pass (*Xuan Guan*)[66] that is not emptiness. Obstinate contemplation of only emptiness is false. Thus all things are completed.

Embrace and abide by the true achievement (*Gong*). Sit quietly everyday with the tongue touching the palate. The eyes watch the tip of the nose and concentrate on the Ancestral Aperture. *Qi* sinks to the bottom of the sea.[67] First count the coming and going of the breaths, ensuring that they are even, continuous and unbroken - as if accumulating the breath and returning it to the root without giving birth to distracting thoughts. Do not stop, let things take their own course, employing the boundless *Yuan Qi* of Heaven and Earth. If the body and form are uneasy and the heart-mind moves, then the spirit will not enter the *Qi* and the body's *Qi* will be consumed and dispersed. Then one's nature will be confused and will lack understanding. Therefore it is said that the body's spirit must not exit. Nothing can reside in the *Ling Tai* (Spirit Platform)[68] and the four gates must be tightly shut. This is the subtle meaning of guarding the center. Constant, unceasing thinking, sexual desire, seeing exotic flowers and exceptional places are all enchanted states, for they disappear immediately after you open your eyes.

---

[66] 玄關 *Xuan Guan*, the "Mysterious Pass" represents the moment *Xing* (the inner nature) and *Ming* (the vital force) come together, or return to a state of oneness. These two (*Xing* and *Ming*) are also known as Dragon and Tiger; Lead and Mercury etc. The mysterious pass is the "door of life and death", the place between being and non-being. It is also a synonym for the *Xuan Pin* (Mysterious Female) and the *Hun Dun*. This is the place transcendence and unity can occur in Daoist practices.
[67] ie: *Dantian*.
[68] *Ling Tai* 灵台: "spirit platform"; is an acu-point on the *Du Mo* just below the 6th thoracic vertebrae, just behind the heart. However *Ling Tai* also refers to the faculties of the spirit and mind associated with the heart and in this context probably refers to the residence of the spirit.

The hand and foot should be harmonious and linked together. The hand should hold *Zi Wu Ba Gua Yin Yang Lian Huan Jue* (Mid-Night and Mid-Day Ba Gua Yin and Yang Linking Rhyme).[69] The left hand is outside and the right hand is inside for yang embracing yin. The right leg is outside and the left leg is inside for yin embracing yang. Sitting in extreme tranquility, the True Qi (*Zhen Qi*) begins to move and the body becomes pleasantly warm. Gradually the brain is strengthened and activated. In front and behind the heart and the two palm centers start to sweat. It is similar to the moment between sleep and waking. The chest cavity is correct (natural). This is the true medicine. It cannot be described by words. After sitting, one should walk a little before doing other things.

Part 6: Women's Aperture Closing Gong – Practice Method for Women

In front of the two eyebrows and behind *Feng Fu* (acu-point DU 16), on the left and right, 0.3 cun above the tips of the two ears, in the center (with the hands crossed), there is a "*Qi* sack" (*Qi Bao*) that links with the

---

[69] *Zi Wu Jue* is a position of the hands used in Daoist practice. The male holds the right hand with the left hand, and the female holds the left hand with the right hand, because the left of the male is yang, and the right hand of the female is yang. So, the yang hand is outside, and yin hand is inside. The thumb of the external yang hand is inside *Hukou* of the yin hand, with the thumbs crisscrossed, like the *Tai Ji* diagram.
Zi Wu Jue can also be a hand form used to calculate the positions and time periods of the 12 Earthly Branches. In this case, the thumb of the left hand is flexed to dig the top part of the middle finger, and the thumb of the right hand goes through the ring of the left thumb and middle finger to the root of the ring finger The right middle finger touches it externally, to hold the two hands.
Zi Wu Ba Gua Yin Yang Lian Huan Jue (Mid-Night and Mid-Day Ba Gua Yin and Yang Linking Rhyme). 子午八卦阴阳连环诀. The Zi Wu cycle is associated with the Pre-Heaven and Post-Heaven arrangement of the trigrams and their relationship to the ten Heavenly Stems and twelve Earthly Branches. Here, *Zi Wu Ba Gua* Linking also references the circulation of the Micro-Cosmic Orbit the transformation of yin and yang and *Jing*, *Qi/Breath* and *Shen* that takes place within that circulation. This is a reflection of the larger heavenly circulation that takes place in the cosmos which is reflected in the cyclical daily, seasonal and sixty year cycles. It is also a metaphor for the inter-transformation of fire and water, Li returning to Qian and Kan returning to Kun to return from the Post-Heaven state to the Pre-Heaven state, and the requisite inner realization that results: one of the goals of Daoist meditation.

Yan Sui Guan ("long marrow tube").[70] This is called *Yu Ding* (Jade Tripod).[71] There is an acu-point 1.3 cun below and behind the navel, in front of the kidneys (in front 70% and behind 30%) and above the two hips that is suspended in the center. It is called *Jin Lu* (Golden Stove). Originally there is no tripod at *Yu Ding* and no stove at *Jin Lu*. When *Qi* is emitted, they become apertures of a subtle and almost indistinct breathing mechanism. In Daoist cultivation practices one must know the location of the Tripod and the Stove. If the heart-mind is capricious and gives rise to distracting thoughts, one must rotate the Wheel of the Law (*Fa Lun*) quickly.[72] In Daoism this is known as *Xiao Zhou Tian* (Small Heavenly Circuit or Micro-Cosmic Orbit). One must think of the *Fa Lun* and inhale *Qi* through the nose so that it descends to *Dantian,* and [guide it] using true intention to *Wei Lu* and *Jia Ji* [until it] reaches *Ni Wan*. Exhale from *Dantian* through the nose, with true intention descending from *Zu Qian* (Ancestral Aperture) to *Jiang Gong* (Crimson Palace) and then to *Qi Xue*, (*Qi* Cave)[73] the intention circulating without end. The True *Qi* gradually will create a warm sensation. After a long time the True *Qi* will emanate and move from the aperture of life and death, flowing to a certain place that you will know. The Scripture of Wisdom and Life (*Hui Ming Jing*)[74] says that the four respirations and two comings and goings refer to this.

---

[70] *Yan Sui Guan* seems to refer to portion of the brain stem that may include the pons, medulla oblongata. The pons is a portion of the hindbrain that connects the cerebral cortex with the medulla oblongata. As a part of the brainstem, the pons helps in the transferring of messages between various parts of the brain and the spinal cord.

[71] *Ding* 鼎: An ancient cooking vessel that was tripodal, with two ear shaped handles.

[72] The *Dharmachakra*: "Wheel of the Law", " Dharma Wheel" or "Wheel of Life", is a symbol that represents the dharma: Buddha's teaching of the eightfold path, the path to enlightenment. *Dharmacakra* is translated as *Fa Lun* in Chinese, and in Daoism is an alternative name for the *Xiao Zhou Tian* (Small Heavenly Circuit or Micro-Cosmic Orbit).

[73] *Zu Qian* 祖窍 (*Ancestral Aperture*) in this case refers to the Upper Ancestral Aperture which is located between the eyebrows. *Jiang Gong* 绛宫 (*Crimson Palace*) is below the heart at the root of the liver and *Qi Xue* 气穴 (Qi Cave) may be the area below navel know as *Qi Hai* (Ren 6), or it may refer to the KID 13 acu-point (3 cun below the navel lateral to *Guan Yuan*: Ren 4). Most likely it is the lower ancestral aperture located in *Dantian*.

[74] The Scripture of Wisdom and Life 慧命经 *Hui Ming Jing* was written by the Chan Monk Liu Hua Yang. It is similar to Daoist alchemical texts that talk about the formation of a

There is another method that takes the Aperture of Life and Death (*Sheng Si Qiao*)[75] as *Zi* (First Earthly Branch), *Jia Ji* as *Mao* (Fourth Earthly Branch, *Ni Wan* as *Wu* (Seventh Earthly Branch), and *Jiang Gong* as *You* (Tenth Earthly Branch). Inhale *Qi* through the nose as you silently recite "*Zi*" with concentration focused on the Aperture of Life and Death, silently recite "*Mao*" with concentration focused on *Jia Ji* and silently recite "*Wu*" with concentration focused on *Ni Wan*. Pause briefly, and then exhale *Qi* through the nose as you silently recite "*Wu*" with concentration focused on *Ni Wan*. Silently recite "*You*" with concentration on *Jiang Gong* and silently recite "*Zi*" with concentration focused on *Qi Xue* and back to the Aperture of Life and Death.

In the cultivation of Daoism in Women, one must first eliminate illness, regulate menstruation and then train themselves to cut off the Red Dragon (menstruation)[76] and finally practice the Small Heavenly Circulation. Excessive menses and irregular menstruation are related to *Ren Mo* and *Dai Mo*, and are caused by blood stasis from excess or deficiency.

---

spiritual embryo. (*The Routledge Encyclopedia of Taoism Volume I:* A-L edited by Fabrizio Pregadio, London and New York: Routledge, 2008, pp.520-21).

[75] Probably *Mingmen*.

[76] Cutting off the "Red Dragon", is a metaphor for cutting off menstruation. In the Daoist alchemical tradition, *Jing* is refined into *Qi/Breath* and *Qi/Breath* into *Shen* which eventually merges with emptiness and the Dao. However the process of life depletes the *Jing*. In men, *Jing* and semen are related, so sexual activity, particularly in excess, depletes the *Jing*. The *Jing* that travels up the spine during the Small Heavenly Circulation is *Jing* that has been transformed and refined. Over time, the Small Heavenly Circulation gives birth to a pearl (the Mysterious Pearl) in the *Dantian*, which is the formation of the elixir which grows (the fetus) and moves upward as *Qi* continues to cycle through the channels. This gives birth to a luminous spirit as the body becomes more yang, returns to the True Yang of the original state, and merges with the Dao. Women lose *Jingqi* not through sexual activity, but through the monthly menses. The breasts are thought to be where the secretions of "perfect yin" originate. These secretions, which are the foundations of breast milk, normally descend into the abdomen and transform into menstrual blood. The breasts then, are one of the key centers for physical and spiritual cultivation in women. Part of the women's practice consists of rubbing the breasts and focusing on the chest area to stimulate secretions which first turn the menses to white (the color of semen) and then ultimately stop them altogether. This practice must be made to coincide with the monthly cycle at the moment *Yang Qi* is about to transform into yin blood. This is explained later in this text. (*Women In Daoism*, by Catherine Despeux and Livia Kohn. Cambridge Mass: Three Pines Press, 2003, pp. 223-227.)

If the menses are not regulated (are irregular) it is necessary to use an herbal formula (a decoction) for dredging the aperture and enlivening the blood.

9 grams	红花	*Hong Hua* (Flos Carthami)
3 grams	桃仁	*Tao Ren* (Semen Persicae)
3 grams	赤芍	*Chi Shao* (Radix Paeoniae Rubra)
6 grams	川芎	*Chuan Xiong* (Rhizoma Ligustici Chuanxiong)
9 grams	生姜	*Sheng Jiang* (Rhizoma Zingiberis Recens)
7 pieces	红枣	*Hong Zao* (Red Fructus Ziziphi Jujubae)
3 stems	老葱	*Lao Cong* (Old Green Onion: Scallion)

First, chop up the ginger green onion, and dates and combine them with the other herbs and simmer in ½ kilo of yellow wine (Huang Jiu), until ½ cup remains and infuse it with a little 麝香 *She Xiang* (Deer Musk). Again bring to a simmer three times and serve. The blood circulation will be smooth and unblocked. The menses will be regular and without any problem. If one is sick with fatigue (weakness), they should take 四物汤 *Si Wu Tang* (Four Agents Decoction).

9 grams	当归	*Dang Gui* (Radix Angelicae Sinensis)
6 grams	白芍	*Bai Shao* (Radix Paeoniae Albae)
6 grams	川芎	*Chuan Xiong* (Rhizoma Ligustici Chuanxiong)
9 grams	生地	*Sheng Di Huang* (Radix Rehmanniae Cruda)
6 grams	人参	*Ren Shen* (Radix Ginseng)
6 grams	白术	*Bai Zhu* (Rhizoma Atractylodis Macrocephalae)
6 grams	柴胡	*Chai Hu* (Radix Bupleuri)
9 grams	白茯苓	*Fu Ling* (Sclerotium Poria)
6 grams	半夏	*Ban Xia* (Rhizoma Pinelliae)
9 grams	香附	*Xiang Fu* (Rhizoma Cyperi)
3 grams	炙甘草	*Zhi Gan Cao* (Radix Glycyrrhizae Praeparata)
3 slices	生姜	*Sheng Jiang* (Rhizoma Zingiberis Recens)

If *Qi* is deficient: add 15 grams of 黄芪 *Huang Qi* (Radix Astragali). Decoct and serve in three doses.

When the blood is sufficient and full, then the Red Dragon can be cut off. Women belong to *Tai Yin* (Greater Yin). Woman's cultivation is based on the menstrual flow. Blood represents *Shao Yin* (Lesser Yin) *Jing Luo* (meridians). *Ren Mo* and *Dai Mo* combine to circulate the flow. Every month, women receive menstruation through one ascension and three harmonies. If the meridians flow smoothly, then menstruation also goes smoothly. At the age of 14, a woman's whole body emits heat so the meridians are unobstructed and clear, so the menses emerge every month.

If one desires to cultivate life, sit in a quiet room, without others coming and going (alone). First sit in meditation, observing the Ancestral Aperture and stopping distracting thoughts. Focus the Mind-Intention carefully on the area between the two breasts. Namely 1.2 cun in the middle of the two breasts, called the *Xue Yuan* (Blood Origin). The Fetus Origin forms the fetus; the Blood Origin gives birth to blood. *Dantian* gives birth to the elixir. Effort should be made at the time periods of midnight and noon. The heart-spirit and intention attentively watch the aperture of the breasts, while the breath is continuous and unbroken. A little goes out (exhalation) and much more comes in (inhalation). At the time of the menses, the menses are transported from the *Dantian* to the breasts. As *Tian Gui*[77] approaches, there are signs of readiness. The woman knows and can prepare in advance because there is perhaps back pain, leg pain, toothache, restlessness, fatigue and poor appetite. This means menstruation is coming. Every 30 days it arrives and True Yin moves. This is the harmony of Heaven.

---

[77] 天癸 *Tian Gui* ("Heavenly Water"): *Tian Gui* refers to a kind of substance necessary for promoting the development and maturity of the reproductive organs. It is formed mainly from the congenital essence we are born with and is also supplemented and nourished by our acquired essence derived from our nutrition. *Tian Gui* functions include the regulation of growth, reproduction, menstruation and pregnancy. The *Su Wen*, one of the seminal texts in Chinese medicine states that when a woman reaches fourteen, "*Tian Gui* reaches (matures), the Conception vessel (*Ren Mo*) is open, the Thoroughfare Vessel (*Chong Mo*) is full and the monthly affair flows down in a timely manner, hence she can have children." This implies that kidney essence (*Jing*) is the foundation of *Tian Gui* which in men produces the sperm and the ability to reproduce. There are alternative thoughts on *Tian Gui*: that it is innate kidney yin-essence; that it is a component of the *Yuan Qi* (the Original *Qi*), or that it is the "moving *Qi* between the kidneys" (*Mingmen*). In modern China *Tian Gui* is sometimes equated with hormones.

At that time one must sit quietly and exhale from the back to the Qian diagram and to the lung, and inhale from the front to the Kun diagram and to the kidney, regulating the breath and concentrating the spirit. Hold the breasts with crossed hands, and lightly rub them 36 times. Employ *Qi* from *Dantian* to faintly inhale for 24 mouthfuls (24 cycles of inhalation and exhalation), still holding the breasts with crossed arms, returning the illumination (looking inward) and regulating respiration. After some time, the true yang will be abundant and the menstrual flow will be cut off. The breasts will shrink to resemble those of a man. At the 26th time period, the *Gong Fu* is finished, meaning that it is in conformity with the required degrees of Heavenly Circuit (Small Heavenly Circulation). For virgin girls it is not necessary to rub and breathe to cut off the Red Dragon. Go straight to the Small Heavenly Circulation *Gong Fu*.

In quiet sitting (meditation), the training, must correctly use the four seasons - when Heaven's *Qi* (the weather) is clear and gentle, avoiding wind, rain and severe cold days and damp, foul and dirty places. Avoid eating meat and cold [food], bitter and sour melons (gourds) and fruits. Within the seven days of menstruation one must cultivate tranquility, and avoid injuring the *Qi*. One must extricate oneself from the blood devil. After half a year, the temperament will change from turbid to clear, and one will be healthy and bright. It is very important to sit [in meditation] at *Zi Hai* (Earthly Branches One and Twelve: 9 to 11 pm and 11 pm to 1 am). After sitting, rub the surface [of the body] with the hands to avoid getting wind-cold. In the female method of cutting off the Red Dragon, determine the date that the menstruation will arrive and two and a half days in advance sit quietly looking inward and menstruation will stop. If it is not complete after two and half days use kneading and breathing to cut off the Red Dragon completely. When the Red Dragon is cut off, the menses should change from bright red to yellow and from yellow to white, and from white to none. From none it changes to *Qi*. Then it is time to do Heavenly Circuit *Gong Fu*. This is the slow cultivation method done at home (ie: not as a monk). If cultivation is done in the temple, one must use the quick method. The medicine for cultivating the Dao is the *Yuan Qi* (Original Qi) of the human body.

The mysterious gates of martial arts cannot be fully expressed and the mysteries of the ancient sages that are passed down will not harm people. I invite the reader to think about it. I cannot dare to say that I fully understand this marvelous Pre-Heaven wisdom, but after being instructed by honest teachers, I can give it to the reader to avoid danger. If the reader likes martial arts, I hope they will cherish it. I hope my poor words will create ties [of friendship] and we can research together.

Chapter Notes

Chapter Notes

PART I

Preface Notes
[1] *Daoism Explained: From the Dream of the Butterfly to the Fishnet Allegory*, by Hans-Georg Moeller, Chicago and La Salle Illinois: Open Court Publishing, 2006. pp. 27-36.

Daoism And Daoist Meditation
[2] *Early Chinese Medical Literature*, translation and study by Donald Harper. New York and London: Kegan Paul International, 1998. p. 47.

[3] A detailed discussion of *qi* and its various meanings is undertaken in Lesson 3.

[4] *Chinese Healing Exercises: The Tradition of Daoyin*, by Livia Kohn Honolulu: University of Hawai'i Press, 2008. p. 8.

[5] *To Live as Long as Heaven and Earth: A Translation and Study of Ge Hong's "Traditions of Divine Transcendents"*, by Robert Ford Campany. Berkeley: University of California Press. 2002. pp. 8-9.

[6] *Qi Gong Essentials for Health Promotion*, by Jiao Guorui. PR China: China Reconstructs Press, p. 61.

[7] 6. Ibid, p. 66.

[8] 7. *T'ai Chi Ch'uan & Meditation* by Da Liu. New York: Schocken Books, 1986. pp. 6-7.

[9] *Chinese Healing Exercises: The Tradition of Daoyin*, by Livia Kohn. Honolulu: University of Hawai'i Press, 2008. p. 184-5.

[10] *Original Tao: Inward Training and the Foundations of Taoist Mysticism* by Harold Roth. New York: Columbia University Press, 1999, pp. 117-18.

Why Meditate?
[11] *The Way and Its Power, A Study of the Tao Te Ching and its Place in Chinese Thought*, by Arthur Waley. New York: Grove Press Inc., 1958, pp. 31-2.

[12] *A Short History of Chinese Philosophy: A Systemic Account of Chinese Thought From Its Origins to the Present Day*, by Fung Yu-Lan. New York; London: The Free Press, 1948 and 1976, p. 105.

[13] *Ling Shu or The Spiritual Pivot*, translated by Wu Jing-Nuan. Washington DC: The Taoist Center, Distributed by University of Hawai'i Press, 1993, p. 39.

[14] *Rooted in Spirit: The Heart of Chinese Medicine*, translation and commentary by Claude Larre, S.J & Elisabeth Rochat de la Vallee. Barrytown, NY: Station Hill Press Inc., 1995, p. 19.

[15] Ibid, p. 23.

[16] *Daoism Explained: From the Dream of the Butterfly to the Fishnet Allegory,* by Hans-Georg Moeller, Chicago and La Salle Illinois: Open Court Publishing, 2006, p.76.

[17] *Vital Nourishment: Departing From Happiness* by Francois Jullien, translated by Arthur Goldhammer. New York: Zone Books, 2007, p. 76.

[18] Ibid. p. 77.

[19] Ibid, p. 37.

[20] Ibid, p. 35.

[21] . Source - Osho Book "The Guest"
http://www.messagefrommasters.com/Stories/Sufi/osho_rabia_hassan_miracles.htm

[22] *Li and Qi in the Yijing* by by Chung-ying Cheng in *Philosophy of the Yi 易: Unity and Dialectics.* Supplement to Volume 36 2009 of the Journal of Chinese Philosophy, edited by Chung-ying Cheng and On-cho Ng. Blackwell Publishing – John Wiley and Sons 2009, p. 92-3.

[23] *A Short History of Chinese Philosophy: A Systemic Account of Chinese Thought From Its Origins to the Present Day,* by Fung Yu-Lan. New York; London: The Free Press, 1948 and 1976, p.25.

[24] Ibid, p. 93.

[25] *Daoism Explained: From the Dream of the Butterfly to the Fishnet Allegory,* by Hans-Georg Moeller, Chicago and La Salle Illinois: Open Court Publishing, 2006, p. 83.

[26] *The Secrets of Chinese Meditation* by Lu K'uan Yu (Charles Luk), Maine: Samuel Weiser Inc. 1969, p. 170.

[27] *Daoist Yoga: Alchemy and Immortality* by Lu K'uan Yu (Charles Luk), Maine: Samuel Weiser Inc. 1973, pp. 27-28.

Lesson 1: The Breath

[1] Wang, Xu and coworkers of the Shanghai Institute of Hypertension had the patients practice *Yan Jing Yi Shen Gong* for 30 minutes twice a day. This qigong is claimed to be especially valuable for therapeutic purposes and delaying senility. The qigong exercise consists of a combination of sitting meditation and gentle physical movements that emphasizes a calm mind, relaxed body, and regular respiration. In 1991, the Shanghai group reported a 20-year controlled study of the anti-aging effects of qigong on 204 hypertensive patients. Subsequently, they reported a 30-year follow-up on 242 hypertensive patients, and more recently, the researchers reported an 18-22 year study of 536 patients.

During the first two months, the blood pressure of all patients dropped in response to the hypotensive drug. Subsequently, and over the period of 20 years, the blood pressures of the qigong group stabilized while that of the control group increased.

Remarkably, during this period the drug dosage for the qigong group could be decreased, while the dosage for the control group had to be increased. http://www.qigonginstitute.org/html/papers/Anti-Aging_Benefits_of_Qigong.html

[2] *Qigong Yangsheng as a complementary therapy in the management of asthma* by I. Reuther and D. Aldridge D. Journal of Alternterative and Complementary Med. 1998 Summer;4(2):173-83.

[3] *The Relaxation Response* (updated-expanded) by Herbert Benson MD. New York: Harper Collins, 2000. First published 1975 by William Morrow and Co. Inc, pp.69-70.

[4] **RESPeRATE** http://www.resperate.com/us/discover/clinicalproof.aspx and http://forum.resperate.com/does-take-effort-t1129-pid-3337.html&s=b4890f258ef8dfa4d086700d85628979#entry3337

[5] *Anatomy Trains: Myofascial Meridians for Manual and Movement Therapists* by Thomas W. Myers, London; New York: Churchill Livingstone, 2001. p. 208.

[6] *Visceral Manipulation,* Jean-Pierre Barral & Pierre Mercier. Seattle: Eastland Press, 1988. p. 11.

[7] *The Body In Question,* Jonathan Miller. New York: Random House, 1978. p. 161.

[8] *The Oxygen Breakthrough: 30 Days to an Illness-Free Life* by Sheldon Saul Hendler, MD, PhD. Pocket Books, 1990. pp.19-20.

[9] Ibid, p. 10.

Lesson 2: Kidney Breathing, Qi and Dantian

[1] *The Oxygen Breakthrough: 30 Days to an Illness-Free Life* by Sheldon Saul Hendler, MD, PhD. Pocket Books, 1990, p. 110.

[2] Ibid. p. 102.

[3] *The Shorter Science & Civilization in China: Vol 1,* Joseph Needham, Cambridge University Press, 1978. p.239.

[4] *Webster's 3rd New International Dictionary,* Springfield, Mass.: G&C : Merriman Co., 1961. p.751.

[5] *Ch'i - A Neo Taoist Approach*, R.G.H. Siu. Cambridge. MA: MIT Press, 1974. p. 257.

[6] *Taoist Meditation: The Mao-Shan tradition of Great Purity*, by Isabelle Robinet, translated by Julian F. Pas and Norman J. Girardot. Albany, NY: State University of New York (SUNY) Press, 1993. Originally published in French as *Meditation Taoiste* (Paris: Dervy Livres, 1979). p. 83.

[7] *Taoism: Growth of a Religion,* by Isabelle Robinet. Translated by Phyllis Brooks. Stanford, Stanford University Press, 1997, pp.7-8.

[8] *Traditional Medicine in Contemporary China: Science, Medicine and Technology in East Asia Vol. 2*, by Nathan Sivin Ann Arbor : Center for Chinese Studies University of Michigan, 1987. pp. 46-7.

[9] *The World of Thought in Ancient China* by Benjamin I. Schwartz, Cambridge Mass: The Belknap press of Harvard University Press, 1985. p.181.

[10] *Ingestion, Digestion and Regestation: the Complexities of Qi Absorption* by Stephen Jackowicz in *Daoist Body Cultivation*, Edited by Livia Kohn. Magdalena, New Mexico: Three Pines Press. 2006. p. 77.

[11] *Foundations of Internal Alchemy: The Taoist Practice of Nei Dan*, by Wang Mu, translated and edited by Fabrizio Pregadio. Mountain View, CA: Golden Elixir Press, 2011, pp. 21-22.

[12] *The Taoist Body* by Kristofer Schipper. Berkely; Los Angeles: University of California Press 1993, p.107.

[13] *Fluid Physiology and Pathology in Traditional Chinese Medicine 2nd Edition*. By Steven Clavey. Churchill Livingstone, 1995, 2003, p. 119.

[14] *The Taoist Body* by Kristofer Schipper, p. 107.

[15] *Qi Gong Essentials for Health Promotion* by Jiao Guorui. PR China: China Reconstructs Press, p. 71.

[16] *The Heart and Essence of Dan-Xi's Methods of Treatment: A Translation of Zhu Dan-Xi's Dan Xi Zhi Fa Xin Yao*, translated by Yang Shou-zhong. Boulder, CO:Blue Poppy Press, 1993, p.xi.

Lesson 3: Quieting the Mind &Gathering the Qi

[1] *The Seven Emotions: Psychology and Health in Ancient China,* by Claude Larre and Elisabeth de la Valle. Cambridge UK: Monkey Press, 1996, pp. 4-5.

[2] *Chuang Tzu: Basic Writings*, translated by Burton Watson New York: Columbia University Press, 1964, p. 54

[3] *Taoist Yoga: Alchemy and Immortality* by Lu K'uan Yu (Charles Luk), Maine: Samuel Weiser Inc., 1973, pp. 10-11.

[4] *Chuang Tzu: Basic Writings*, translated by Burton Watson New York: Columbia University Press, 1964. p. 124

[5] *Traditional Medicine in Contemporary China: Science, Medicine and Technology in East Asia Vol. 2*, by Nathan Sivin. Ann Arbor: Center for Chinese Studies University of Michigan, 1987. p.230.

[6] *In Praise of Blandness: Proceeding From Chinese Thought and Aesthetics*, by Francois Jullien, translated by Paula M. Varsano. New York: Zone Books, 2004, p. 27.

[7] Ibid, p. 42.

[8] Ibid. p. 79.

[9] Ibid, p. 129.

[10] *Sources Of Chinese Tradition vol. 1*, Wm. Theodore de Barry ed. New York: Columbia University Press, 1960. p.74.

[11] Ibid.

[12] *Vital Nourishment: Departing From Happiness* by Francois Jullien, translated by Arthur Goldhammer. New York: Zone Books, 2007. P. 93.

[13] *The Way and Its Power, A Study of the Tao Te Ching and its Place in Chinese Thought*, by Arthur Waley. New York: Grove Press Inc., 1958. pp. 153.

[14] Ibid, p. 118

[15] Ibid, p. 154.

[16] *Original Tao: Inward Training and the Foundations of Taoist Mysticism* by Harold Roth, New York,: Columbia University Press, 1999, p. 92.

[17] *The Way and Its Power, A Study of the Tao Te Ching and its Place in Chinese Thought*, by Arthur Waley. New York: Grove Press Inc., 1958, p. 141.

[18] Ibid., p. 142.

[19] *Fathoming the Cosmos and Ordering the World: The Yijing and its Evolution in China*, Richard J. Smith, University of Virginia Press, 2008, pp. 92-3.

[20] *Chuang Tzu: Basic Writings*, translated by Burton Watson New York: Columbia University Press, 1964, p. 140.

[21] *Daoism Explained: From the Dream of the Butterfly to the Fishnet Allegory*, by Hans-Georg Moeller, Chicago and La Salle Illinois: Open Court Publishing, 2006, pp. 60-61.

[22] Ibid, p. 61.

[23] *The Essentials of Buddhist Meditation*, by Sramana Zhiyi (Chih-i) translated by Bhikshu Dharmamitra. Seattle WA: Kalavinka Press, 1992-2008, pp. 89-91.

[24] Ibid, p. 91.

[25] *Master of the Three Ways: Reflections of a Chinese Sage on Living a Satisfying Life,* by Hung Ying-ming, Translated By William Scott Wilson. Boston: Shambala, 2012, p. 86.

Lesson 4: Returning to Emptiness – Wu Ji

[1] *A Short History of Chinese Philosophy: A Systemic Account of Chinese Thought From Its Origins to the Present Day,* by Fung Yu-Lan. New York; London: The Free Press, 1948 and 1976, p. 131.

[2] Ibid, p. 132.

[3] Ibid, p. 131.

[4] *Li, Qi and Shu: An Introduction to Science and Civilization in China,* by Ho Peng Yoke. Seattle: University of Washington Press, 1987, p. 12.

[5] *The Way and Its Power, A Study of the Tao Te Ching and its Place in Chinese Thought,* by Arthur Waley. New York: Grove Press Inc., 1958, p. 195.

[6] *Heaven and Earth in Early Han Thought* (chapters three, four and five of the *Hainanzi*) John S. Major. Albany: State University of New York Press, 1993, p.32.

Lesson 5: Wu Ji and Song - Relaxation

[1] *Original Tao: Inward Training and the Foundations of Taoist Mysticism* by Harold Roth, New York,: Columbia University Press, 1999, pp. 109-110.

Lesson 6: Dissolving & Clearing Blockages

[1] *All Disease Comes From the Heart: The Pivotal Role of the Emotions in Classical Chinese Medicine,* by Heiner Fruehauf. www.classicalchinesemedicine.org/wp-content/.../emotions_Fruehauf.pdf, p. 6.

[2] Ibid.

[3] *The Seven Emotions: Psychology and Health in Ancient China,* by Claude Larre and Elisabeth de la Valle. Cambridge UK: Monkey Press, 1996, p. 113.

[4] *The Classic of the Way and Virtue: A New translation of the Tao-te-Ching of Lao Zi as Interpreted by Wang Bi,* translated by Richard John Lynn. New York: Columbia University Press, 1999, p.51.

[5] Ibid, pp.51-2.

[6] *Ba Gua Zhang* by Jiang Rong Jiao, Translated by Huang Guo-Qi and Edited by Tom Bisio.

Lesson 7: The Three Treasures & the Circulation of Water and Fire

[1] *Wenlin Software for Learning Chinese.* Copyright 1997-2007, Wenlin Institute Inc. www.wenlin.com

[2] *Qi Gong Teachings of a Taoist Immortal: The Eight Essential Exercises of Master Li Ching-Yun*, by Stuart Alve Olson, Rochester Vermont: Healing Arts Press, 2002, p. 13.

[3] *Rooted in Spirit: The Heart of Chinese Medicine*, translation and commentary by Claude Larre, S.J & Elisabeth Rochat de la Vallee. Barrytown, NY: Station Hill Press Inc., 1995, p. 30.

[4] *Ling Shu or The Spiritual Pivot,* translated by Wu Jing-Nuan. Washington DC: The Taoist Center - Distributed by University of Hawai'i Press, 1993, p. 39.

[5] *Rooted in Spirit: The Heart of Chinese Medicine,* p. 16.

[6] *Vital Nourishment: Departing From Happiness* by Francois Jullien, translated by Arthur Goldhammer. New York: Zone Books, 2007, pp. 84-85.

[7] *Qi Gong Essentials for Health Promotion* by Jiao Guorui. PR China: China Reconstructs Press, p. 73.

[8] *Foundations of Internal Alchemy: The Taoist Practice of Nei Dan,* by Wang Mu, translated and edited by Fabrizio Pregadio. Mountain View, CA: Golden Elixir Press, 2011, pp. 51-52.

[9] *Science and Civilization in China: Volume 5, Chemistry and Chemical Technology; Part 5, Spagyrical Discovery and Invention: Physiological Alchemy* By Joseph Needham, Cambridge University Press Cambridge 1983;1986 and 2000, p. 49.

[10] *Rooted in Spirit: The Heart of Chinese Medicine,* p. 66-67.

[11] *Science and Civilization in China: Volume 5,* p. 63.

[12] *An Exposition of the Eight Extraordinary Vessels: Acupuncture, Alchemy & Herbal Medicine,* by Charles Chace and Miki Shima. Seattle WA: Eastland Press, 2010, p. 78.

[13] *A Dictionary of Chinese Symbols: Hidden Symbols in Chinese Life and Thought,* Wofram Eberhard, trans. From German by G.L. Campbell. New York & London: Routledge & Kegan Paul, 1986 and 1996, p.272.

[14] *T'ai Chi Ch'uan & Meditation* by Da Liu. New York: Schocken Books, 1986, pp.28-9.

[15] *The Way and Its Power, A Study of the Tao Te Ching and its Place in Chinese Thought,* by Arthur Waley. New York: Grove Press Inc., 1958 p. 149.

[16] Ibid, 56-7.

[17] *The Way of Qigong: The Art and Science of Chinese Energy Healing* by Ken Cohen. New York: Random house - Ballantine Books, 1997, p. 122.

Lesson Eight: Golden Fluid & The Micro-Cosmic Orbit

[1] *Taoist Meditation: The Mao-Shan Tradition of Great Purity*, by Isabelle Robinet, translated by Julian F. Pas and Norman J. Girardot. Albany, NY: State University of New York (SUNY) Press, 1993. Originally published in French as *Meditation Taoiste* (Paris: Dervy Livres, 1979), p. 91.

[2] *Taoist Yoga: Alchemy and Immortality* by Lu K'uan Yu (Charles Luk), Maine: Samuel Weiser Inc., 1973, pp. 10-11.

[3] *Power Eating Program: You Are How You Eat*, by Lino Stanchich. Asheville, NC: Healthy Products Inc. 1989, pp.3-4.

[4] *Fire Pathognomy Due to Internal Injury in Chinese Medicine*, by Tian He Lu translated by Huang Guo Qi.

[5] *An Exposition of the Eight Extraordinary Vessels: Acupuncture, Alchemy & Herbal Medicine*, by Charles Chace and Miki Shima. Seattle WA: Eastland Press, 2010, p. 70.

[6] Ibid, p. 146.

[7] Ibid, p. 70.

[8] *Taoist Meditation: The Mao-Shan Tradition of Great Purity*, by Isabelle Robinet, translated by Julian F. Pas and Norman J. Girardot. Albany, NY: State University of New York (SUNY) Press, 1993. Originally published in French as *Meditation Taoiste* (Paris: Dervy Livres, 1979), p. 87.

[9] *Vital Nourishment: Departing From Happiness* by Francois Jullien, translated by Arthur Goldhammer. New York: Zone Books, 2007, p. 31.

[10] http://en.wikipedia.org/wiki/Hypothalamus
http://en.wikipedia.org/wiki/Endocrine_system

[11] *Fire Pathognomy Due to Internal Injury in Chinese Medicine*, by Tian He Lu translated by Huang Guo Qi.

[12] *Taoist Meditation: The Mao-Shan Tradition of Great Purity*, by Isabelle Robinet, translated by Julian F. Pas and Norman J. Girardot. Albany, NY: State University of New York (SUNY) Press, 1993. Originally published in French as *Meditation Taoiste* (Paris: Dervy Livres, 1979), p. 91.

[13] *Original Tao: Inward Training and the Foundations of Taoist Mysticism* by Harold Roth, New York,: Columbia University Press, 1999, p. 66.

[14] *A Dictionary of Chinese Symbols: Hidden Symbols in Chinese Life and Thought*, Woforam Eberhard, trans. From German by G.L. Campbell. New York & London: Routledge & Kegan Paul, 1986 and 1996, p. 295.

[15] *An Exposition of the Eight Extraordinary Vessels: Acupuncture, Alchemy & Herbal Medicine*, by Charles Chace and Miki Shima. Seattle WA: Eastland Press, 2010, p. 71.

[16] *The Complete System of Self Healing: Internal Exercise,* by Dr. Stephen T. Chang. San Francisco: Tao Publishing 1986, pp.93-98

[17] *The Complete System of Self Healing: Internal Exercise,* by Dr. Stephen T. Chang, p. 113.

[18] *Women In Daoism,* by Catherine Despeux and Livia Kohn. Cambridge Mass: Three Pines Press, 2003, p. 192.

[19] Ibid, p. 190.

Lesson Nine: Golden Fluid Returning to Dan Tian Meditation

[1] *Fire Pathognomy Due to Internal Injury in Chinese Medicine,* by Tian He Lu translated by Huang Guo Qi.

[2] http://www.chinapage.com/poet-e/sushi2e.html#006

[3] *Selected poems of Su Tung P'o* translated by Burton Watson. Port Townsend, WA: Copper Canon Press. 1994, p. 60.

[4] Time Magazine. CHINA: Tortoise-Pigeon-Dog. Monday, May. 15, 1933
http://www.time.com/time/magazine/article/0,9171,745510,00.html

[5] Ibid.

[6] *Qi Gong Teachings of a Taoist Immortal: The Eight Essential Exercises of Master Li Ching-Yun,* by Stuart Alve Olson, Rochester Vermont: Healing Arts Press, 2002, pp. 30-4.

[7] Time Magazine. CHINA: Tortoise-Pigeon-Dog.

[8] *Xiuzhentu: Diagram of Cultivating Truth,* translated by Mikael Ikivesi, 2009, p. 31.

[9] *Chinese Qigong Outgoing-Qi Therapy* by Bi Yongsheng. Trans. By Yu Wenping and John R. Black. Jinan, China: Shandong Science and Technology Press, 1992, pp. 109-110.

[10] *Nei Gong: The Authentic Classic, A Translation of the Nei Gong Zhen Chuan,* translated by Tom Bisio, Huang Guo-Qi and Joshua Paynter. Boulder,Co: Outskirts Press, 2011, p. 3

[11] http://en.wikipedia.org/wiki/Water_wheel
http://en.wikipedia.org/wiki/File:Undershot_water_wheel_schematic.svg

[12] *Holding Yin, Embracing Yang: Three Taoist classics on Meditation, Breath Regulation, Sexual Yoga and the Circulation of Internal Energy,* Translated by Eva Wong, Boston: Shambhala, 2005, pp. 15-16.

[13] *Holding Yin, Embracing Yang: Three Taoist Classics on Meditation, Breath Regulation, Sexual Yoga and the Circulation of Internal Energy,* Translated by Eva Wong, Boston: Shambhala, 2005, p. 16.

Beyond the Nine Lessons – The Macro-Cosmic Orbit

[1] *Chuang Tzu: Basic Writings,* translated by Burton Watson New York: Columbia University Press, 1964, pp.73-4.

[2] *The Essentials of Ba Gua Zhang,* by Gao Ji Wu and Tom Bisio. New York: Trip Tych Enterprises LLC, 2007, p. 108.

[3] *Xing Yi Nei Gong: Xing Yi Health Maintenance and Internal Strength Development,* compiled and edited by Dan Miller and Tim Cartmell. Pacific Grove, CA: High View Publications, 1994, p. 114.

[4] *Taoist Yoga: Alchemy and Immortality* by Lu K'uan Yu (Charles Luk), Maine: Samuel Weiser Inc., 1973, p. 21.

[5] *Nei Gong: The Authentic Classic, A Translation of the Nei Gong Zhen Chuan,* translated by Tom Bisio, Huang Guo-Qi and Joshua Paynter. Boulder,Co: Outskirts Press, 2011, p.21.

Daoist Nourishing Life Longevity Methods

[1] *Alchemy, Medicine & Religion in the China of A.D. 320: The Nei Pien of Ko Hung,* translated and edited by James R. Ware. New York: Dover Publications, 1966, p. 223.

[2] Ibid, 223-4.

[3] *Disputers of the Tao: Philosophical Argument in Ancient China,* By A.C. Graham. Chicago: Open Court Publishing Company,1989, pp. 352.

[4] *Practical Ways to Good Health Through Chinese Traditional Medicine,* Beijing: China Reconstructs Press, 1989, p. 67

[5] *Disputers of the Tao: Philosophical Argument in Ancient China,* By A.C. Graham. Chicago: Open Court Publishing Company,1989, pp. 353.

[6] Ibid.

[7] *Practical Ways to Good Health Through Chinese Traditional Medicine,* Beijing: China Reconstructs Press, 1989, p. 67

[8] *Disputers of the Tao,* pp. 353-4.

[9] *Promoting Health During the Four Seasons,* translated and introduced by Heiner Fruehauf, Ph.D., L.Ac., Institute for Traditional Medicine, Portland, OR. Introduction edited and amended by Subhuti Dharmananda, Ph.D., Institute for Traditional Medicine, Portland, OR. http://www.itmonline.org/articles/four_seasons/four_seasons.htm Ibid.

[10] *The Mystery of Longevity,* by Liu Zhengcai. Beijing: Foreign Language Press. 1990 and 1996, p. 34.

[11] *Transforming Emotions with Chinese Medicine: An Ethnographic Account From Contemporary China,* by Yanhua Zhang. Albany, NY: SUNY Press 2007, pp. 40-41.

[12] *Ling Shu or The Spiritual Pivot,* translated by Wu Jing-Nuan. Washington DC: The Taoist Center - Distributed by University of Hawai'i Press, 1993, p. 39

[13] *Transforming Emotions with Chinese Medicine: An Ethnographic Account From Contemporary China,* by Yanhua Zhang, p. 41

[14] *Yellow Emperor's Canon of Internal Medicine,* Bing Wang, translated by Nelson Liansheng Wu and Andrew Qi Wu. China Science and Technology Press, p. 24.

[15] Ibid.

[16] *Li Dong-Yuan's Treatise on the Spleen and Stomach: A Translation of the Pi Wei Lun.* Translated and annotated by Bob Flaws. Boulder, CO: Blue Poppy Press, 2004, p. 297

[17] *The Tao of Health and Longevity* (revised and expanded Edition) by Da Liu New York: Marlowe and Co. 1978, 1990, pp. 48-50.

PART II

Cracking the Code: Understanding Daoist Meditation
[1] *The World Upside-Down: Essays on Taoist Internal Alchemy,* Isabelle Robinet, Edited and Translated by Fabrizio Pregadio, Mountain View CA: Golden Elixir Press, 2011, p. 33.

[2] *Picturing the True Form: Daoist Visual Culture in Traditional China,* Shih-shan Susan Huang, Harvard East Asian Monographs 342. Harvard University Asia Center Cambidge Mass: Harvard University Press, 2012, p. 8.

[3] Ibid, p. 11.

The Dao De Jing and Daoist Meditation: The Hidden Message Within the Text
[1] *Taoism: Growth of a Religion,* by Isabelle Robinet. Translated by Phyllis Brooks. Stanford, Stanford University Press, 1997, p. 26.

[2] http://plato.stanford.edu/entries/laozi/

[3] *Ho-Shang-Kung's Commentary on Lao-Tse,* translated and annotated by Eduard Erkes. Switzerland: Press of Artibus Asiae Ascona (First published in Journal Artibus Saiae),1950, p. 13.

[4] Ibid, pp. 13-15.

[5] Ibid, p.14.

[6] Ibid, pp.14-15.

[7] *The Secret Teachings of the Tao Te Ching,* by Mantak Chia and Tao Huang. Rochester Vermont: Destiny Books, 2002 and 2005, p. 10.

[8] *Disputers of the Tao: Philosophical Argument in Ancient China,* By A.C. Graham. Chicago: Open Court Publishing Company,1989, p. 220.

[9] *Ho-Shang-Kung's Commentary on Lao-Tse,* translated and annotated by Eduard Erkes. Switzerland: Press of Artibus Asiae Ascona (First published in Journal Artibus Saiae),1950, p. 15.

[10] Ibid, p. 16.

[11] Ibid.

[12] *The Silent Transformations*, by Francois Jullien. Translated by Micahel Richardson and Krzysztof Fijalkowski. London, New York, Calcutta: Seagull Books, 2011, p. 39.

[13] Ibid, p. 33.

[14] *Ho-Shang-Kung's Commentary on Lao-Tse*, translated and annotated by Eduard Erkes, p.16.

[15] Ibid.

[16] Ibid, p. 20.

[17] Ibid.

[18] *The Secret Teachings of the Tao Te Ching*, pp. 34-5.

[19] *In Praise of Blandness: Proceeding From Chinese Thought and Aesthetics*, by Francois Jullien, translated by Paula M. Varsano. New York: Zone Books, 2004, p.51.

[20] Ibid.

[21] *Ho-Shang-Kung's Commentary on Lao-Tse*, translated and annotated by Eduard Erkes, p. 21.

[22] *Two Visions of The Way: A Study of Wang Pi and the Ho-shang Kung Commentaries on the Lao Tzu*, by Alan K.L. Chan. Albany: State University of New York Press, 1991, pp. 139-140.

[23] *Lao-tzu's Taoteching: with Selected Commentaries of the Past 2000 Years*, translated by Red Pine (Bill Porter). Townsend WA: Copper Canyon Press, 2009, p.13.

[24] *Two Visions of The Way*, p. 140.

[25] *Ho-Shang-Kung's Commentary on Lao-Tse*, translated and annotated by Eduard Erkes, p. 22.

[26] *The Way and Its Power, A Study of the Tao Te Ching and its Place in Chinese Thought*, by Arthur Waley. New York: Grove Press Inc., 1958, p. 57.

[27] *Ho-Shang-Kung's Commentary on Lao-Tse*, translated and annotated by Eduard Erkes, p.25.

[28] Ibid, pp.25-7.

[29] *Comments on the Hun and Po,* by Cheng Zhi-Qing in *Blue Poppy Essays 1988,* by Bob Flaws, Charles Chace and Zhang Ting-liang et al. Boulder, CO: Blue Poppy Press, 1988, pp. 3-4.

[30] *The Shambhala Guide to Taoism* by Eva Wong, Boston & London: Shambhala Publications Inc. 1997, p. 201.

[31] http://plato.stanford.edu/entries/laozi/

[32] *Two Visions of The Way*, p. 143.

[33] *Ho-Shang-Kung's Commentary on Lao-Tse*, translated and annotated by Eduard Erkes, p. 26.

[34] Ibid.

[35] Ibid, p. 97.

[36] *The Way and Its Power, A Study of the Tao Te Ching and its Place in Chinese Thought,* by Arthur Waley, p. 209.

[37] *Ho-Shang-Kung's Commentary on Lao-Tse*, translated and annotated by Eduard Erkes, p. 97.

[38] *The Way and Its Power, A Study of the Tao Te Ching and its Place in Chinese Thought,* by Arthur Waley, p. 209.

[39] *Daoism Explained: From the Dream of the Butterfly to the Fishnet Allegory,* by Hans-Georg Moeller, Chicago and La Salle Illinois: Open Court Publishing, 2006, p. 76.

[40] *Two Visions of The Way*, p. 144.

[41] *Ho-Shang-Kung's Commentary on Lao-Tse*, translated and annotated by Eduard Erkes, p.28.

[42] Ibid, p.28.

[43] Ibid, p.29.

[44] Ibid, p. 28.

[45] *Daoism Explained: From the Dream of the Butterfly to the Fishnet Allegory*, p. 27.

[46] *Ho-Shang-Kung's Commentary on Lao-Tse*, translated and annotated by Eduard Erkes, p. 30.

[47] *The Way and Its Power, A Study of the Tao Te Ching and its Place in Chinese Thought,* by Arthur Waley, p. 156.

[48] *Ho-Shang-Kung's Commentary on Lao-Tse*, translated and annotated by Eduard Erkes, p. 146.

[49] *Lao-tzu's Taoteching: with Selected Commentaries of the Past 2000 Years,* translated by Red Pine (Bill Porter). Townsend WA: Copper Canyon Press, 2009, p. 25.

[50] *Cultivating Perfection: Mysticism and Self-transformation in Early Quanzhen Daoism*, by Louis Komjathy. Leiden; Boston: Brill, 2007, pp.164-65.

[51] Ibid, p. 165.

[52] *Ho-Shang-Kung's Commentary on Lao-Tse*, translated and annotated by Eduard Erkes, p. 24.

[53] Ibid, pp.130-31.

[54] *A Treatise on Efficacy: Between Western and Chinese Thinking*, by Francois Jullien, translated by Janet Lloyd, Honolulu: University of Hawai'i Press, 2004, p. 170.

[55] *Ho-Shang-Kung's Commentary on Lao-Tse*, translated and annotated by Eduard Erkes, p. 23.

[56] *A Treatise on Efficacy: Between Western and Chinese Thinking*, by Francois Jullien, p. 171.

[57] *Ho-Shang-Kung's Commentary on Lao-Tse*, translated and annotated by Eduard Erkes, p.24.

[58] Ibid.

[59] Ibid.

[60] *Ho-Shang-Kung's Commentary on Lao-Tse*, translated and annotated by Eduard Erkes, p.104.

[61] Ibid, p.105

[62] Ibid.

[63] *Ho-Shang-Kung's Commentary on Lao-Tse*, translated and annotated by Eduard Erkes, p. 80.

[64] Ibid.

[65] *Two Visions of The Way*, p. 126.

[66] *Two Visions of The Way*, p. 126.

[67] *Two Visions of The Way*, p. 127.

[68] *The Classic of the Way and Virtue: A New Translation of the Tao-Te Ching of Lao Zi as Interpreted by Wang Bi*, translated by Richard John Lynn. New York: Columbia University Press, 1999, p. 135.

[69] *Ho-Shang-Kung's Commentary on Lao-Tse*, translated and annotated by Eduard Erkes, p. 81.

Diagram of the Inner Circulation of Qi/Breath: Nei Jing Tu
[1] *Mountains and Water in Chinese Art*, by Karin Albert
http://www.venuscomm.com/montainsandwater.html
This article was first published in Bonsai Clubs International, Sept./Oct. 1988.

[2] *Daoism Explained: From the Dream of the Butterfly to the Fishnet Allegory*, by Hans-Georg Moeller, Chicago and La Salle Illinois: Open Court Publishing, 2006, p. 115.

[3] *The Great Image Has No Form, or On the Nonobject Through Painting* by Francois Jullien, Translated by Jane Marie Todd. University of Chicago Press 2009, p. 42.

[4] *Taoism: Growth of a Religion,* by Isablle Robinet. Tranlated by Phyllis Brooks. Stanford: Stanford University Press, 1997, p. 224.

[5] *Nei Jing Tu, a Daoist Diagram of the Internal Circulation of Man* by David Teh-Yu Wang. The Journal of the Walters Art Gallery 49-50:141-158. 1992. p. 151.

[6] *Nei Gong: The Authentic Classic, A Translation of the Nei Gong Zhen Chuan*, translated by Tom Bisio, Huang Guo-Qi and Joshua Paynter. Boulder,Co: Outskirts Press, 2011, p. 53.

[7] *Taoism: Growth of a Religion,* by Isabelle Robinet. Translated by Phyllis Brooks. Stanford, Stanford University Press, 1997, p. 143.

[8] *The Taoist Body* by Kristofer Schipper - Berkely, Los Angeles: University of California Press 1993, p. 107.

[9] *Fluid Physiology and Pathology in Traditional Chinese Medicine* 2nd Edition, by Steven Clavey. Australia: Churchill Livingstone, 2003, p. 119.

[10] *The Way of Qigong: The Art and Science of Chinese Energy Healing* by Ken Cohen. NewYork: Random House – Ballantine Books, 1997, p. 153.

[11] *Taoism and the Arts of China,* by Stephen Little, with Shawn Eichman; with essays by Patricia Ebrey et als. The Art institute of Chicago, 2000, p. 134.

[12] *Nei Gong: The Authentic Classic, A Translation of the Nei Gong Zhen Chuan*, translated by Tom Bisio, Huang Guo Qi and Joshua Paynter. Boulder,CO: Outskirts Press, 2011, pp. 10-11.

[13] Ibid.

[14] *Nei Jing Tu, a Daoist Diagram of the Internal Circulation of Man* by David Teh-Yu Wang. The Journal of the Walters Art Gallery 49-50:141-158. 1992. p. 147.

[15] *Nei Jing Tu, a Daoist Diagram of the Internal Circulation of Man* by David Teh-Yu Wang. The Journal of the Walters Art Gallery 49-50:141-158. 1992. p. 150.

[16] *Heaven and Earth in Early Han Thought* (chapters three, four and five of the *Hainanzi*) John S. Major. Albany: State University of New York Press, 1993, p. 32.

[17] Ibid, pp. 32-7

[18] Ibid. p. 37

[19] *Taoism: Growth of a Religion,* by Isabelle Robinet. Translated by Phyllis Brooks. Stanford, Stanford University Press, 1997, p. 94.

[20] *Nei Jing Tu, a Daoist Diagram of the Internal Circulation of Man* by David Teh-Yu Wang. The Journal of the Walters Art Gallery 49-50:141-158. 1992, p. 145.

[21] *The Forge and the Crucible: the Origins and Structures of Alchemy* (2nd Edition), by Mircea Eliade. University of Chicago Press, 1956 and 1962, p. 117-118.

[22] Ibid.

[23] Ibid, p. 150.

[24] *The Treatment of Psycho-Emotional Disturbance by Acupuncture with Particular Reference to the Du Mai* by Peter Deadman and Mazin Al-Khafaji. Journal of Chinese Medicine: number 46, September 1994.

[25] Ibid.

[26] *Taoism and the Arts of China,* By Stephen Little, with Shawn Eichman; with essays by Patricia Ebrey et als. The Art institute of Chicago, 2000, p. 134.

[27] *Nei Jing Tu, a Daoist Diagram of the Internal Circulation of Man* by David Teh-Yu Wang, p. 145.

[28] *Foundations of Internal Alchemy: The Taoist Practice of Nei Dan*, by Wang Mu, translated and edited by Fabrizio Pregadio. Mountain View, CA: Golden Elixir Press, 2011, pp. 6-7.

Keys to the Code: Understanding Daoist Symbolism

[1] *Science and Civilization in China: Volume 5, Chemistry and Chemical Technology; Part 5, Spagyrical Discovery and Invention: Physiological Alchemy* By Joseph Needham, Cambridge University Press Cambridge 1983;1986 and 2000, pp. 53, 55 and 60.

[2] *The Seal of the Unity of the Three: A Study and Translation of the Cantong Qi, the Source of the Taoist Way of the Golden Elixir,* translated by Fabrizio Pregadio, Mountain View CA: Golden Elixir Press, 2011, p. 129.

[3] Ibid.

[4] Ibid, p.129 and 260.

[5] *Strategy and Change: An Examination of Military Strategy, the I-Ching, and Ba Gua Zhang,* by Tom Bisio. Denver, CO: Outskirts Press, 2010, p. 138.

[6] *The Taoist Classics: The Collected Translations of Thomas Cleary, Vol. 2.* Boston: Shambala, 2003, p. 26.

[7] *Strategy and Change: An Examination of Military Strategy, the I-Ching, and Ba Gua Zhang,* by Tom Bisio. Denver, CO: Outskirts Press, 2010, p. 137.

[8] *The Taoist Classics: The Collected Translations of Thomas Cleary*, Vol. 2. Boston: Shambala, 2003, p. 26.

[9] *History of Chinese Philosophy* (Routledge History of World Philosophies vol. 3), Edited by Bob Mou. London and New York: Routledge 2009, p. 285.

[10] *Survey Of Traditional Chinese Medicine*, Larre, Schatz et als. Paris: Institut Ricci & Columbia, Maryland: Traditional Acupuncture Foundation, 1986. p. 115.

[11] *Ling Shu or The Spiritual Pivot*, translated by Wu Jing-Nuan. Washington DC: The Taoist Center – Distributed by University of Hawai'I Press, 1993, p. 39.

[12] *Comments on the Hun and Po* by Cheng Zhi-Qing in *Blue Poppy Essays 1988* by Bob Flaws, Zhang Ting-liang, Charles Chace et al. Boulder, CO: 1988, p. 4.

[13] Farzeen Baldrian-Hussein in *The Encyclopedia of Taoism*, Fabrizio Pregadio, ed., Routledge Press. http://en.wikipedia.org/wiki/Hun_and_po

[14] *Rooted in Spirit: The Heart of Chinese Medicine*, translation and commentary by Claude Larre, S.J & Elisabeth Rochat de la Vallee. Barrytown, NY: Station Hill Press Inc., 1995, p. 38.

[15] *Comments on the Hun and Po* by Cheng Zhi-Qing in *Blue Poppy Essays 1988*, p. 6.

[16] *Rooted in Spirit: The Heart of Chinese Medicine*, p. 37.

[17] Ibid, p. 38.

[18] *Wandering Spirits* - Sample Chapter www.ucpress.edu/content/chapters/10876.ch01.pdf

[19] Farzeen Baldrian-Hussein, http://en.wikipedia.org/wiki/Hun_and_po

[20] *Applied Channel Theory in Chinese Medicine: Wang Ju-Yi's Lectures on Applied Channel Therapeutics* by Wang Ju-Yi and Jason D. Robertson. Seattle: Eastland Press, 2008, p. 148.

[21] *Rooted in Spirit: The Heart of Chinese Medicine*, p. 51.

[22] *The Forge and the Crucible: the Origins and Structures of Alchemy* (2nd Edition), by Mircea Eliade. University of Chicago Press, 1956 and 1962, p.116.

[23] *Science and Civilization in China: Volume 5, Chemistry and Chemical Technology; Part 5, Spagyrical Discovery and Invention: Physiological Alchemy* By Joseph Needham, Cambridge University Press Cambridge 1983;1986 and 2000, p. 333.

[24] Ibid. p. 104.

[25] *Foundations of Internal Alchemy: The Taoist Practice of Nei Dan*, by Wang Mu, translated and edited by Fabrizio Pregadio. Mountain View, CA: Golden Elixir Press, 2011, p. 86.

[26] Ibid. pp. 74-77.

[27] Ibid. p. 85.

[28] *The Secret of the Golden Flower: a Chinese Book of Life*, translated and explained by Richard Wilhelm, commentary by C.G. Jung. New York: Harcourt, Brace and World Inc. 1931 and 1962, pp. 13-17

[29] *Li Dong-Yuan's Treatise on the Spleen and Stomach: A Translation of the Pi Wei Lun.* Translated and annotated by Bob Flaws. Boulder, CO: Blue Poppy Press, 2004, p. 227.

[30] Ibid. p. 227-28.

[31] *Developing Clarity and Stillness: The Scripture for Daily Internal Practice.* By Louis Komjathy. Posted on February 1, 2004. Originally published in The Dragon's Mouth Winter 2002/2003: 9-13. http://www.daoistcenter.org/basic.html

[32] Source: Fabrizio Pregadio, "Jindan." In Fabrizio Pregadio, ed., *The Encyclopedia of Taoism* (London: Routledge, 2007), vol. 1, pp. 551-55. http://www.goldenelixir.com/publications/eot_jindan.html

[33] *Taoism and the Arts of China,* By Stephen Little, with Shawn Eichman; with essays by Patricia Ebrey et als. The Art institute of Chicago, 2000, p. 389.

[34] *The Seal of the Unity of the Three: A Study and Translation of the Cantong Qi, the Source of the Taoist Way of the Golden Elixir*, translated by Fabrizio Pregadio, Mountain View CA: Golden Elixir Press, 2011, pp. 57-8.

[35] *Developing Clarity and Stillness: The Scripture for Daily Internal Practice.* By Louis Komjathy. Posted on February 1, 2004. Originally published in The Dragon's Mouth Winter 2002/2003: 9-13.
http://www.daoistcenter.org/basic.html

[36] *Nourishing the Essence of Life: The Outer, Inner and Secret Teachings of Taoism,* Translated with and Introduction by Eva Wong. Boston: Shambhala, 2004, pp.9-11.

[37] *The World Upside-Down: Essays on Taoist Internal Alchemy,* by Isabelle Robinet, Edited and Translated by Fabrizio Pregadio, Mountain View CA: Golden Elixir Press, 2011, p.47.

[38] *The Classic of the Way of Virtue: a New translation of the Tao-te-Ching of Lao Zi as Interpreted by Wang Bi,* translated by Richard John Lynn. New York: Columbia University Press, 1999, p. 135.

[39] *The World Upside-Down: Essays on Taoist Internal Alchemy,* by Isabelle Robinet, p.50.

[40] *The Numerology of the I Ching: A Sourcebook of Symbols, Structures and Traditional Wisdom,* by Master Alfred Huang. Rochester VT: Inner Traditions International, 2000, p.22.

[41] *The World Upside-Down: Essays on Taoist Internal Alchemy,* by Isabelle Robinet, p.52.

[42] *Introduction to the Study of the Classic of Change (I hsueh ch'i-meng),* by Chu His. Translated by Joseph Adler. Global Scholarly Publication, 2002 – Brigham Young University – Provo Utah, p. 7.

[43] *Awakening to Reality: The "Regulated Verses" of the Wuzhen Pian, a Taoist Classic of Internal Alchemy*, Translated with introduction and notes by Fabrizio Pregadio, Mountain View CA: Golden Elixir Press, 2009, p.64.

[44] Ibid.

[45] Ibid, p. 65.

[46] *The Numerology of the I Ching: A Sourcebook of Symbols, Structures and Traditional Wisdom*, by Master Alfred Huang. Rochester VT: Inner Traditions International, 2000, pp. 29-30.

[47] *The World Upside-Down: Essays on Taoist Internal Alchemy*, by Isabelle Robinet, p. 53.

[48] Ibid, p. 54.

[49] *The Origins of Ba Gua Zhang*, by Kang Ge Wu and Dan Miller. Pa Kua Chang Journal, Vol 3, No. 4 May/June 1993 High View Publications. pp. 27-9.

[50] *Chinese Numbers: Significance, Symbolism and Traditions*, by Evelyn Lip, Times Editions Pte Ltd. Singapore, 1992 and Union City CA, Heian International Inc., p. 65

[51] *Introduction to the Study of the Classic of Change (I hsueh ch'i-meng)*, by Chu His. Translated by Joseph Adler. Global Scholarly Publication, 2002 – Brigham Young University – Provo Utah, p. 10.

[52] *Buddhism and Taoism Face To Face: Scripture, Ritual and Iconographic Exchange in Medieval China*, by Christine Mollier. Honolulu: University of Hawai'I Press, 2008, p.135.

[53] *Chinese Mathematical Astrology: Reaching Out to the Stars* by Ho Peng Yoke. London and NewYork: Routledge – Needham Research Institute Series, 2003, pp.23-4.

[54] *Progressive and Regressive Time Cycles in Taoist Rituals* by Kristofer Schipper and Wang Hsiu Huei - in *Time, Science and Society in China and the West; the Study of Time V*, Edited by J.T. Fraser, N. Lawrence and F. C. Haber. University of Mass Press. © 1966, J.T. Fraser, p. 199.

[55] *The World Upside-Down: Essays on Taoist Internal Alchemy*, by Isabelle Robinet, p. 58-9.

[56] *The Taoist Classics: The Collected Translations of Thomas Cleary, Vol. 2*. Boston: Shambala, 2003.

[57] *Rooted in Spirit: The Heart of Chinese Medicine*, translation and commentary by Claude Larre, S.J & Elisabeth Rochat de la Vallee. Barrytown, NY: Station Hill Press Inc., 1995, pp. 58-61.

[58] *The Taoist Body* by Kristofer Schipper - Berkely, Los Angeles: University of California Press 1993, p. 210.

[59] *Zhuanzi: The Essential Writings with Selections from Traditional Commentaries*, translated by Brook Ziporyn. Indianapolis IN: Hackett Publishing Co., 2009, p. 171.

[60] *Applied Channel Theory in Chinese Medicine: Wang Ju-Yi's Lectures on Applied Channel Therapeutics* by Wang Ju-Yi and Jason D. Robertson. Seattle: Eastland Press, 2008, p. 289.

[61] Ibid.

[62] Ibid.

[63] *The Essentials of Ba Gua Zhang*, by Gao Ji Wu and Tom Bisio. New York: Trip Tych Enterprises LLC, 2007, p. 324.

[64] *Liang Zhen Pu Eight Diagram Palm*, Li Zi Ming, compiled and edited by Vincent Black. pp. High View Publications: Pacific Grove, CA, 1993, pp.56-57.

[65] *Foundations of Internal Alchemy: The Taoist Practice of Nei Dan*, by Wang Mu, translated and edited by Fabrizio Pregadio. Mountain View, CA: Golden Elixir Press, 2011, p. 31.

[66] *Chuang Tzu: The Inner Chapters*, translated by A.C. Graham. Indianapolis, Indiana: Hackett Publishing Co. Inc., 1981, 2002, p. 62.

[67] *The Taoist Body* by Kristofer Schipper - Berkely, Los Angeles: University of California Press 1993, pp. 210-12.

[68] http://Hackettpublishing.com/zhuangzi3.3
Additional Comments to Passage 3:3 in the Zhuangzi, by Brook Ziporyn

[69] Ibid.

[70] *Zhuanzi: The Essential Writings with Selections from Traditional Commentaries*, translated by Brook Ziporyn. Indianapolis IN: Hackett Publishing Co., 2009, p. 22.

[71] *Vital Nourishment: Departing From Happiness* by Francois Jullien, translated by Arthur Goldhammer. New York: Zone Books, 2007, p. 31.

[72] *The Taoist Body* by Kristofer Schipper - Berkely, Los Angeles: University of California Press 1993, pp. 210-12.

Daoist Meditation and the Image of the Gen Diagram

[1] *The I Ching: A Biography*, by Richard J. Smith. Princeton & Oxford: Princeton University Press, 2012, p. 7.

[2] *The Complete I-Ching*, by Alfred Huang. Rochester, VT: Inner Traditions International, 1998, p. 415.

[3] *Strategy and Change: An Examination of Military Strategy, the I-Ching, and Ba Gua Zhang*, by Tom Bisio. Denver, CO: Outskirts Press, 2010, p. 212.

[4] *Zhouyi the Book of Changes*, a new translation with commentary by Richard Rutt. London and New York: Routledge, 2002.

[5] *Yijing Wondering and Wandering*, by Jane Schorre and Carrin Dunne, Houston Texas: Arts of China Seminars, 2003, p. 148.

[6] *Yi Jing*, by Wu Jing-Nuan. Washington D.C.: The Daoist Center, 1991, p.186.

[7] *Wenlin Software for Learning Chinese.* Copyright 1997-2007, Wenlin Institute Inc. www.wenlin.com

[8] *Yi Jing*, by Wu Jing-Nuan, p. 186.

[9] *Wenlin Software for Learning Chinese.*

[10] *The Classic of the Changes: A New Translation of the I Ching as Interpreted by Wang Bi,* translated by Richard John Lynn. New York: Columbia University Press, 1994, p. 466.

[11] *The Classic of the Changes: A New Translation of the I Ching as Interpreted by Wang Bi,* p. 466.

[12] Ibid.

[13] *Yi Jing*, by Wu Jing-Nuan, p. 186.

[14] *The Classic of the Changes: A New Translation of the I Ching as Interpreted by Wang Bi,* p. 468.

[15] *The Complete I-Ching* p. 416.

[16] *The I Ching: or Book of Changes,* Richard Wilhelm and Cary F. Baynes. New York: Bollingen Series XIX Princeton University Press, 1950. 24th printing: 1990, p. 655.

[17] *The Living I Ching: Using Ancient Chinese Wisdom to Shape Your Life,* by Deng Ming-Dao. San Francisco: Harper-Collins, 2006, p. 297.

[18] *Ho-Shang-Kung's Commentary on Lao-Tse,* translated and annotated by Eduard Erkes. Switzerland: Press of Artibus Asiae Ascona. First published in Journal Artibus Saiae. 1950, p. 115.

[19] Ibid, pp. 115-16.

[20] *The Complete I-Ching* p. 413.

[21] *Fathoming the Cosmos and Ordering the World: The Yi Jing and Its Evolution in China,* by Richard J. Smith. Charlottesville NC and London: University of Virginia Press, 2008, p. 166.

[22] Ibid.

[23] *The I Ching Handbook: Decision Making With and Without Divination,* by Mondo Secter, Berkeley, CA: North Atlantic Books, 2002, p. 57.

[24] *The Classic of the Changes: A New Translation of the I Ching* as interpreted by Wang Bi, translated by Richard John Lynn. New York: Columbia University Press, 1994, p. 380.

[25] *The Complete I-Ching,* by Alfred Huang. Rochester, VT: Inner Traditions International, 1998, p. 327.

[26] *The Book of Changes and the Unchanging Truth,* by Hua-Ching Ni. Santa Monica, CA: Seven Star Communications, 1997, p. 444.

[27] *The Classic of the Changes: A New Translation of the I Ching* as interpreted by Wang Bi, translated by Richard John Lynn. New York: Columbia University Press, 1994, p. 381.

The Message in the Code

[1] *Developing Clarity and Stillness: The Scripture for Daily Internal Practice.* By Louis Komjathy. Posted on February 1, 2004. Originally published in The Dragon's Mouth Winter 2002/2003: 9-13. http://www.daoistcenter.org/basic.html

[2] *Taoist Meditation: Methods for Cultivatign a Healthy Mind and Body,* Translated by Thomas Cleary. Boston: Shambhala Publications Inc., 2000. p. 122.

Appendix 1: Body Configurations for Daoist Meditation & Nei Gong

[1] *Nei Gong: The Authentic Classic, A Translation of the Nei Gong Zhen Chuan,* translated by Tom Bisio, Huang Guo Qi and Joshua Paynter. Boulder, Co: Outskirts Press, 2011, pp. 44-45.

[2] *Nei Gong: The Authentic Classic, A Translation of the Nei Gong Zhen Chuan,* translated by Tom Bisio, Huang Guo Qi and Joshua Paynter. Boulder, Co: Outskirts Press, 2011. 53.

[3] Ibid, p. 55.

[4] Ibid, p. 57.

[5] Ibid.

[6] *The Book of Changes and the Unchanging Truth,* by Hua-Ching Ni. Santa Monica, CA: Seven Star Communications, 1997, p. 357.

[7] Ibid, p.357-58.

Bibliography

Bibliography

A Dictionary of Chinese Symbols: Hidden Symbols in Chinese Life and Thought, Wofram Eberhard, trans. From German by G.L. Campbell. New York & London: Routledge & Kegan Paul, 1986 and 1996.

A Tooth From the Tiger's Mouth: How to Treat Your Injuries with Powerful Healing Secrets of the Great Chinese Warriors by Tom Bisio. New York: Simon and Schuster Fireside Book, 2004.

A Treatise on Efficacy: Between Western and Chinese Thinking, by Francois Jullien, translated by Janet Lloyd, Honolulu: University of Hawai'i Press, 2004.

All Disease Comes From the Heart: The Pivotal Role of the Emotions in Classical Chinese Medicine, by Heiner Fruehauf. classicalchinesemedicine.org/wpcontent/.../emotions_Fruehauf.pdf.

A Short History of Chinese Philosophy: A Systemic Account of Chinese Thought From Its Origins to the Present Day, by Fung Yu-Lan. New York; London: The Free Press, 1948 and 1976.

A Study of Taoist Acupuncture by Liu Zheng Cai et Als. Boulder, CO: Blue Poppy Press, 1999.

Alchemy, Medicine & Religion in the China of A.D. 320: The Nei Pien of Ko Hung, translated and edited by James R. Ware. New York: Dover Publications, 1966.

Anatomy Trains: Myofascial Meridians for Manual and Movement Therapists by Thomas W. Myers, London; New York: Churchill Livingstone, 2001.

An Exposition of the Eight Extraordinary Vessels: Acupuncture, Alchemy & Herbal Medicine, by Charles Chace and Miki Shima. Seattle WA: Eastland Press, 2010.

Applied Channel Theory in Chinese Medicine: Wang Ju-Yi's Lectures on Applied Channel Therapeutics by Wang Ju-Yi and Jason D. Robertson. Seattle: Eastland Press, 2008.

Art of the Bedchamber: The Chinese Sexual Yoga Classic Including Woman's Solo Meditation Texts, Douglas Wile. Albany: State University of New York Press, 1992.

Awakening to Reality: The "Regulated Verses" of the Wuzhen Pian, a Taoist Classic of Internal Alchemy, Translated with introduction and notes by Fabrizio Pregadio, Mountain View CA: Golden Elixir Press, 2009.

Ba Gua Zhang by Jiang Rong Jiao. Translated by Huang Guo-Qi and Edited by Tom Bisio.

Breathing-Control Lowers Blood Pressure, E Grossman, A Grossman, MH Schein, R Zimlichman and B Gavish. Nature Publishing Group: Journal of Human Hypertension (2001) 15, pp. 263–269.

Buddhism and Taoism Face To Face: Scripture, Ritual and Iconographic Exchange in Medieval China, by Christine Mollier. Honolulu: University of Hawai'I Press, 2008.

Cheng Branch Gao Style Bagua Palm by Liu Shu Xing, Ge Guo Liang and Li Xue Yi, translated by Huang Guo Qi.

Ch'i: A Neo Taoist Approach, R.G.H. Siu. Cambridge. MA: MIT Press, 1974.

Chinese Healing Exercises: The Tradition of Daoyin, by Livia Kohn Honolulu: University of Hawai'i Press, 2008.

Chinese Mathematical Astrology: Reaching Out to the Stars by Ho Peng Yoke. London and NewYork: Routledge – Needham Research Institute Series, 2003.

Chinese Numbers: Significance, Symbolism and Traditions, by Evelyn Lip, Times Editions Pte Ltd. Singapore, 1992 and Union City CA, Heian International Inc.

Chinese Qigong. A Practical English-Chinese Library of Traditional Chinese Medicine, Publishing House of Shanghai College of Traditional Chinese Medicine. 1988.

Chinese Qigong Essentials by Cen Yuefang. Beijing: New World Press, 1996.

Chinese Qi Gong Illustrated by Yu Gongbao. Beijing: New World Press, 1995.

Chinese Qigong Outgoing Qi Therapy by Bi Yongsheng. Trans. By Yu Wen Ping and John R. Black. Jinan, China: Shandong Science and Technology Press, 1992.

Chuang Tzu: Basic Writings, translated by Burton Watson New York: Columbia University Press, 1964.

Chuang Tzu: The Inner Chapters, translated by A.C. Graham. Indianapolis, Indiana: Hackett Publishing Co. Inc., 1981, 2002.

Comments on the Hun and Po by Cheng Zhi-Qing in *Blue Poppy Essays 1988* by Bob Flaws, Zhang Ting-liang, Charles Chace et al. Boulder, CO: 1988.

Cultivating Perfection: Mysticism and Self-transformation in Early Quanzhen Daoism, by Louis Komjathy. Leiden; Boston: Brill, 2007.

Cultivating Stillness: A Taoist Manual for Transforming Body and Mind, Translated by Eva Wong, Boston and London: Shambhala, 1992.

Daoist Body Cultivation, Edited by Livia Kohn. Magdalena, New Mexico: Three Pines Press. 2006.

Daoism Explained: From the Dream of the Butterfly to the Fishnet Allegory, by Hans-Georg Moeller, Chicago and La Salle Illinois: Open Court Publishing, 2006.

Developing Clarity and Stillness: The Scripture for Daily Internal Practice. By Louis Komjathy. Posted on February 1, 2004. Originally published in The Dragon's Mouth Winter 2002/2003: pp. 9-13.
http://www.daoistcenter.org/basic.html

Disputers of the Tao: Philosophical Argument in Ancient China, By A.C. Graham. Chicago: Open Court Publishing Company,1989.

Early Chinese Medical Literature, translation and study by Donald Harper. New York and London: Kegan Paul International, 1998. p. 47.

Encyclopedia of Taoism, Vols, I & II by Fabrizio Pregadio. Routledge, 2008.

Essentials of Xing Yi Quan by Wang Li with Li Gui Chang and Chen Cheng Fu. Translated by Huang Guo-Qi and edited by Tom Bisio

Fathoming the Cosmos and Ordering the World: The Yijing and its Evolution in China, by Richard J. Smith. University of Virginia Press, 2008.

Fire Pathognomy Due to Internal Injury in Chinese Medicine, by Tian He Lu translated by Huang Guo Qi.

Fluid Physiology and Pathology in Traditional Chinese Medicine 2nd Edition. By Steven Clavey. Churchill Livingstone, 1995, 2003.

Foundations of Internal Alchemy: The Taoist Practice of Nei Dan, by Wang Mu, translated and edited by Fabrizio Pregadio. Mountain View, CA: Golden Elixir Press, 2011.

Grasping the Wind: An Exploration into the Meaning of Chinese Acupuncture Point Names by Andrew ellis, Nigel Wiseman, Ken Boss. Brookline, Mass: Paradigm Publications, 1989.

Harmonizing Yin and Yang: The Dragon- Tiger Classic, Translated by Eva Wong. Boston & London: Shambhala Publications Inc., 1997.

Heaven and Earth in Early Han Thought (chapters three, four and five of the *Hainanzi*) John S. Major. Albany: State University of New York Press, 1993.

History of Chinese Philosophy (Routledge History of World Philosophies vol. 3), Edited by Bob Mou. London and New York: Routledge 2009.

Ho-Shang-Kung's Commentary on Lao-Tse, translated and annotated by Eduard Erkes. Switzerland: Press of Artibus Asiae Ascona. First published in Journal Artibus Saiae. 1950.

Holding Yin, Embracing Yang: Three Taoist classics on Meditation, Breath Regulation, Sexual Yoga and the Circulation of Internal Energy, Translated by Eva Wong, Boston: Shambhala, 2005.

Huangdi Neijing Lingshu: Books I-III with commentary, Vol.1., Nguyen Van Nghi MD, Tran Viet Dzung MD and Christine Recours-Nguyen MD. Published in English by Jung Tao Productions, Sugar Grove, North Carolina, 2005.

Hua Yo T'ai Chi Chuan: The Kung Fu of Six Combinations and Eight Methods (Liu He Ba Fa) by Kahn Foxx

In Praise of Blandness: Proceeding From Chinese Thought and Aesthetics, by Francois Jullien, translated by Paula M. Varsano. New York: Zone Books, 2004.

Introduction to the Study of the Classic of Change (I hsueh ch'i-meng), by Chu Hsi. Translated by Joseph Adler. Global Scholarly Publication, 2002 – Brigham Young University – Provo Utah.

Lao-tzu's Taoteching: with Selected Commentaries of the Past 2000 Years, translated by Red Pine (Bill Porter). Townsend WA: Copper Canyon Press, 2009.

La Voie Du Tao: Un Autre Chemin De L'Etre. Gallery Guide to the Exposition at the Galleries Nationales, at the Grand Palais, Paris: 29 Mars to 5 Juillet 2010. Paris: Editions de la Reunion des Musees Nautionaux, 2010.

Li, Qi and Shu: An Introduction to Science and Civilization in China, by Ho Peng Yoke. Seattle: University of Washington Press, 1987.

Li and Qi in the Yijing by Chung-ying Cheng in *Philosophy of the Yi 易: Unity and Dialectics*. Supplement to Volume 36 2009 of the Journal of Chinese Philosophy, edited by Chung-ying Cheng and On-cho Ng. Blackwell Publishing - John Wiley and Sons, 2009.

Liang Zhen Pu Eight Diagram Palm, Li Zi Ming, compiled and edited by Vincent Black. pp. High View Publications: Pacific Grove, CA, 1993.

Li Dong-Yuan's Treatise on the Spleen and Stomach: A Translation of the Pi Wei Lun. Translated and annotated by Bob Flaws. Boulder, CO: Blue Poppy Press, 2004.

Ling Bai Tong Zhi Neng Nei Gong Shu, Wang Li Ping; translated by Richard Liao. 2012.

Ling Shu or The Spiritual Pivot, translated by Wu Jing-Nuan. Washington DC: The Taoist Center – Distributed by University of Hawai'I Press, 1993.

Master of the Three Ways: Reflections of a Chinese Sage on Living a Satisfying Life, by Hung Ying-ming, Translated By William Scott Wilson. Boston: Shambala, 2012.

Multifaceted Health Benefits of Medical Qigong (PDF 69KB) - Kenneth M. Sancier PhD and Devatara Holman MS. MA. LAc Originally Published in: Journal of Alternative and Complementary Medicine (2004) Vol 10, No. 1

Nei Gong: The Authentic Classic, A Translation of the Nei Gong Zhen Chuan, translated by Tom Bisio, Huang Guo Qi and Joshua Paynter. Boulder, Co: Outskirts Press, 2011.

Nei Jing Tu, a Daoist Diagram of the Internal Circulation of Man by David Teh-Yu Wang. The Journal of the Walters Art Gallery 49-50:141-158. 1992.

Nourishing the Essence of Life: The Outer, Inner and Secret Teachings of Taoism, Translated with and Introduction by Eva Wong. Boston: Shambhala, 2004.

Original Tao: Inward Training and the Foundations of Taoist Mysticism by Harold Roth, New York,: Columbia University Press, 1999.

Picturing the True Form: Daoist Visual Culture in Traditional China, Shih-shan Susan Huang, Harvard East Asian Monographs 342. Harvard University Asia Center Cambidge Mass: Harvard University Press, 2012.

Power Eating Program: You Are How You Eat, by Lino Stanchich. Asheville, NC: Healthy Prodcuts Inc. 1989.

Practical Ways to Good Health Through Chinese Traditional Medicine, Beijing: China Reconstructs Press, 1989.

Progressive and Regressive Time Cycles in Taoist Rituals by Kristofer Schipper and Wang Hsiu Huei - in *Time, Science and Society in China and the West; the Study of Time V*, Edied by J.T. Fraser, N. Lawrence and F. C. Haber. University of Mass Press. © 1966, J.T. Fraser.

Promoting Health During the Four Seasons, translated and introduced by Heiner Fruehauf, Ph.D., L.Ac., Institute for Traditional Medicine, Portland, OR. Introduction edited and amended by Subhuti Dharmananda, Ph.D., Institute for Traditional Medicine, Portland, OR. http://www.itmonline.org/articles/four_seasons/four_seasons.htm Ibid.

Qi Gong Essentials for Health Promotion by Jiao Guorui. PR China: China Reconstructs Press.

Qi Gong for Treating Common Ailments: The Essential Guide to Self-Healing by Xue Xiangcai. Boston: YMMA Publication Center, 2000.

Qi Gong Teachings of a Taoist Immortal: The Eight Essential Exercises of Master Li Ching-Yun, by Stuart Alve Olson, Rochester Vermont: Healing Arts Press, 2002.

Qi Gong The Secret Of Youth: Da Mo's Muscle/Tendon Changing and Marrow/Brain Washing Classics. By Dr. Yang Jwing-Ming. Boston: YMAA Publication Center, 2000.

Qigong Yangsheng as a Complementary Therapy in the Management of Asthma by I. Reuther and D. Aldridge D. Journal of Alternative and Complementary Med. 1998 Summer;4(2):173-83.

Rooted in Spirit: The Heart of Chinese Medicine, translation and commentary by Claude Larre, S.J & Elisabeth Rochat de la Vallée. Barrytown, NY: Station Hill Press Inc., 1995.

Rubbing the Abdomen to Aid the Stomach, by Zeng Qingnan & Liu Daoqing *Qi Magazine* Issue 72 Jul/Aug/Sept 2004. Publisher: Tse Qigong Centre, Editor: Michael Tse pp. 14-15

Science and Civilization in China: Volume 5, Chemistry and Chemical Technology; Part 5, Spagyrical Discovery and Invention: Physiological Alchemy By Joseph Needham, Cambridge University Press Cambridge 1983;1986 and 2000.

Selected poems of Su Tung P'o translated by Burton Watson. Port Townsend, WA: Copper Canon Press. 1994.

Sources Of Chinese Tradition vol. 1, Wm. Theodore de Barry ed. New York: Columbia University Press, 1960.

Strategy and Change: An Examination of Military Strategy, the I-Ching, and Ba Gua Zhang, by Tom Bisio. Denver, CO: Outskirts Press, 2010.

Survey Of Traditional Chinese Medicine, Larre, Schatz et als. Paris: Institut Ricci & Columbia, Maryland: Traditional Acupuncture Foundation, 1986.

T'ai Chi Ch'uan & Meditation by Da Liu. New York: Schocken Books, 1986.

T'ai Chi Ch'uan & I Ching by Da Liu. New York: Harper and Row Publishers, 1972.

Tao Te Ching, Lao Tzu. Introduction and Translation by D. C. Lau. Penguin Books. First Published in 1963.

Tao Te Ching by Stephen Mitchell. New York, Harper and Row, 1988.

Tao: The Subtle Universal Law and the Integral Way of Life by Ni Hua Ching. Malibu California: The Shrine of the Eternal Breath of Tao, 1979.

Taoism and the Arts of China, By Stephen Little, with Shawn Eichman; with essays by Patricia Ebrey et als. The Art institute of Chicago, 2000.

Taoism: Growth of a Religion, by Isabelle Robinet. Translated by Phyllis Brooks. Stanford, Stanford University Press, 1997.

Taoist Meditation: The Mao-Shan Tradition of Great Purity, by Isabelle Robinet, translated by Julian F. Pas and Norman J. Girardot. Albany, NY: State University of New York (SUNY) Press, 1993. Originally published in French as *Meditation Taoiste* (Paris: Dervy Livres, 1979).

Taoist Yoga: Alchemy and Immortality by Lu K'uan Yu (Charles Luk), Maine: Samuel Weiser Inc., 1973.

The Attacking Hands of Ba Gua Zhang, by Gao Ji Wu with Tom Bisio, Photos by Valerie Ghent. New York: Trip Tych Enterprises LLC, 2010.

The Body In Question, Jonathan Miller. New York: Random House, 1978. p. 161.

The Book of Changes and the Unchanging Truth, by Hua-Ching Ni. Santa Monica, CA: Seven Star Communications, 1997.

The Chinese Heart: Chinese Medicine and Stress Management by Dr. Miao Ching Chiang, Beijing: Foreign Language Press, 2009.

The Classic of the Changes: A New Translation of the I Ching as interpreted by Wang Bi, translated by Richard John Lynn. New York: Columbia University Press, 1994.

The Classic of the Way and Virtue: A New translation of the Tao-te-Ching of Lao Zi as Interpreted by Wang Bi, translated by Richard John Lynn. New York: Columbia University Press, 1999.

The Complete Book of Taoist Health and Healing: Guarding the Three Treasures by Daniel Reid. Boston: Shambhala, 1994.

The Complete I-Ching, by Alfred Huang. Rochester, VT: Inner Traditions International, 1998.

The Complete System of Self Healing: Internal Exercise, by Dr. Stephen T. Chang. San Francisco: Tao Publishing 1986.

The Daodejing of Laozi, translation and commentary by Philip J. Ivanhoe. Indianapolis: Hackett Publishing Company Inc. 2003.

The Essentials of Ba Gua Zhang, by Gao Ji Wu and Tom Bisio. New York: Trip Tych Enterprises LLC, 2007.

The Essentials of Buddhist Meditation, by Sramana Zhiyi (Chih-i) translated by Bhikshu Dharmamitra. Seattle WA: Kalavinka Press, 1992-2008.

The Forge and the Crucible: the Origins and Structures of Alchemy (2nd Edition), by Mircea Eliade. University of Chicago Press, 1956 and 1962.

The Great Image Has No Form, or On the Nonobject Through Painting, by Francois Jullien, translated by Jane Marie Todd. University of Chicago Press 2009.

The Great Tao by Stephen T. Chang. San Francisco: Tao Publishing 1985. San Francisco: Tao Publishing 1986.

The Heart and Essence of Dan-xi's Methods of Treatment: A Translation of Zhu Dan-xi's Dan Xi Zhi Fa Xin Yao, translated by Yang Shou-zhong. Boulder, CO: Blue Poppy Press, 1993.

The I Ching: or Book of Changes, Richard Wilhelm and Cary F. Baynes. New York: Bollingen Series XIX Princeton University Press, 1950. 24th printing: 1990.

The I Ching: A Biography, by Richard J. Smith. Princeton& Oxford: Princeton University Press, 2012.

The I Ching Handbook: Decision Making With and Without Divination, by Mondo Secter, Berkeley, CA: North Atlantic Books, 2002.

The Living I Ching: Using Ancient Chinese Wisdom to Shape Your Life, by Deng Ming-Dao. San Francisco: Harper-Collins, 2006.

The Method of Holding the Three Ones: A Taoist Manual of Meditation of the Fourth Century A.D., by Poul Anderson. Studies on Asian Topics no 1. London: Curzon Press 1980.

The Mystery of Longevity, by Liu Zhengcai. Beijing: Foreign Language Press. 190 and 1996.

The Numerology of the I Ching: A Sourcebook of Symbols, Structures and Traditional Wisdom, by Master Alfred Huang. Rochester VT: Inner Traditions International, 2000.

The Oxygen Breakthrough: 30 Days to an Illness-Free Life by Sheldon Saul Hendler, MD, PhD. Pocket Books, 1990.

The Relaxation Response (updated-expanded) by Herbert Benson MD. New York: Harper Collins, 2000. First published 1975 by William Morrow and Co. Inc.

The Seal of the Unity of the Three: A Study and Translation of the Cantong Qi, the Source of the Taoist Way of the Golden Elixir, translated by Fabrizio Pregadio, Mountain View CA: Golden Elixir Press, 2011.

The Secret Teachings of the Tao Te Ching, by Mantak Chia and Tao Huang. Rochester Vermont: Destiny Books, 2002 and 2005.

The Secrets of Chinese Meditation by Lu K'uan Yu (Charles Luk), Maine: Samuel Weiser Inc. 1969.

The Secret of the Golden Flower: a Chinese Book of Life, translated and explained by Richard Wilhelm, commentary by C.G. Jung. New York: Harcourt, Brace and World Inc. 1931 and 1962.

The Seven Emotions: Psychology and Health in Ancient China, by Claude Larre and Elisabeth de la Vallée. Cambridge UK: Monkey Press, 1996.

The Shambhala Guide to Taoism by Eva Wong, Boston & London: Shambhala Publications Inc. 1997.

The Shorter Science & Civilization in China: Vol 1, Joseph Needham, Cambridge University Press, 1978.

The Silent Transformations, by Francois Jullien. Translated by Micahel Richardson and Krzysztof Fijalkowski. London, New York, Calcutta: Seagull Books, 2011.

The Taoist Classics: The Collected Translations of Thomas Cleary, Vol. 2. Boston: Shambala, 2003.

The Tao of Health and Longevity (revised and expanded Edition) by Da Liu New York: Marlowe and Co. 1978, 1990. Pp. 48-50.)

The Tao of Health Longevity and Immortality: The Teachings of the Immortals Chung and Lu, Translated by Eva Wong. Boston & London: Shambhala Publications Inc., 2000.

The Tao of Meditation: Way to Enlightenment, by Jou Tsung Hwa. Scottsdale AZ: Tai Chi Foundation, 1983 (1st Printing) and 2000 (6th Printing).

The Tao of Natural Breathing: For Health, Wellbeing and Inner Growth by Dennis Lewis, Berkeley CA: Rodmell Press 1997, 2006.

The Taoist Body by Kristofer Schipper. Berkely, Los Angeles: University of California Press 1993.

The Treatment of Psycho-Emotional Disturbance by Acupuncture with Particular Reference to the Du Mai by Peter Deadman and Mazin Al-Khafaji. Journal of Chinese Medicine: number 46, September 1994.

The Way and Its Power, A Study of the Tao Te Ching and its Place in Chinese Thought, by Arthur Waley. New York: Grove Press Inc., 1958.

The Way of Qigong: The Art and Science of Chinese Energy Healing by Ken Cohen. New York: Random House – Ballantine Books, 1997.

The World of Thought in Ancient China by Benjamin I. Schwartz, Cambridge Mass: The Belknap press of Harvard University Press, 1985.

The World Upside-Down: Essays on Taoist Internal Alchemy, Isabelle Robinet, Edited and Translated by Fabrizio Pregadio, Mountain View CA: Golden Elixir Press, 2011.

To Live as Long as Heaven and Earth: A Translation and Study of Ge Hong's "Traditions of Divine Transcendents", by Robert Ford Campany Berkeley: University of California Press. 2002.

Traditional Medicine in Contemporary China: Science, Medicine and Technology in East Asia Vol. 2, by Nathan Sivin Ann Arbor : Center for Chinese Studies University of Michigan, 1987.

Treasured Qi Gong of Traditional Medical School by Huang Runtian. Kowloon: Hai Feng Publishing Co., 1994.

Two Visions of The Way: A Study of Wang Pi and the Ho-shang Kung Commentaries on the Lao Tzu, by Alan K.L. Chan. Albany: State University of New York Press, 1991.

Visceral Manipulation, by Jean-Pierre Barral & Pierre Mercier. Seattle: Eastland Press, 1988.

Visual Representations of the Body in Chinese Medical and Daoist Texts from the Song to the Qing Period (tenth to nineteenth century). By Catherine Despeux, Translated by Penelope Barrett. *Asian Medicine,* January 2005, vol. 1, no. 1, pp. 10-52(43).

Vital Nourishment: Departing From Happiness by Francois Jullien, translated by Arthur Goldhammer. New York: Zone Books, 2007.

Webster's 3rd New International Dictionary, Springfield, MA: G&C Merriman Co., 1961. p.751.

Wenlin Software for Learning Chinese. Copyright 1997-2007, Wenlin Institute Inc. www.wenlin.com

Women In Daoism, by Catherine Despeux and Livia Kohn. Cambridge Mass: Three Pines Press, 2003.

Wu Ji Qi Gong and the Secret of Immortality by Stephen Elliot with Dr. Meng Sheng Lin. Allen, Texas: Coherence Press, 2010.

Xing Yi Nei Gong: Xing Yi Health Maintenance and Internal Strength Development, compiled and edited by Dan Miller and Tim Cartmell. Pacific Grove, CA: High View Publications, 1994.

Xiuzhentu: Diagram of Cultivating Truth, translated by Mikael Ikivesi, 2009.

Yellow Emperor's Canon of Internal Medicine, compiled (Tang Dynasty) by Wang Bing, Translated into English by Nelson Liansheng Wu and Andrew Qi Wu. Beijing: China Science and Technology Press, 1997.

Yi Jing, by Wu Jing-Nuan. Washington D.C.: The Daoist Center, 1991.

Yijing Wondering and Wandering, by Jane Schorre and Carrin Dunne, Houston Texas: Arts of China Seminars, 2003.

Yin and Yang in Classical Texts, by Elisabeth Rochat de La Valée. Monkey Press, 2006.

Zhouyi the Book of Changes, a new translation with commentary by Richard Rutt. London and New York: Routledge, 2002.

Zhuanzi: The Essential Writings with Selections from Traditional Commentaries, translated by Brook Ziporyn. Indianapolis IN: Hackett Publishing Co., 2009.

Web Sources

Chinese Alchemy
http://www.themystica.com/mystica/articles/~alchemy/chinese_alchemy.html

Chinese Painting
Mountains and Water in Chinese Art, by Karin Albert
http://www.venuscomm.com/montainsandwater.html
This article was first published in Bonsai Clubs International, Sept./Oct. 1988.

Chinese Religion – Trinity Edu
http://www.trinity.edu/rnadeau/asianreligions/LectureNotes/Chinese Religions/Yinyangsouls and spirits.htm

Fabrizio Pregadio
goldenelixir.com
http://www.goldenelixir.com/publications/eot_jindan.html

Lao Zi
http://plato.stanford.edu/entries/laozi/

Nei Jing Tu
http://en.wikipedia.org/wiki/Neijing_Tu
http://wapedia.mobi/en/Neijing_Tu#3.

Osho Book "The Guest"
http://www.messagefrommasters.com/Stories/Sufi/osho_rabia_hassan_miracles.htm

Qi Gong and Health
Multifaceted Health Benefits of Medical Qigong. File Format: PDF/Adobe
by KM Sancier. J. Alt Compl Med. 2004; 10(1):163-166. by. Kenneth M. Sancier, Ph.D. Devatara Holman MS, MA, LAc ...
www.qigonginstitute.org/.../Multifaceted_Benefits_Medical_Qigong.pdf
- http://www.qigonginstitute.org/html/papers/Anti-Aging_Benefits_of_Qigong.html

RESPeRATE
http://www.resperate.com/us/discover/clinicalproof.aspx

http://forum.resperate.com/does-take-effort-t1129-pid-3337.html&s=b4890f258ef8dfa4d086700d85628979#entry3337

Su Shi Poetry (Su Dong Po)
http://www.chinapage.com/poet-e/sushi2e.html#006

Time Magazine CHINA: Tortoise-Pigeon-Dog. Monday, May. 15, 1933
http://www.time.com/time/magazine/article/0,9171,745510,00.html
Wandering Spirits - Sample Chapter
www.ucpress.edu/content/chapters/10876.ch01.pdf

Wikipedia
http://en.wikipedia.org/wiki/Endocrine_system
http://en.wikipedia.org/wiki/Hun_and_po
http://en.wikipedia.org/wiki/Hypothalamus
http://en.wikipedia.org/wiki/Li_Ching-Yuen
http://en.wikipedia.org/wiki/Water_wheel
http://en.wikipedia.org/wiki/File:Undershot_water_wheel_schematic.svg

Other Books from Outskirts Press by Tom Bisio

Available from Outskirts Press:
http://outskirtspress.com/bookstore/
or purchase on amazon.com

Ba Gua Circle Walking Nei Gong: The Meridian Opening Palms of Ba Gua Zhang by Tom Bisio

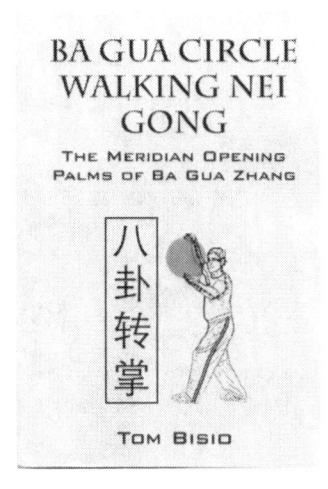

Here's another significant book by Tom Bisio. He is probably doing more than anyone else in English to chronicle a consistent style and approach to Bagua training, especially within the Gao branch of the style. This book concentrates on the Ding Shi, the walking palms with stationary upper body positions. These form much of the core of Bagua.

Drawing on his own knowledge as an acupuncturist, conversations and lessons from Zhao Da Yuan, along with notes taken from the famous Li Zi Ming, Tom has produced a book not only of tips on how to walk the Ding Shi (the same as in his DVDs) but also which meridians correspond to which postures. There is much information about the cycle of energy in the body and its relation to Bagua. There is a lot of information here and this can only be a valuable supplement to any Bagua student's training. Topics include the Channels, Micro-cosmic orbit, the functions and locations of the channels, walking the Bagua posts and "the rarely taught Bagua Energy Accepting Palm, in which vital force (qi) is absorbed from the natural environment."

Review from Plum Publications (plumpub.com)

Every Bagua Practitioner Should Own This Book!!

This is by far the most useful book on bagua I've read. Most books on the martial arts give you the author's theories on various aspects of their art, with little practical application, or different exercises or techniques that are hard to get anything out of without the feedback of an instructor. Bisio's book is a great departure from this - it gives you enough information to understand the significance of Bagua circle walking neigong in terms of Traditional Chinese Medicine and, to a lesser extent, Daoist alchemy. It also gives practical instructions for circle walking, and detailed instructions for getting each posture right. I'm somewhat skeptical about the possibility of learning circle walking from a book, but if that's your goal this books provides instructions which are clearer and more straightforward than the dozen other bagua books I have on my shelf - although you might want to get his video series to see how it looks in motion. (Ideally, of course, find a qualified master to learn from - but I understand most places in the world aren't overflowing with good bagua schools. Or even bad ones.)

I've been to a number of Bagua schools where fixed palm walking is treated as a warm up that you rush through before you get to the "good stuff" of palm changes, forms and applications - sometimes teaching them in a weekend workshop, or not at all. When I started learning bagua I spent several months learning fixed palm walking, where most classes consisted of me walking around a tree for a couple of hours, with my master correcting my posture every now and then. Its not sexy, or even particularly interesting, but it creates a foundation you need to do anything more complex well. Bisio gives a good understanding of why fixed palm walking is so fundamental in Bagua, and gives instructions that even people who have been studying for a while should find worthwhile. The correlation between postures and qi meridians alone is more than worth the price.

amazon.com review

At the Very Top

I am 67 and have studied internal martial arts, as well as other Bodymind approaches, all my life. I have read most of what has been published on these topics, though it is rarer and rarer now that I find a book which really gives me something. This book, as well as others by Tom Bisio, is among the ones that do. I have corresponded with Tom, though I have not yet met him. As well as being extraordinarily knowledgeable and accomplished, Tom is also humble and seems to me pretty much free of the ego trips that unfortunately are so common in the martial arts. He is also unusual in that he genuinely wants to share all he knows, making it as clear and accessible as possible without (it seems to me) holding anything back. In this book on Bagua walking, he goes into great depth (as is appropriate, and also rare) about the precise details of posture. If you do not know this, I am telling you: that is the million-dollar secret in the internal martial arts. Getting the correct posture, then maintaining this while moving: that's the ticket! (As to the fighting, learning techniques is just to keep you interested while you move with good posture; combat skill comes through intuitively sensing relationship, not by learning techniques.)

Anyway, Tom gives as good instruction as one can get in a book, and this particular walking practice is second to none for health and meditation, and as a solid foundation for fighting if you are so inclined. Check out his web site too; good stuff there.

amazon.com review

Nei Gong: The Authentic Classic
A Translation of the Nei Gong Zhen Chuan
translated by Tom Bisio, Huang Guo-Qi and Joshua Paynter

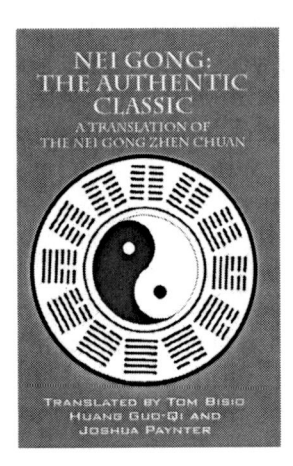

Mr. Bisio has crafted something which sits at the intersection of the scholarly and the practical: it will certainly aid martial/internal artists with alignments and combat strategy, while readers interested in the esoteric side of the internal arts will gain access into the alchemy that is present in these practices and Yi Jing scholars may find a very useful and different take on interpretation of the trigrams.
-amazon.com review

The book is an invaluable supplement to training with a teacher and may bridge many gaps and questions marks for students in regard to structure, shen fa, fa jing/fa li and issuing, intent, san ti shi and many other difficult to grasp concepts in the art, strategy and medicinal attributes and applications of nei gong, in particular for students of Xing yi, yet valuable to an open minded student of any internal art. This classic can also serve as indispensable tool to teachers in order to help articulate difficult ideas in a new light, or as a companion guide and as part of an essential reading list and resource to students outside of actual practice. As one's knowledge of the art expands, the value of this text/translation will increase over the years.

To any naysayers about the practical value of this book I say, look again. The section on San ti shi alone is a treasure trove. The authors are highly accomplished in their respective fields and Dr. Bisio's knowledge and skill in both Bagua and Xing yi are well respected. In the end, this really is a user's manual, if viewed properly. No, this is not a manual on how to throw a proper punch like Dempsey's classic but the translated songs really do give profound practical insight, overview and resource to anyone invested in the lifelong practice that is nei gong; keep it close.
-amazon.com review

Strategy and Change: An Examination of Military Strategy, the I-Ching and Ba Gua Zhang by Tom Bisio

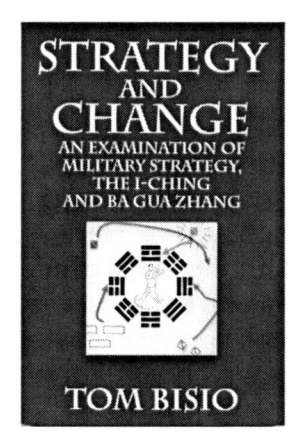

What is remarkable about Tom Bisio's approach to Ba Gua Zhang, as exemplified in Strategy and Change, is his lucid and pragmatic explication of the relationship of internal energy and body states to external situations of crisis. His approach is holistic, not linear, so one can enter this book at any point and find insight. By relating internal flow of energy to external battle plans from military thinkers as diverse as Sun Tzu to Mao Ze Dong and Belisarius to Clausewitz, Strategy and Change offers numerous examples of how spontaneously deploying internalized strategies consistently overcomes traditional martial maneuvers. For me, the real benefit of this book is its application to the strategic moments we all face daily, of holding and releasing power in the body with mindfulness, whether negotiating in business, competing in sports, disciplining one's self (or one's kids!), or any circumstance where one's self goes out into the world with intent, not necessarily to conquer but to persuade and prevail without resentment or backlash. I highly recommend this book of strategy, which so compellingly demonstrates the Daoist principles of transforming conflict into creative tension and the emotional resolution and satisfaction of achieving victories that free us to move forward by leaving behind only the soft echo of self.
   -amazon.com review

   This is an in-depth contemplation on the meaning of strategy with a wealth of examples from both Western and Eastern Military history. Using such sources as Sun Zi, Liddel, Francoise Jullien, and our own Kang Ge Wu, the author shows many correlates between martial arts and the wide ranging application of strategy in both war and daily life. We share many of Mr. Bisio's views and have also had Bagua instructors who see little correlation between the I Ching, for example, and the concepts of Bagua in actual practice. However, we feel there is a wider activity here than one may first suspect. Asians, long familiar with these sources, already think along these strategic avenues. But as Kung Fu becomes a shared art in the world, the original source materials bear investigation. It's not a matter so much of keeping alive the thoughts of previous generations as examining the underpinnings of the most basic ideas. Tom Bisio supplies many examples from famous military histories: Hannibal to Cao Cao, then correlates them to martial arts examples which add life and immediacy to the concepts. Like Musashi, we can see the connection

between beating one man and employing ten thousand troops. He takes these examples and correlates them to that mysterious and perennial source of wisdom, the I-Ching. Should start some people thinking and the stories, mostly unknown to non-Asians, are the very stuff of the martial inheritance.
 -Ted Mancuso Plum Publications (plumpub.com)

This book clarifies many of the strategic concepts and subtleties of both Baguazhang and the internal arts. The author does this through a clever use of examples and analogy, drawn from both historic instances of warfare in the West and the East, as well as classic military doctrine. In other words, there being infinite areas to direct concentration towards, Mr. Bisio does an excellent job of describing the actual paths of strategic thought the practitioner may take to address any given situation of conflict.

I really like this book; it's easy to read, and for the practitioner it elucidates many of the finer points of training that may be missed with the prerequisite focus on form, internal principle, and mind/body training.
 -amazon.com review

CPSIA information can be obtained at www.ICGtesting.com
Printed in the USA
LVOW09s1750170416

484034LV00016B/308/P